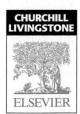

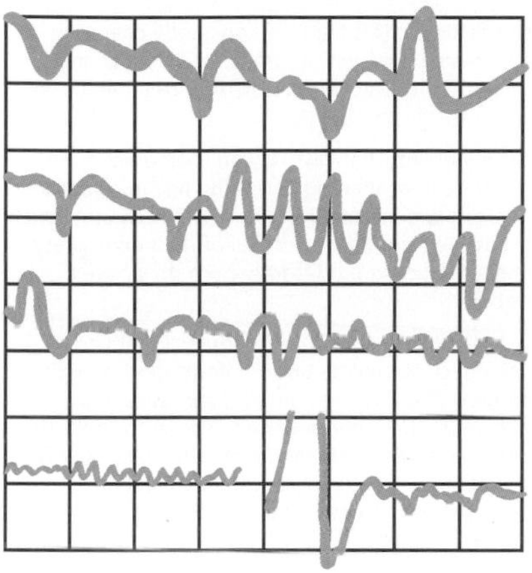

150 ECG Problems

FOURTH EDITION

John R. Hampton
DM MA DPhil FRCP FFPM FESC
Emeritus Professor of Cardiology,
University of Nottingham, UK

CHURCHILL LIVINGSTONE
ELSEVIER
EDINBURGH LONDON NEW YORK OXFORD PHILADELPHIA ST LOUIS SYDNEY TORONTO 2013

CHURCHILL LIVINGSTONE
ELSEVIER

First edition 1997
Second edition 2003
Third edition 2008
Fourth edition 2013

ISBN 978-0-7020-4645-2
International ISBN 978-0-7020-4671-1
e-book ISBN 978-0-7020-5245-3

British Library Cataloguing in Publication Data
A catalogue record for this book is available from the British Library

Library of Congress Cataloging in Publication Data
A catalog record for this book is available from the Library of Congress

Printed in China

Preface

Learning about ECG interpretation from books such as *The ECG Made Easy* or *The ECG in Practice* is fine as far as it goes, but it never goes far enough. As with most of medicine there is no substitute for experience, and to make the best use of the ECG there is no substitute for reviewing large numbers of them. ECGs need to be interpreted in the context of the patient from whom they were recorded. You need to learn to appreciate the variations of normality and of the patterns associated with different diseases, and to think about how the ECG can help patient management.

Although no book can be a substitute for practical experience, *150 ECG Problems* goes a stage nearer the clinical world than books that simply aim to teach ECG interpretation. It presents 150 clinical problems in the shape of simple case histories, together with the relevant ECG. It then invites the reader to interpret the ECG in the light of the clinical evidence provided, and to decide on a course of action before looking at the answer. Having seen the answers, the reader may feel the need for more information, so each one is cross-referenced to *The ECG Made Easy* and/or *The ECG in Practice*.

The ECGs in *150 ECG Problems* range from the simple to the complex. About one-third of the problems are of a standard that a medical student should be able to cope with, and should be answered correctly by anyone who has read *The ECG Made Easy*. A junior doctor, specialist nurse or paramedic should get another third right, if they have read *The ECG in Practice*. The remainder should challenge the MRCP candidate. As a very rough guide to the level of difficulty of each problem, each answer is graded using stars (see the summary box of each answer): one star represents the easiest records, and three stars the most difficult.

The ECGs are arranged in random order, not in order of difficulty, to maintain the reader's interest. Readers are invited to attempt their own interpretation before looking at the star rating – after all, in a real-life situation one never knows which patient will be easy and which will be difficult to diagnose or treat.

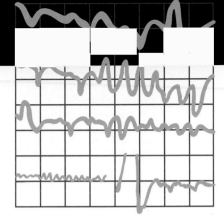

In this fourth edition there are many new ECGs, mainly to provide examples that reproduce more clearly. However, to maintain the "real world"

approach, some technically poor records have deliberately been included. The balance between easy, moderately difficult and very difficult records has been maintained.

I am extremely grateful to Alison Gale, my copy-editor, and to Rich Cutler of Helius. Their patience, understanding and attention to detail made the preparation of this new edition an easy and satisfying experience for me.

John Hampton
Nottingham, 2013

Cross-references

The symbols

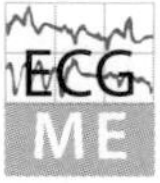

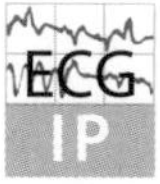

indicate cross-references to useful information in the books *The ECG Made Easy*, 8th edn, and *The ECG in Practice*, 6th edn, respectively.

Introduction: making the most of the ECG

Recording and reporting an ECG should never be an end in itself. The ECG is a basic and valuable tool in the investigation of cardiac problems, and it can be helpful in the case of non-cardiac problems too, but it must always be viewed in the context of the patient from whom the record came. The ECG must never be a substitute for taking a proper medical history and carrying out a careful physical examination. Because it is simple, harmless and cheap, the ECG is usually the first investigation in a patient with possible cardiac disease and it may be followed by the plain chest X-ray, the echocardiogram, radionuclide studies, CT and MR imaging, and cardiac catheterization and angiography – but none of these are substitutes. The ECG, a recording of the electrical activity of the heart, gives information that can be obtained in no other way. However, even though it is irreplaceable, it is not infallible.

ECGs are recorded from a wide variety of patients, in an attempt to help with a wide variety of possible diagnoses. An ECG is frequently recorded in the course of 'health screening', but here it must be regarded with considerable caution. It can not be assumed that individuals who present themselves for screening are asymptomatic – the process may be being used as a substitute for a consultation with a doctor. The ECG itself may cause difficulties of interpretation, for there are a dozen or more normal variants. Minor abnormalities, such as nonspecific ST segment or T wave changes, will have diagnostic and prognostic significance if the individual has symptoms that may be cardiac in origin, but these changes can be of no importance in totally healthy people. It is rare for an ECG to demonstrate anything of importance in a totally healthy individual, although in athletes the detection of abnormalities suggesting asymptomatic hypertrophic cardiomyopathy is important.

In patients with chest pain, the ECG is important but sometimes misleading. It is essential to remember that the ECG can remain normal for some hours after the onset of a myocardial infarction. Too often patients are sent home from an A & E department because their ECG is normal, despite a reasonably convincing story of ischaemic chest pain. Under such circumstances the ECG should be repeated several times to see if changes are appearing, and patient management should depend on the plasma troponin level rather than on the ECG. Nevertheless the ECG is important for deciding treatment in a patient with chest pain, for the management of a patient with myocardial infarction with ST segment elevation is quite different from that of a patient whose ECG shows a non-ST segment elevation infarction.

Patients with intermittent chest pain that could be angina frequently have completely normal ECGs at rest – and then the exercise test can be valuable. The exercise test is to some extent being replaced by myocardial perfusion scanning for the diagnosis of coronary disease because its predictive accuracy depends on the likelihood of the patient having angina, because there can be false negative or false positive results, and because exercise tests are sometimes unreliable in women. Remember that an exercise test is safe, but not totally safe, because arrhythmias (including ventricular fibrillation) may be induced. Nevertheless the exercise test has the great advantage of showing a patient's exercise tolerance, and also showing what limits his capability.

The ECG also has a role in the investigation of patients with breathlessness, for it can show changes associated with heart disease (e.g. an old myocardial infarction) or with chronic chest disease. Evidence of left ventricular hypertrophy may point to hypertension, mitral regurgitation or aortic stenosis or regurgitation, and right ventricular hypertrophy may be the result of pulmonary emboli or mitral stenosis – however, all of these should have been detected during the examination of the patient. The ECG is not a good tool for grading the hypertrophy of the different heart chambers. It is particularly important to remember that the ECG cannot demonstrate heart failure: it may suggest a condition that may cause heart failure, but is impossible to determine from an ECG whether a patient is in heart failure or not. However, in the presence of a completely normal ECG, heart failure is certainly unlikely.

There are characteristic ECG appearances in several conditions that are not primarily cardiac – for example with severe electrolyte derangement. ECG monitoring is not an acceptable way of following electrolyte changes in conditions such as diabetic ketoacidosis, but at least any abnormalities may prompt the appropriate biochemical tests. The ECG has, however, become important in the development of new drugs, for any drug that causes QT prolongation – and this is by no means uncommon – may cause sudden death due to ventricular tachycardia.

It is in the investigation and management of patients with possible arrhythmias that the ECG is of paramount importance. Patients may complain of palpitations or dizziness and syncope as a result of rhythm disturbances, and there is no way of identifying these with certainty other than with an ECG. Dizziness and syncope can be the result of rhythms that are either too fast or too slow for an effective cardiac output, or of slow rhythms associated with disorders of conduction. There may be little in the patient's history to point specifically to a cardiac problem when dizziness or collapse is the main symptom, but an appropriately abnormal ECG may immediately point to the right diagnosis. When a patient complains of palpitations there is a clearly a heart problem of some sort, and it is usually possible to come close to a diagnosis by taking a careful history – the patient with extrasystoles will describe the heart 'jumping out of the chest' or something equally unlikely, and the problem will be worse when lying down at night, and after smoking and alcohol. The patient with a true paroxysmal tachycardia will describe the sudden onset (and sometimes the sudden cessation) of the rapid heartbeat, and if the attack is associated with chest pain, dizziness or breathlessness then the presence of a paroxysmal tachycardia becomes highly likely.

Few patients will have their arrhythmia at the time they are seen, but the ECG can still give valuable clues to its nature. A patient whose ECG shows bifascicular block, or first degree atrioventricular block together with left bundle branch block, may have intermittent complete block and Stokes–Adams attacks. A patient whose ECG shows pre-excitation (the Wolff–Parkinson–White or Lown–Ganong–Levine syndromes) is at risk of paroxysmal arrhythmias – though many people with these ECG patterns never have any problems at all. A patient with a prolonged QT syndrome, as a result of either a congenital defect or drug treatment, is at risk of torsade de pointes ventricular tachycardia. Under all these circumstances, ambulatory ECG recording, by one of a variety of techniques, may demonstrate the true nature of the arrhythmia that causes the symptoms – but it must be remembered that many, if not most, arrhythmias will be seen transiently in completely healthy people and only when an abnormal ECG corresponds to symptoms can one be certain that the two are related.

So the way to approach the ECG, and this book – and indeed any medical situation – is to start with the patient. If you cannot make a reasonable diagnosis from the history, and to a lesser extent the examination, the chances of doing so as a result of investigations are not great. The role of the ECG and of more complex investigations is to help differentiate between the various possible diagnoses suggested by talking to, and examining, the patient. The clinical scenarios given with each ECG in this book are of necessity brief, but think about them, ask yourself what the diagnosis might be, and then describe and report on the ECG. That is the way to make the most of the ECG.

ECG 1

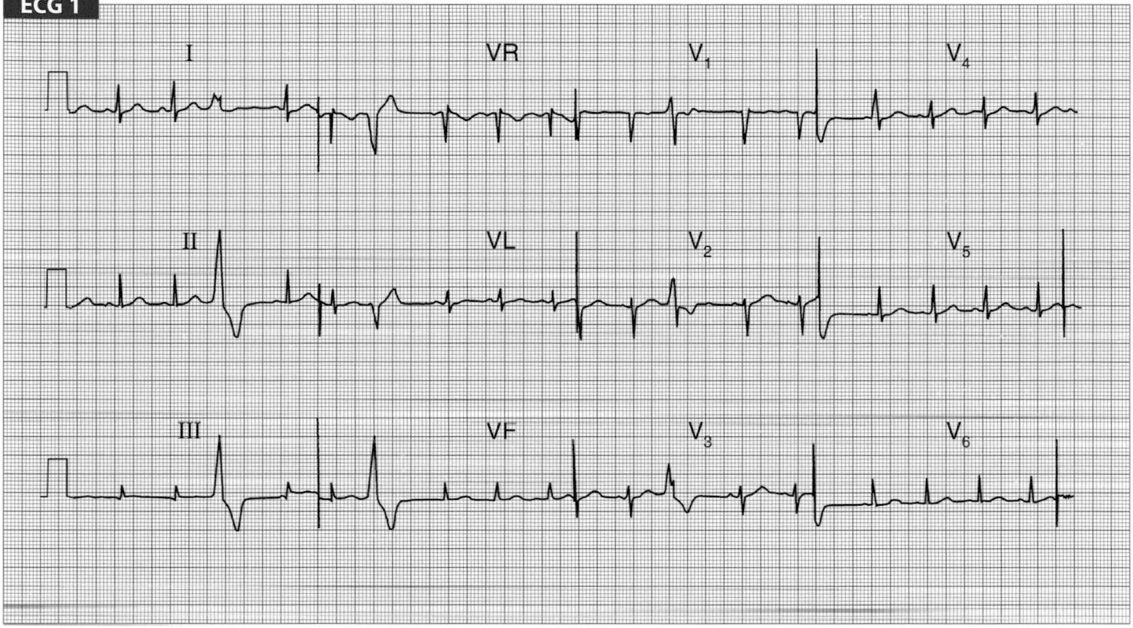

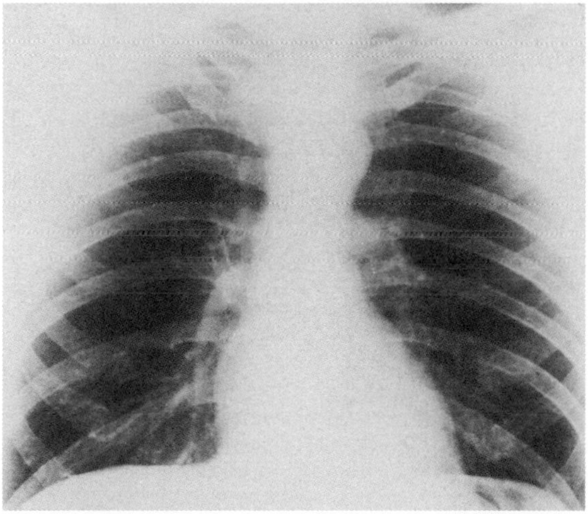

This ECG was recorded from a 20-year-old student who complained of an irregular heartbeat. Apart from an irregular pulse, her heart was clinically normal. What do the ECG and chest X-ray show and what would you do?

ANSWER 1

The ECG shows:

- Sinus rhythm, rate 100/min
- Ventricular extrasystoles
- Normal axis
- Normal QRS complexes and T waves

The chest X-ray is normal.

Clinical interpretation

The extrasystoles are fairly frequent but the ECG is otherwise normal.

What to do

Ventricular extrasystoles are very common. In large groups of people, there is a correlation between the presence of extrasystoles and heart disease of many types. However, in young people who are otherwise asymptomatic and whose hearts are otherwise normal, the chances of a significant cardiac problem are very low.

In a young woman it is worth checking the haemoglobin level. An echocardiogram might set her mind at rest, but is not essential. The important thing is to advise her not to smoke and to avoid alcohol, coffee and tea.

Summary ★

Sinus rhythm with ventricular extrasystoles.

ECG ME See p. 64, 108, 8E

ECG IP See p. 7, 6E

ECG 2

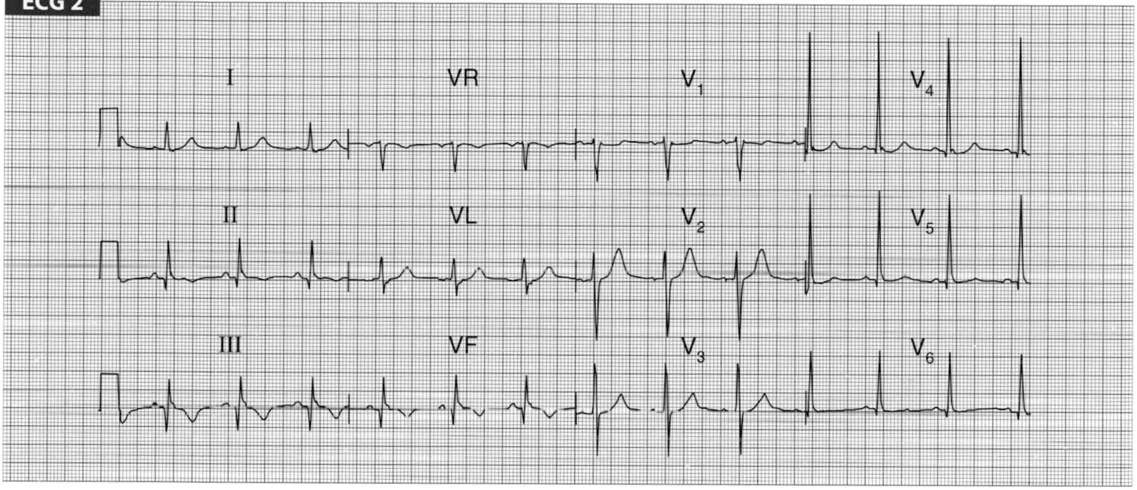

A 60-year-old man was seen as an outpatient, complaining of rather vague central chest pain on exertion. He had never had pain at rest. What does this ECG show and what would you do next?

ANSWER 2

The ECG shows:

- Sinus rhythm, rate 77/min
- Normal PR interval
- Normal axis
- Prominent and deep Q waves in leads II, III and VF, indicating an inferior infarction. There are also small Q waves in leads V_5–V_6, but these may be septal
- ST segments normal, with no elevation in the leads showing Q waves
- Inverted T waves in leads II, III and VF

Clinical interpretation

The Q waves in the inferior leads, together with inverted T waves, point to an old inferior myocardial infarction.

What to do

The patient seems to have had a myocardial infarction at some point in the past, and by implication his vague chest pain may be due to angina. Attention must be paid to risk factors (smoking, blood pressure, plasma cholesterol), and he probably needs long-term treatment with aspirin and a statin. An exercise test or a perfusion scan will be the best way of deciding whether he has coronary disease that merits angiography.

Summary ★

Old inferior myocardial infarction.

ECG ME See p. 91, 8E

ECG IP See p. 215, 6E

ECG 3

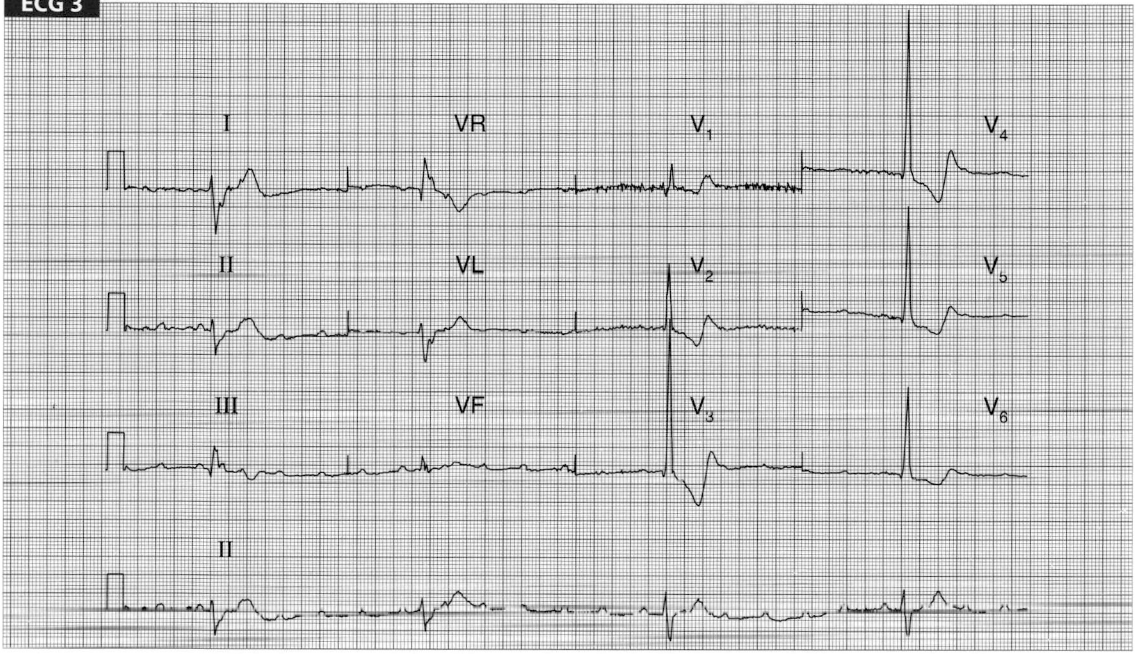

An 80-year-old woman, who had previously had a few attacks of dizziness, fell and broke her hip. She was found to have a slow pulse, and this is her ECG. The surgeons want to operate as soon as possible but the anaesthetist is unhappy. What does the ECG show and what should be done?

ANSWER 3

The ECG shows:

- P wave rate 130/min
- Complete heart block
- Ventricular (QRS complex) rate 23/min
- The ventricular 'escape' rhythm has wide QRS complexes and abnormal T waves

No further interpretation of the ECG is possible.

Clinical interpretation

In complete heart block there is no relationship between the P waves (here with a rate of 120/min) and the QRS complexes.

What to do

In the absence of a history suggesting a myocardial infarction, this woman almost certainly has chronic heart block: the fall may or may not have been due to a Stokes–Adams attack. She needs a permanent pacemaker, ideally immediately. If permanent pacing is not possible immediately, a temporary pacemaker will be needed preoperatively.

Summary ★
Complete (third degree) heart block.

ECG ME See p. 41, 8E

ECG IP See p. 179, 6E

ECG 4

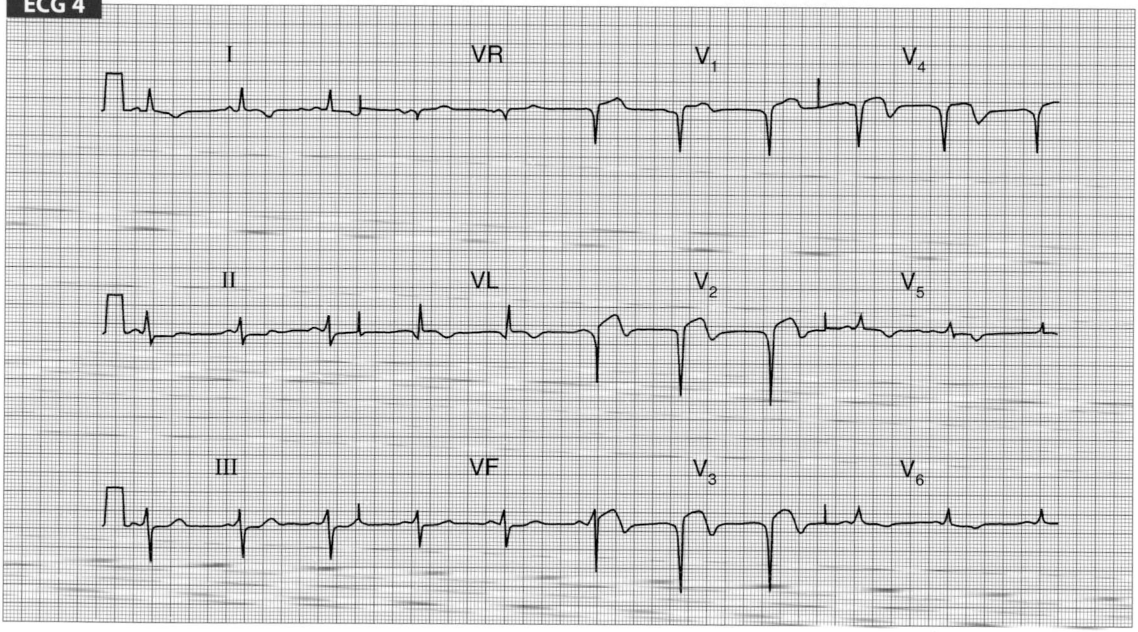

A 50-year-old man is seen in the A & E department with severe central chest pain which has been present for 18 h. What does this ECG show and what would you do?

ANSWER 4

The ECG shows:

- Sinus rhythm, rate 64/min
- Normal axis
- Q waves in leads V_2–V_4
- Raised ST segments in leads V_2–V_4
- Inverted T waves in leads I, VL, V_2–V_6

Clinical interpretation

This is a classic acute ST segment elevation anterior myocardial infarction (STEMI).

What to do

More than 18 h have elapsed since the onset of pain, so this patient is outside the conventional limit for thrombolysis or percutaneous coronary intervention (PCI). Nevertheless, if he is still in pain and still looks unwell, PCI or thrombolytic treatment should be given unless there are good reasons not to do so. In any case, he should be given pain relief and aspirin, and must be admitted to hospital for observation.

Summary ★
Acute anterior STEMI.

ECG ME See p. 91, 92, 8E

ECG IP See p. 217, 6E

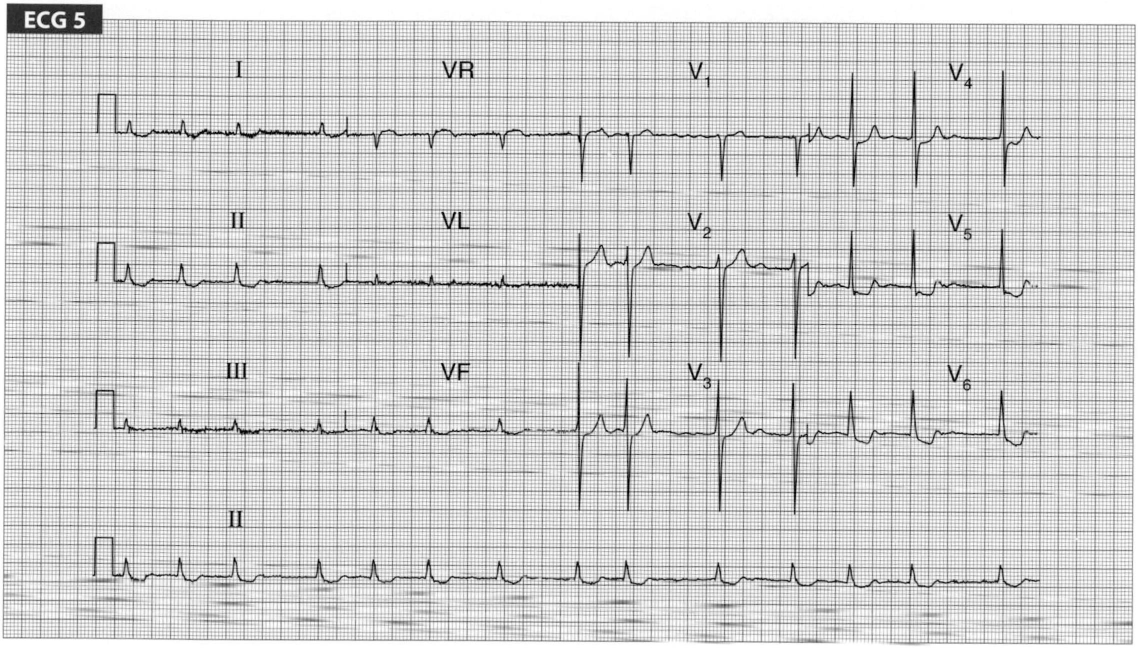

This ECG was recorded from a 60-year-old woman with rheumatic heart disease. She had been in heart failure, but this had been treated and she was no longer breathless. What does the ECG show and what question might you ask her?

ANSWER 5

The ECG shows:

- Atrial fibrillation with a ventricular rate of about 80/min
- Normal axis
- Normal QRS complexes
- Downward-sloping ST segments, best seen in leads V_5–V_6
- Prominent U waves in leads V_2–V_3

Clinical interpretation

The downward-sloping ST segments (the 'reverse tick') indicate that digoxin has been given. The ventricular rate seems well controlled. The prominent U waves in leads V_2–V_3 are probably normal: U waves due to hypokalaemia are associated with flattened T waves.

What to do

Ask the patient about her appetite: the earliest symptom of digoxin toxicity is appetite loss, followed by nausea and vomiting. If the patient is being treated with diuretics, check the serum potassium level – a low potassium level potentiates the effects of digoxin. If in doubt, the serum digoxin level is easily measured.

Summary ★★

Atrial fibrillation with digoxin effect.

ECG ME See p. 76, 101, 8E

ECG IP See p. 335, 6E

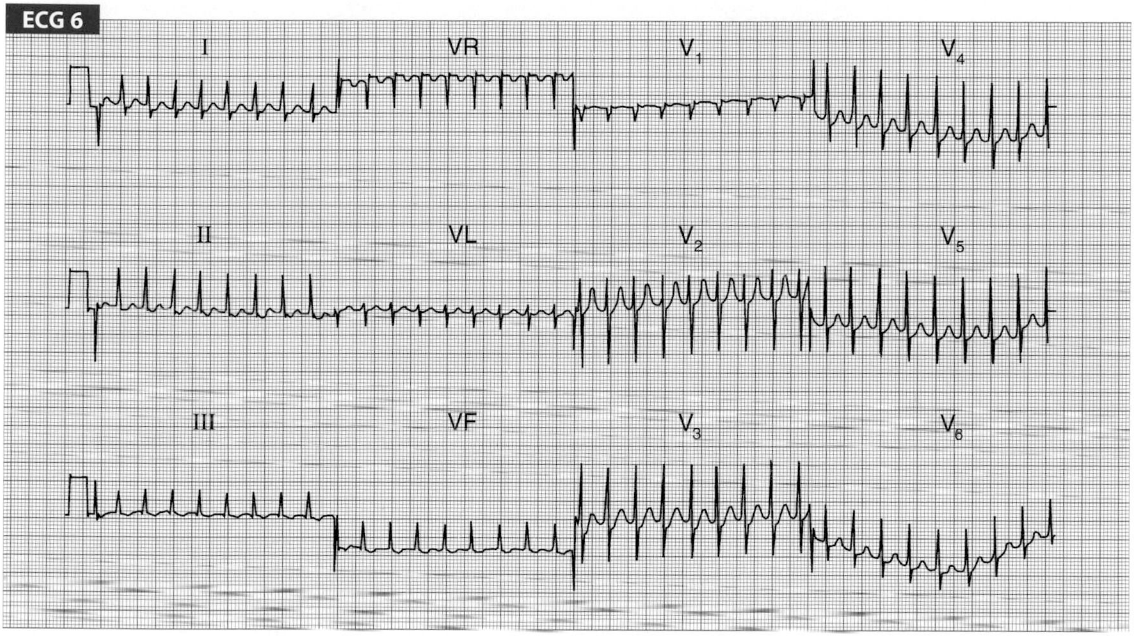

A 26-year-old woman, who has complained of palpitations in the past, is admitted to hospital via the A & E department with palpitations. What does the ECG show and what should you do?

ANSWER 6

The ECG shows:

- Narrow complex tachycardia, rate about 200/min
- No P waves visible
- Normal axis
- Regular QRS complexes
- Normal QRS complexcs, ST segments and T waves

Clinical interpretation

This is a supraventricular tachycardia, and since no P waves are visible this is a junctional, or atrioventricular nodal re-entry, tachycardia (AVNRT).

What to do

AVNRT is the commonest form of paroxysmal tachycardia in young people, and presumably explains her previous episodes of palpitations. Attacks of AVNRT may be terminated by any of the manoeuvres that lead to vagal stimulation – Valsalva's manoeuvre, carotid sinus pressure, or immersion of the face in cold water. If these are unsuccessful, intravenous adenosine should be given by bolus injection. Adenosine has a very short half-life, but can cause flushing and occasionally an asthmatic attack. If adenosine proves unsuccessful, verapamil 5–10 mg given by bolus injection will usually restore sinus rhythm. Otherwise, DC cardioversion is indicated.

Summary ★

Atrioventricular nodal re-entry (junctional) tachycardia (AVNRT).

ECG ME See p. 81, 8E

ECG IP See p. 109, 6E

ECG 7

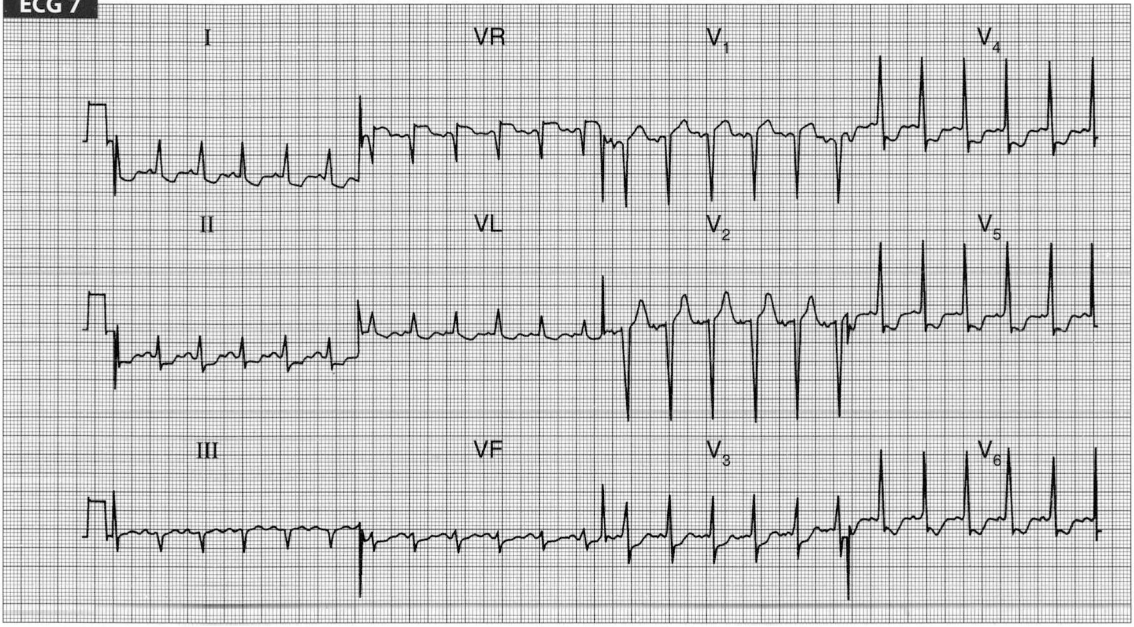

This ECG was recorded in the A & E department from a 55-year-old man who had had chest pain at rest for 6 h. There were no abnormal physical findings, and his plasma troponin level was normal. What does the trace show, and how would you manage him?

ANSWER 7

The ECG shows:

- Sinus rhythm, rate 130/min
- Normal axis
- Normal QRS complexes
- ST segment depression – slightly upward-sloping in lead V_3, downward-sloping in leads I, VL, V_4–V_6

Clinical interpretation

This ECG shows anterior and lateral ischaemia without evidence of infarction. Taken with the clinical history, the diagnosis is clearly 'unstable' angina.

What to do

There is no evidence that he would benefit from thrombolysis: percutaneous coronary intervention (PCI) would probably be the treatment of choice. Immediately, however, he needs a beta-blocker to bring his heart rate down. Although the normal troponin level suggests that he has not (yet) had a myocardial infarction, in view of the length of the history it would be prudent to treat him with aspirin, heparin and a statin.

Summary ★

Anterolateral ischaemia.

ECG ME See p. 144, 8E

ECG IP See p. 212, 6E

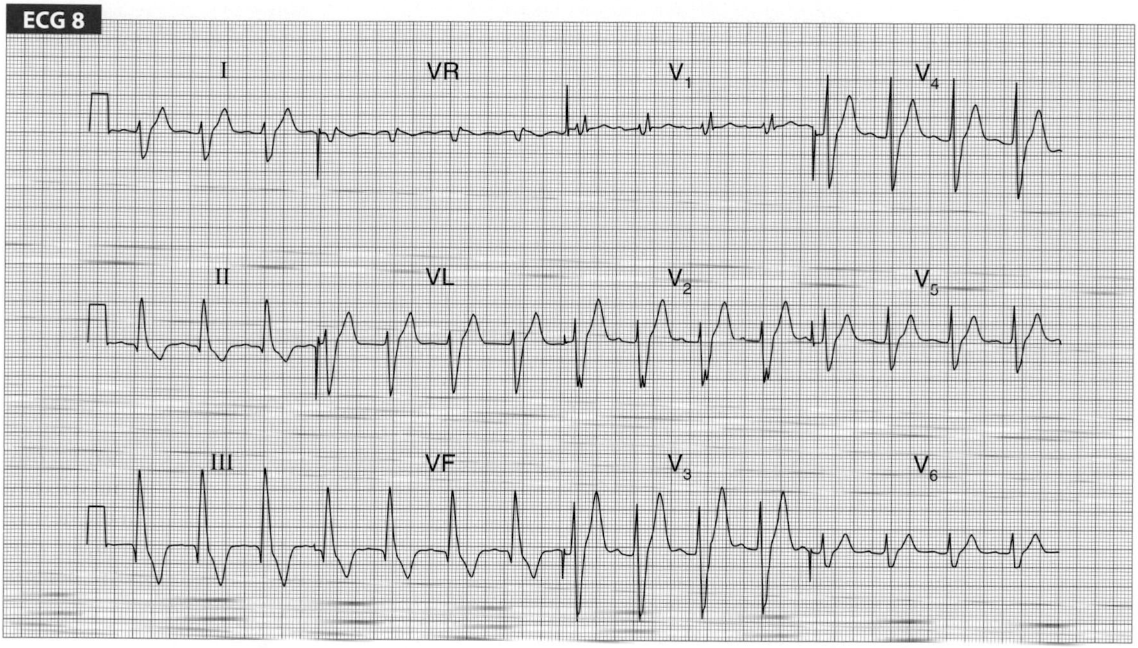

An 80-year-old woman complained of breathlessness and frequent attacks of dizziness. This was her ECG when she attended the clinic. She lived alone, and it seemed unlikely that she could cope with an ambulatory recorder. What does the ECG show, what might the dizziness be due to, and how would you manage her?

ANSWER 8

The ECG shows:

- Sinus rhythm, rate 90/min
- Right axis deviation
- Right bundle branch block (RBBB)

Clinical interpretation

The right axis deviation suggests left posterior hemiblock, and, combined with RBBB, this suggests bifascicular block. The patient is therefore at risk of complete (third degree) block, which could cause a Stokes–Adams attack.

What to do

This woman was admitted to hospital and monitored, and had a severe attack of dizziness and fainting. During this attack, another ECG was recorded (see below). This ECG shows complete heart block with a ventricular rate of about 15/min. The patient was immediately given a permanent pacemaker.

See p. 41, 43, 51, 8E ECG ME

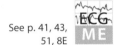

See p. 89, 6E ECG IP

Summary ★★★

Left posterior hemiblock and RBBB – bifascicular block, followed by complete heart block (see ECG below).

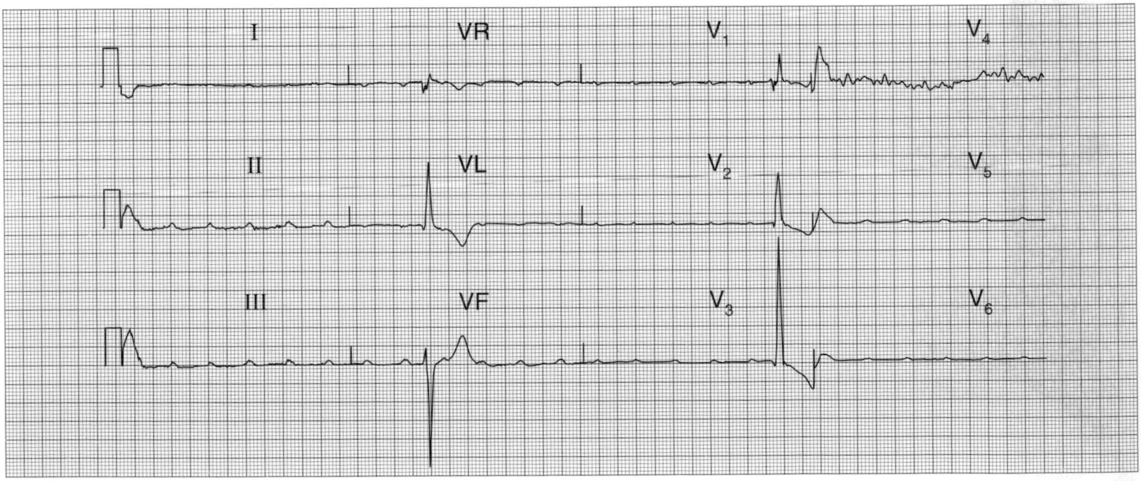

ECG 9

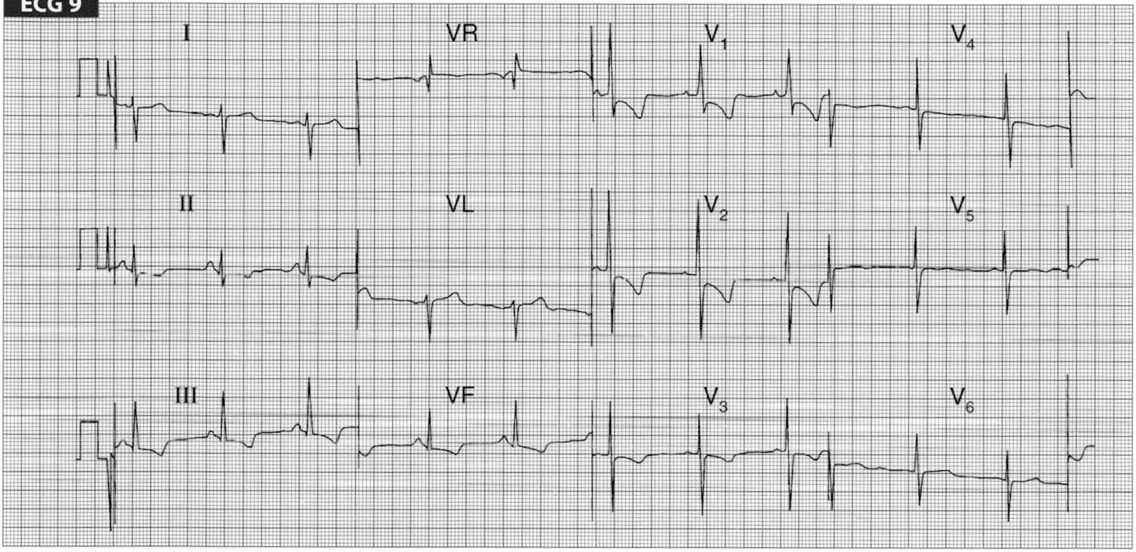

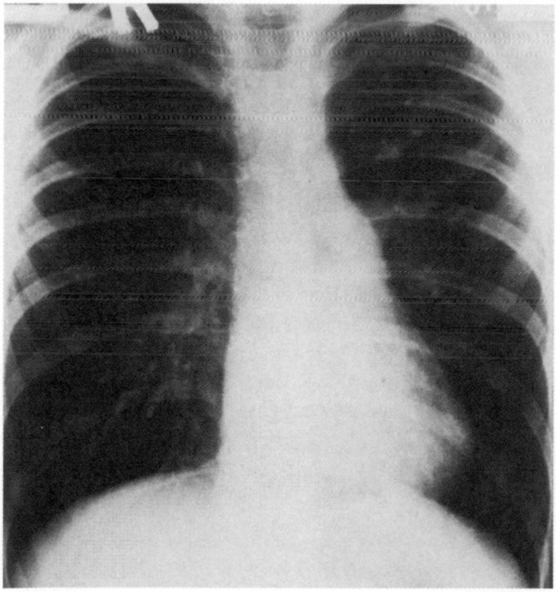

A 40-year-old woman is referred to the outpatient department because of increasing breathlessness. What do this ECG and chest X-ray show, what physical signs might you expect, and what might be the underlying problem? What might you do?

ANSWER 9

The ECG shows:

- Sinus rhythm, rate 65/min
- Peaked P waves, best seen in lead II
- Right axis deviation
- Dominant R waves in lead V_1
- Deep S waves in lead V_6
- Inverted T waves in leads II, III, VF, V_1–V_3

The chest X-ray shows a slightly enlarged heart with a high cardiac apex and a prominent main pulmonary artery, suggesting right ventricular hypertrophy.

Clinical interpretation

This combination of right axis deviation, dominant R waves in lead V_1 and inverted T waves spreading from the right side of the heart is classic of severe right ventricular hypertrophy. Right ventricular hypertrophy can result from congenital heart disease, or from pulmonary hypertension which may be idiopathic, secondary to mitral valve disease, lung disease, or pulmonary embolism. The physical signs of right ventricular hypertrophy are a left parasternal heave and a displaced but diffuse apex beat. There may be a loud pulmonary second sound. The jugular venous pressure may be elevated, and a 'flicking A' wave in the jugular venous pulse is characteristic of pulmonary hypertension.

What to do

The two main causes of pulmonary hypertension of this degree in a 40-year-old woman are recurrent pulmonary emboli, and idiopathic (primary) pulmonary hypertension. Clinically, it is difficult to differentiate between the two, but a lung scan and CT pulmonary angiography will help. In either case, anticoagulants are indicated. In fact, this patient had primary pulmonary hypertension and treatment with high dose calcium channel blockers, prostanoids, endothelin receptor antagonists (bosentan) and phosphodiesterase inhibitors was tried, without success. Eventually she needed heart and lung transplantation.

See p. 87, 8E ECG ME

See p. 305, 6E ECG IP

Summary ★

Severe right ventricular hypertrophy.

ECG 10

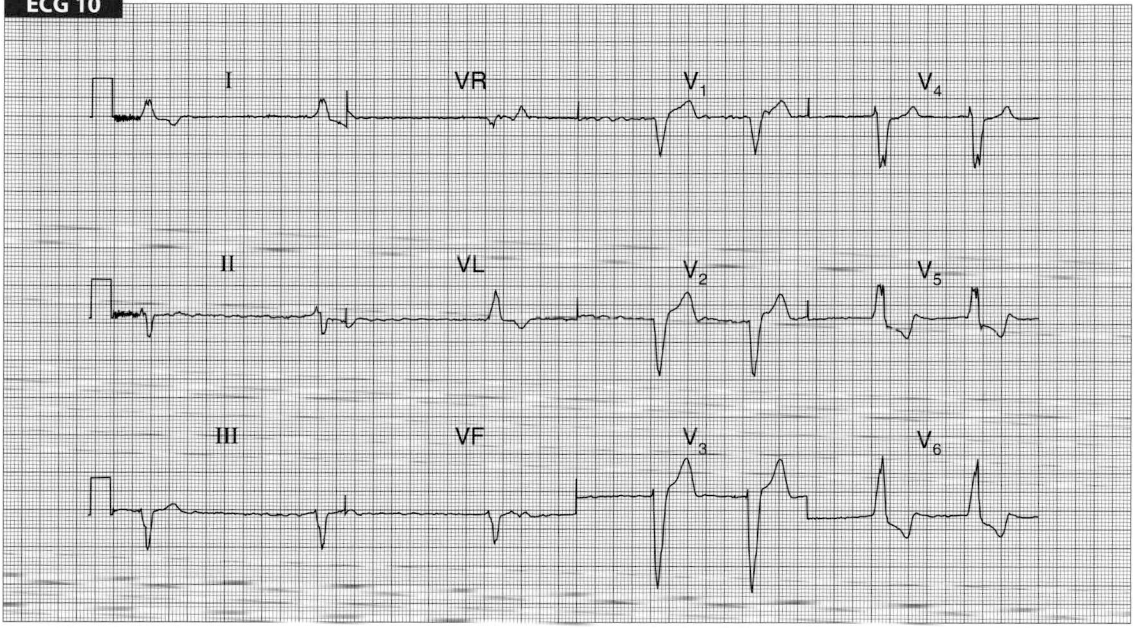

This ECG was recorded from an 80-year-old man who complained of breathlessness and ankle swelling which had become slowly worse over the preceding few months. He had had no chest pain and was on no treatment. He had a slow pulse, and signs of heart failure. What does the ECG show and how would you manage him?

ANSWER 10

The ECG shows:

- Atrial fibrillation with a ventricular rate of about 40/min
- Left axis deviation
- Left bundle branch block (LBBB)

Clinical interpretation

When an ECG shows LBBB, no further interpretation is usually possible. Here there is atrial fibrillation, and the ventricular response is very slow, suggesting that there is conduction delay in the His bundle as well as in the left bundle branch. Alternatively he may be taking too much digoxin.

What to do

It is always important to establish the cause of heart failure. In this patient the slow ventricular rate may be at least part of the problem. The most important causes of LBBB are ischaemia, aortic stenosis and cardiomyopathy. In this patient an echocardiogram will show whether he has significant valve disease and how impaired his left ventricular function is. In the absence of pain, coronary angiography is probably not indicated. The heart failure needs to be treated with diuretics and an angiotensin-converting enzyme inhibitor, but digoxin must be avoided as it may slow the ventricular response still further. He almost certainly needs a permanent pacemaker.

Summary ★

Atrial fibrillation and LBBB.

ECG ME See p. 45, 76, 8E

ECG IP See p. 127, 6E

ECG 11

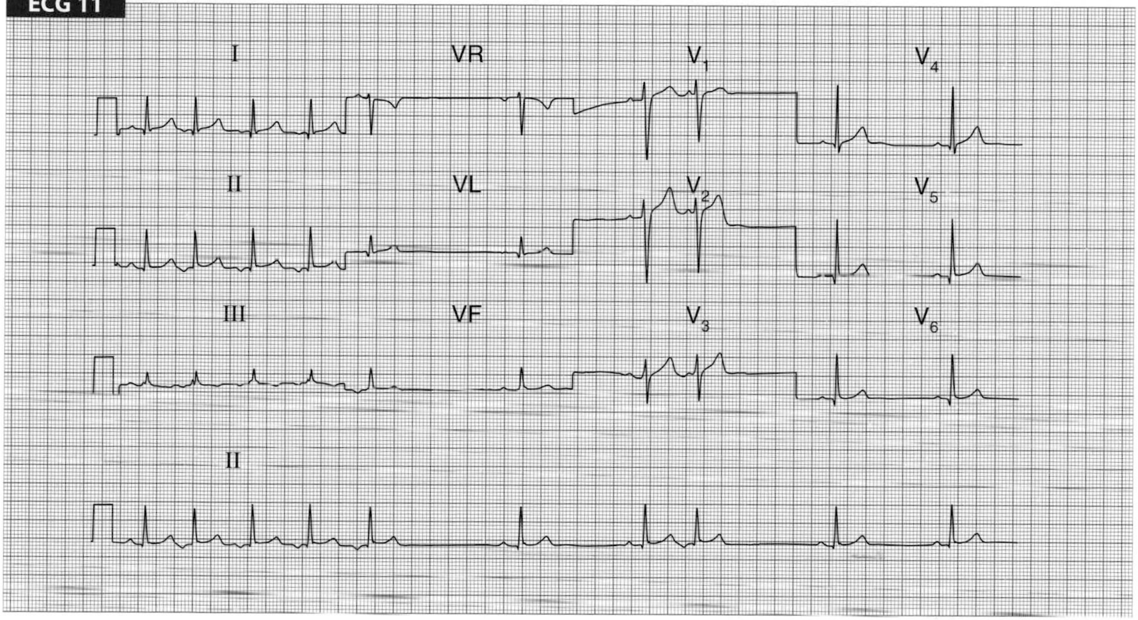

This ECG came from a 40-year-old woman who complained of palpitations, which were present when the recording was made. What abnormality does it show?

ANSWER 11

The ECG shows:

- Lead II rhythm strip of the ECG
- The first beat has a normal P wave and is normal (i.e. a sinus beat)
- The next four beats, at about 100/min, have abnormal (inverted) P waves, and this is an atrial tachycardia
- After a pause the next two beats have normal P waves and are in sinus rhythm at about 60/min
- After two sinus beats there is an extrasystole with an inverted P wave; this is an atrial extrasystole
- Normal axis
- The QRS complexes, ST segments and T waves are normal

Clinical interpretation

Since the patient had her symptoms at the time of the recording, we can be confident that the ECG findings explain them. Atrial extrasystoles are not a manifestation of cardiac disease, but the atrial tachycardia may be and will need treating on symptomatic grounds.

What to do

Ensure that there is no other evidence of heart disease. She should stop smoking and avoid alcohol, coffee and tea. A beta-blocker will probably prevent the tachycardia.

Summary ★
Sinus rhythm with atrial tachycardia and one atrial extrasystole.

ECG ME See p. 66, 8E

ECG IP See p. 107, 6E

ECG 12

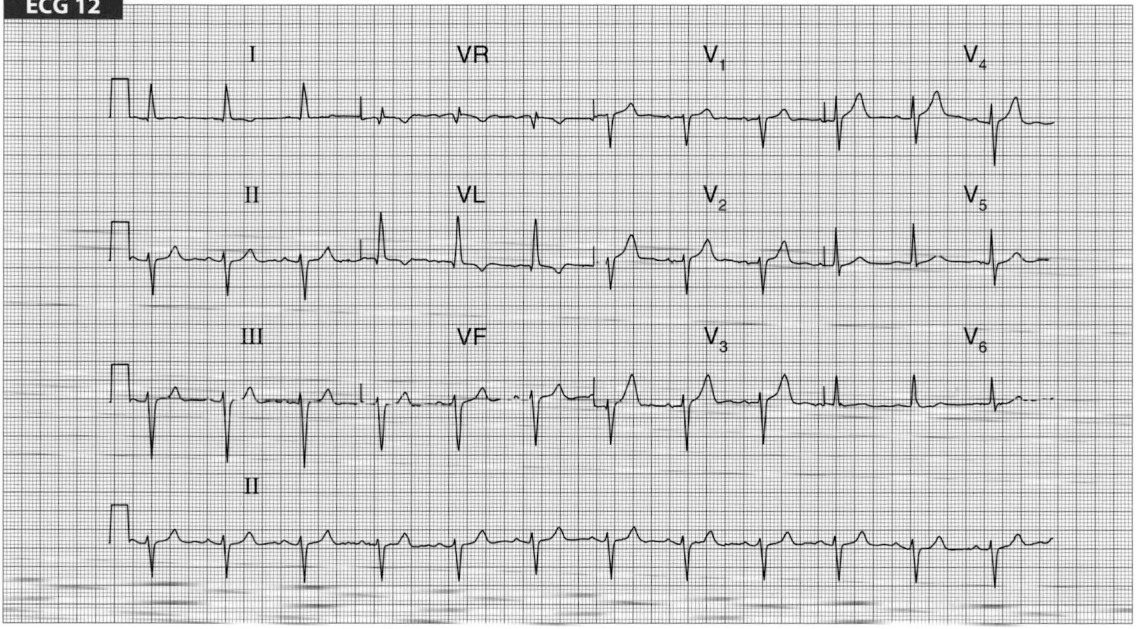

A 70-year-old man had had high blood pressure for many years, but it was now well controlled at 140/85. He had no symptoms, and no abnormalities were detected on physical examination. This ECG was recorded during a routine follow-up appointment. Does it give any cause for concern, and if so, what would you do?

ANSWER 12

The ECG shows:

- Sinus rhythm, rate 73/min
- Normal PR interval
- Left axis deviation (left anterior hemiblock)
- Normal QRS complexes
- T wave inversion in leads I and VL

Clinical interpretation

The left axis deviation indicates a conduction defect in the anterior fascicle of the left bundle branch – left anterior hemiblock. This is due to fibrosis, almost certainly the result of long-standing hypertension. The T wave inversion in the lateral leads (I and VL) probably indicates left ventricular hypertrophy, although the QRS complex in lead V_6 is not unusually tall and the 'voltage criteria' for left ventricular hypertrophy are not met. It is, therefore, possible that the T wave inversion is due to ischaemia.

What to do

This man clearly has 'target organ' (heart) damage as the result of his hypertension. An echocardiogram should be recorded to assess his left ventricular thickness and function, because the prognosis is worse if there is left ventricular hypertrophy or if there is any reduction in function. The presence of other risk factors, such as diabetes and hypercholesterolaemia, must be checked and, if necessary, treated. If there is any suggestion of angina, an exercise test should be performed, but if he really is completely asymptomatic this is probably not essential. Careful control of his blood pressure is the key to management, and since there is evidence of cardiac damage, an angiotensin-converting enzyme inhibitor should be the basis of treatment.

Summary ★★

Left anterior hemiblock and either left ventricular hypertrophy or ischaemia.

ECG ME See p. 49, 8E

ECG IP See p. 85, 6E

ECG 13

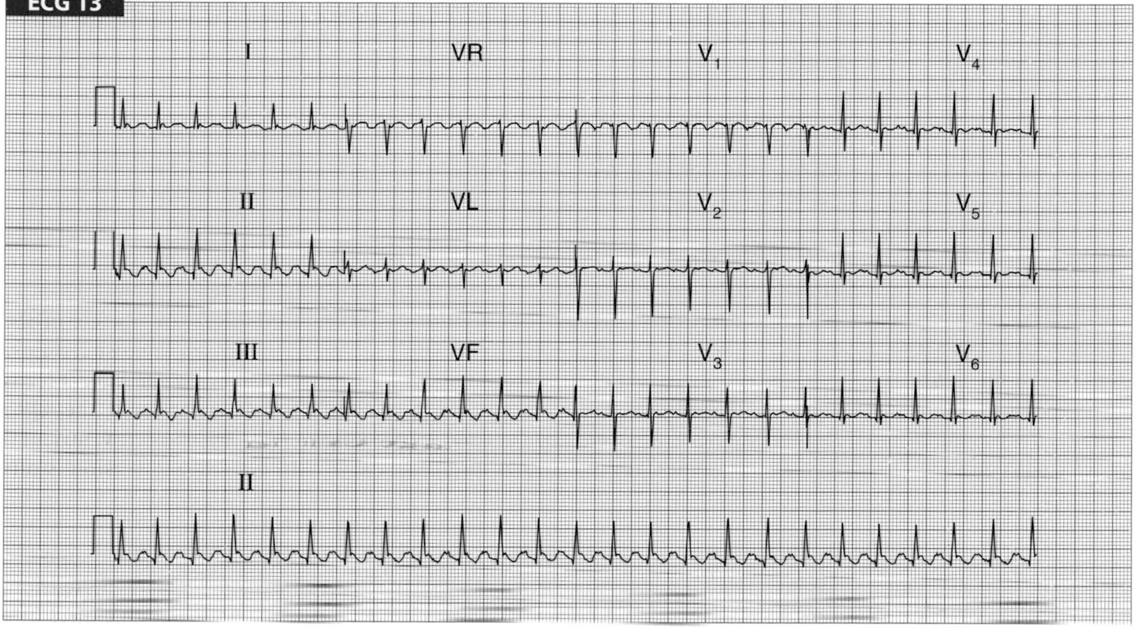

This ECG was recorded from a 40-year-old man who was admitted to hospital as an emergency, with the sudden onset of the symptoms and signs of severe left ventricular failure. What does it show and what would you do?

ANSWER 13

The ECG shows:

- Atrial flutter with 2:1 block (best seen in leads II, III, VF)
- Normal axis
- Normal QRS complexes
- The T waves are difficult to identify because of the flutter waves

Clinical interpretation

The sudden onset of atrial flutter presumably explains the heart failure. There is nothing on the ECG to suggest a cause for the arrhythmia.

What to do

When an arrhythmia causes severe heart failure, immediate treatment is more important than establishing the underlying diagnosis. Carotid sinus pressure and adenosine may increase the degree of block, but are unlikely to convert the heart to sinus rhythm. It is worth trying intravenous flecainide, but a patient with severely compromised circulation is best promptly treated with DC cardioversion. In the long term, ablation therapy to prevent further episodes of atrial flutter may be needed.

Summary ★
Atrial flutter with 2:1 block.

ECG ME See p. 67, 8E

ECG IP See p. 117, 6E

ECG 14

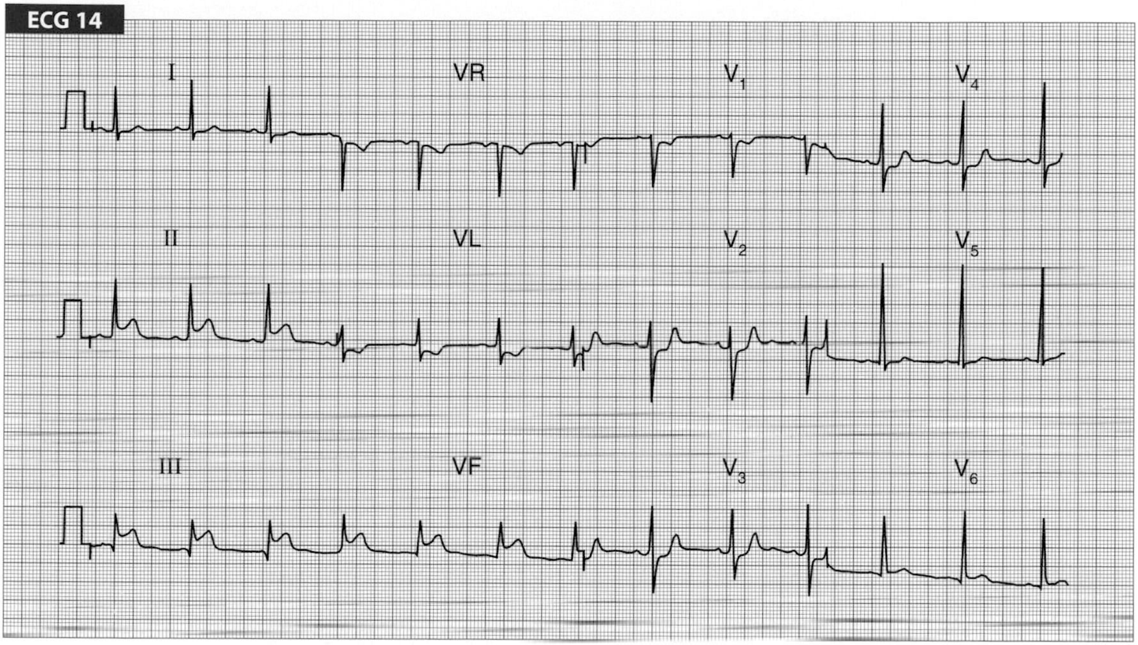

A 50-year-old man is admitted to hospital as an emergency, having had chest pain characteristic of a myocardial infarction for 4 h. Apart from the features associated with pain there are no abnormal physical findings. What does this ECG show and what would you do?

ANSWER 14

The ECG shows:

- Sinus rhythm, rate 72/min
- Normal axis
- Small Q waves in lead III
- Elevated ST segments in leads II, III, VF, with upright T waves
- Suggestion of ST segment depression in leads V_2–V_3
- T wave inversion in lead VL

Clinical interpretation

A classic ECG of an acute inferior myocardial infarction, with lead VL indicating ischaemia. The rate of development of Q waves is very variable: compare this record with ECG 32, which came from a patient with a similar duration of symptoms.

What to do

Pain relief must take priority. In the absence of contraindications (i.e. risk of bleeding from any important site), the patient should be given aspirin and then percutaneous coronary intervention (PCI) or a thrombolytic agent.

Summary ★
Acute inferior myocardial infarction.

ECG ME See p. 91, 8E

ECG IP See p. 215, 6E

ECG 15

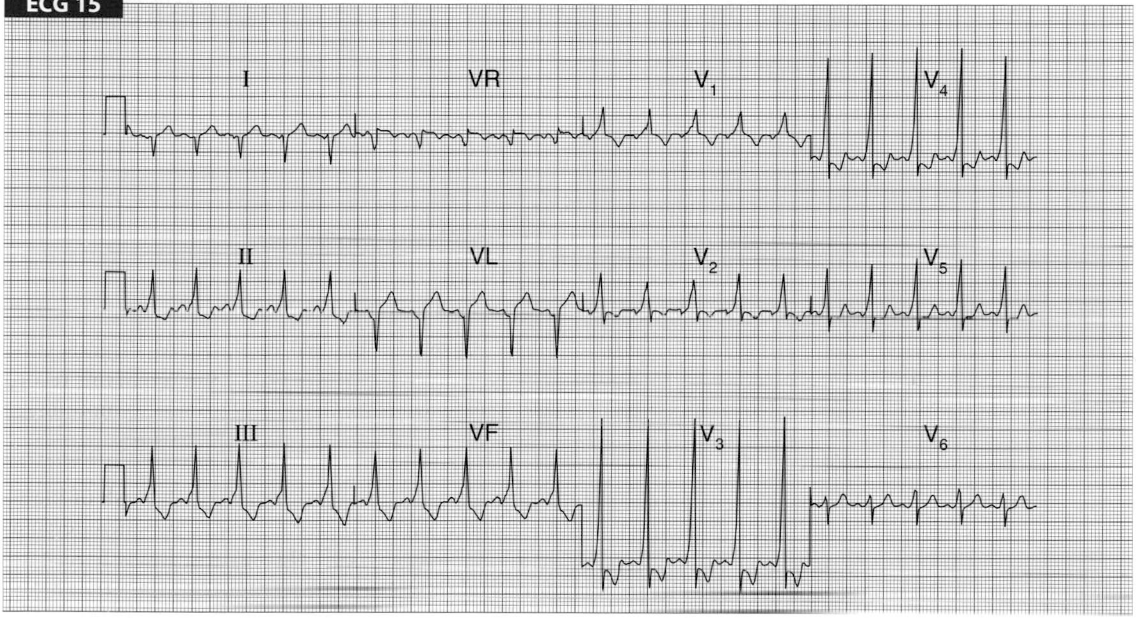

A 20-year-old student complains of palpitations. Attacks occur about once per year. They start suddenly, his heart feels very fast and regular, and he quickly feels breathless and faint. The attacks stop suddenly after a few minutes. There are no abnormalities on examination, and this is his ECG. What would you do?

ANSWER 15

The ECG shows:

- Sinus rhythm, rate 56/min
- Short PR interval, most obvious in the chest leads
- Normal axis
- Wide QRS complexes (136 ms)
- Slurred upstroke of the QRS complex (delta wave)
- Dominant R wave in lead V_1

Clinical interpretation

This ECG is classic of Wolff–Parkinson–White (WPW) syndrome. The resemblance to the ECG of right ventricular hypertrophy is because this is WPW type A, with a left-sided accessory pathway.

What to do

The patient gives a clear story of a paroxysmal tachycardia, and during attacks he feels dizzy, so the circulation is clearly compromised. The attacks are infrequent, so there is little point in recording an ambulatory ECG. The patient needs immediate referral to an electrophysiologist for ablation of the aberrant conducting pathway.

Summary ★

The WPW syndrome type A.

ECG ME See p. 79, 8E

ECG IP See p. 69, 6E

ECG 16

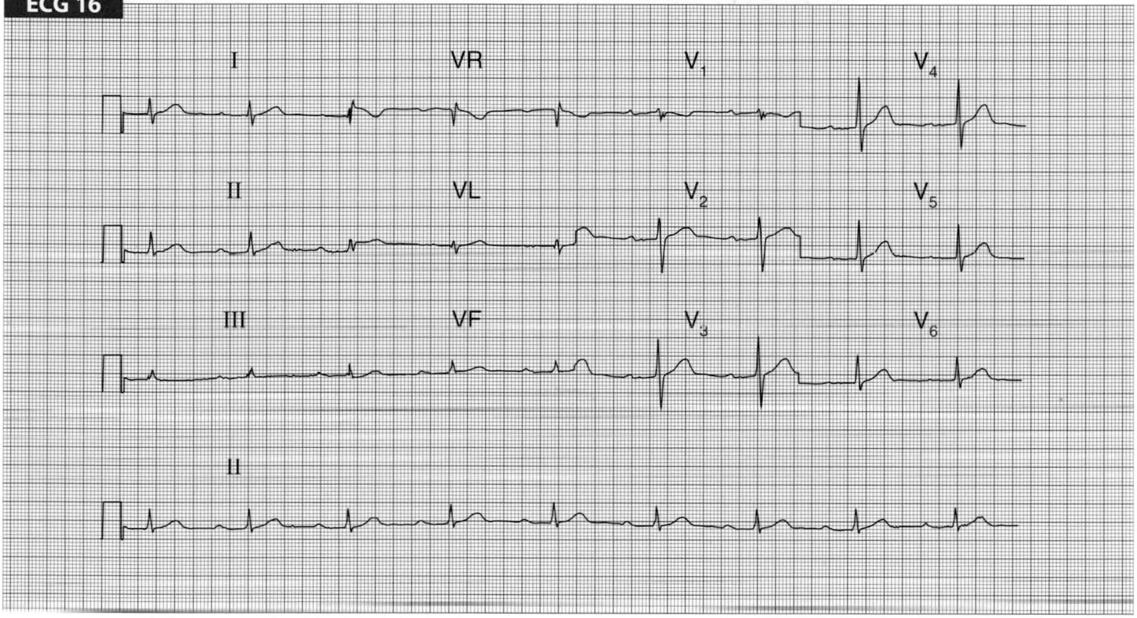

This ECG was recorded from a 75-year-old woman who complained of attacks of dizziness. It shows one abnormality: what is its significance?

ANSWER 16

The ECG shows:

- Sinus rhythm, 55/min
- Prolonged PR interval of 320 ms
- Normal axis
- RSR^1 pattern in lead V_1, with normal QRS complex duration: partial right bundle branch block (RBBB)
- Normal ST segments and T waves

Clinical interpretation

Sinus rhythm with first degree block. The partial RBBB is probably not significant.

What to do

First degree block does not cause any haemodynamic impairment, and by itself is of little significance. However, when a patient has symptoms (in this case dizziness) which might be due to a bradycardia, there may be episodes of second or third degree block, or possibly Stokes–Adams attacks, associated with a slow ventricular rate. The appropriate action is therefore to request an ambulatory ECG, recorded over 24 h, in the hope that the patient will have one of her attacks of dizziness during this time. It would then be possible to see whether the dizziness was associated with a change in heart rhythm. First degree block itself is not an indication for permanent pacing or for any other intervention.

Summary ★★

Sinus rhythm with first degree block.

ECG ME See p. 37, 8E

ECG IP See p. 184, 6E

ECG 17

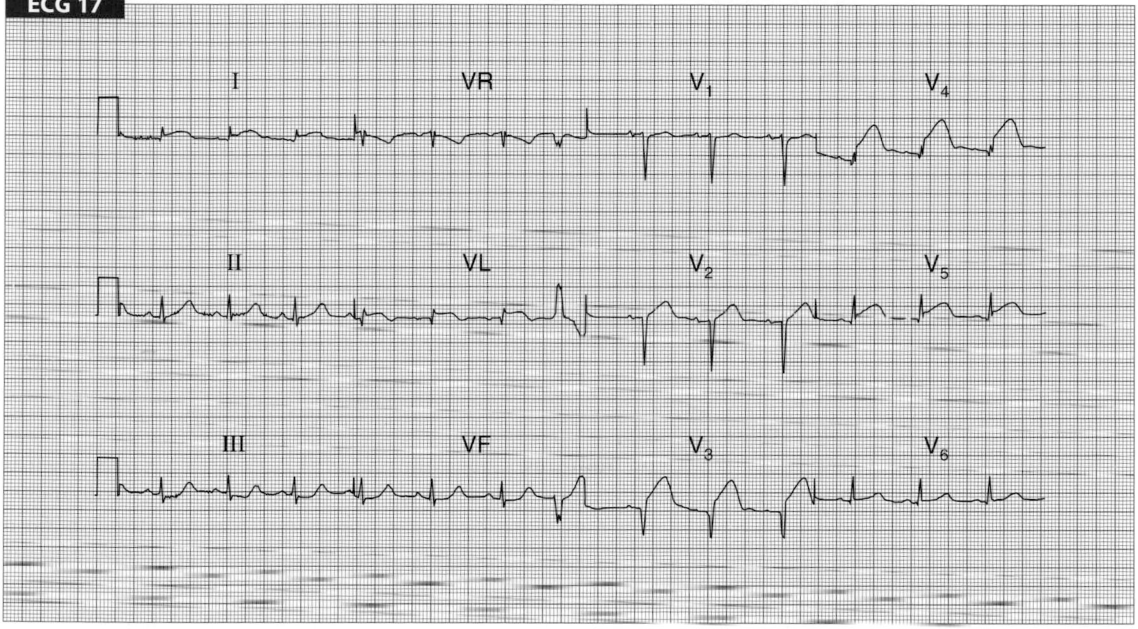

This ECG was recorded in the A & E department from a 60-year-old man who had had severe central chest pain for 1 h. What does it show and what would you do?

ANSWER 17

The ECG shows:

- Sinus rhythm, rate 82/min
- One ventricular extrasystole
- Normal axis
- Q waves in leads V_2–V_3; small Q waves in leads VL, V_4
- Raised ST segments in leads I, VL, V_3–V_6

Clinical interpretation

This is an acute anterolateral ST segment elevation myocardial infarction (STEMI). Although a Q wave is well developed in lead V_3, the changes are entirely consistent with the story of pain for 1 h.

What to do

This patient needs pain relief with diamorphine. The ECG shows ST segments raised by more than 2 mm in several leads, so he needs immediate percutaneous coronary intervention (PCI) or thrombolysis once any risk of excessive bleeding has been excluded. This treatment should not be delayed by waiting for a chest X-ray or any other investigations. Ventricular extrasystoles do not need treating.

Summary ★
Acute anterolateral STEMI.

ECG ME See p. 91, 8E

ECG IP See p. 217, 6E

ECG 18

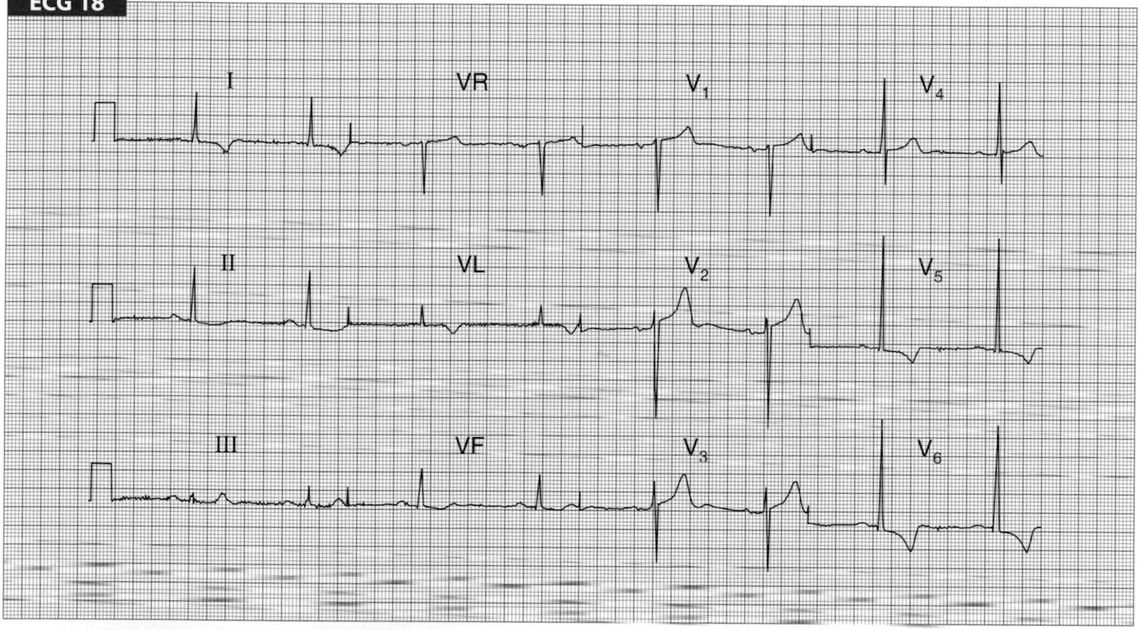

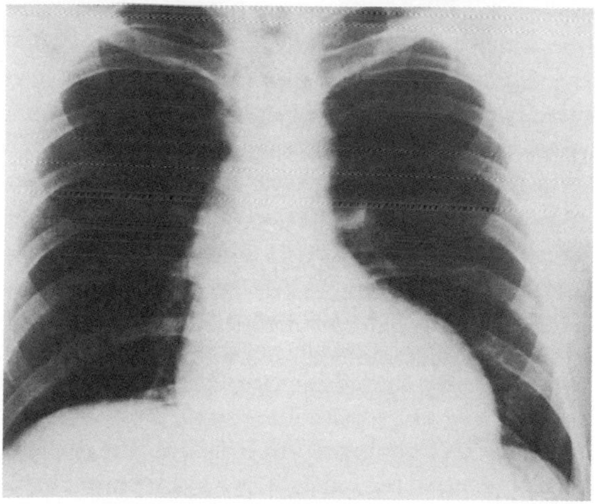

A 70-year-old retired orthopaedic surgeon telephones to say that he always gets dizzy playing golf. You find that he has a systolic heart murmur. His ECG and chest X-ray are shown. What is the diagnosis and what do you do next?

ANSWER 18

The ECG shows:

- Sinus rhythm, rate 48/min
- Normal axis
- QRS complex duration normal, but the R wave height in lead V_5 is 30 mm, and the S wave depth in lead V_2 is 25 mm
- Inverted T waves in leads I, VL, V_5–V_6

The chest X-ray shows an enlarged left ventricle with 'post-stenotic' dilatation of the ascending aorta (arrowed).

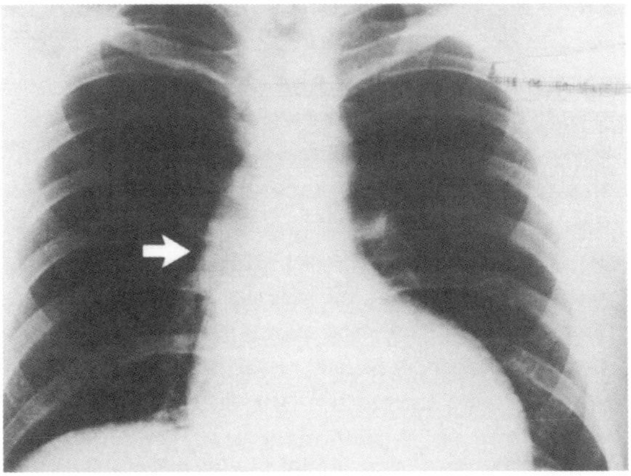

Clinical interpretation

This is the classic ECG appearance of left ventricular hypertrophy.

What to do

See p. 118, 8E ECG ME

The combination of dizziness on exercise, a systolic murmur, and evidence of left ventricular hypertrophy suggests significant aortic stenosis. The next step is an echocardiogram: in this patient it showed a gradient across the aortic valve of 140 mmHg, indicating severe stenosis. He needed an urgent aortic valve replacement.

See p. 295, 6E ECG IP

Summary ★

Left ventricular hypertrophy.

ECG 19

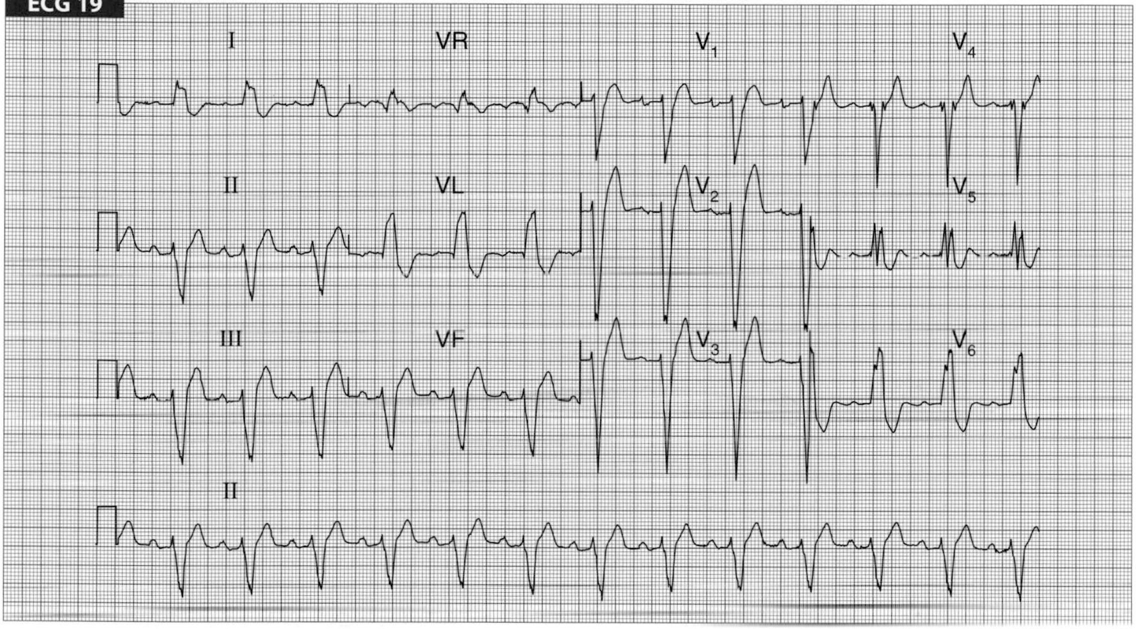

A 75-year-old woman complained of central chest discomfort on climbing hills, together with dizziness; on one occasion she had 'fainted' while climbing stairs. What abnormality does this ECG show and what physical signs would you look for?

ANSWER 19

The ECG shows:

- Sinus rhythm, rate 79/min
- Left axis deviation
- Broad QRS complexes (192 ms)
- 'M' pattern in lead V_6
- Inverted T waves in leads I, VL, V_6

Clinical interpretation

This is the characteristic pattern of left bundle branch block (LBBB). The ECG cannot be interpreted further.

What to do

A patient who has chest pain that could be angina, and who has dizziness and syncope on exertion, probably has severe aortic stenosis – this was the case with this woman. Clinically she had a slow rising pulse, a blood pressure of 100/80, and a slightly enlarged heart. There was a loud ejection systolic murmur, best heard at the upper right sternal edge and radiating to both carotids. The diagnosis was confirmed by an echocardiogram, which showed a gradient across the aortic valve of about 100 mmHg. A cardiac catheter was necessary to exclude coronary disease. She then had an aortic valve replacement, and made a complete recovery.

Summary ★
Sinus rhythm with LBBB.

ECG ME See p. 43, 8E

ECG IP See p. 297, 6E

ECG 20

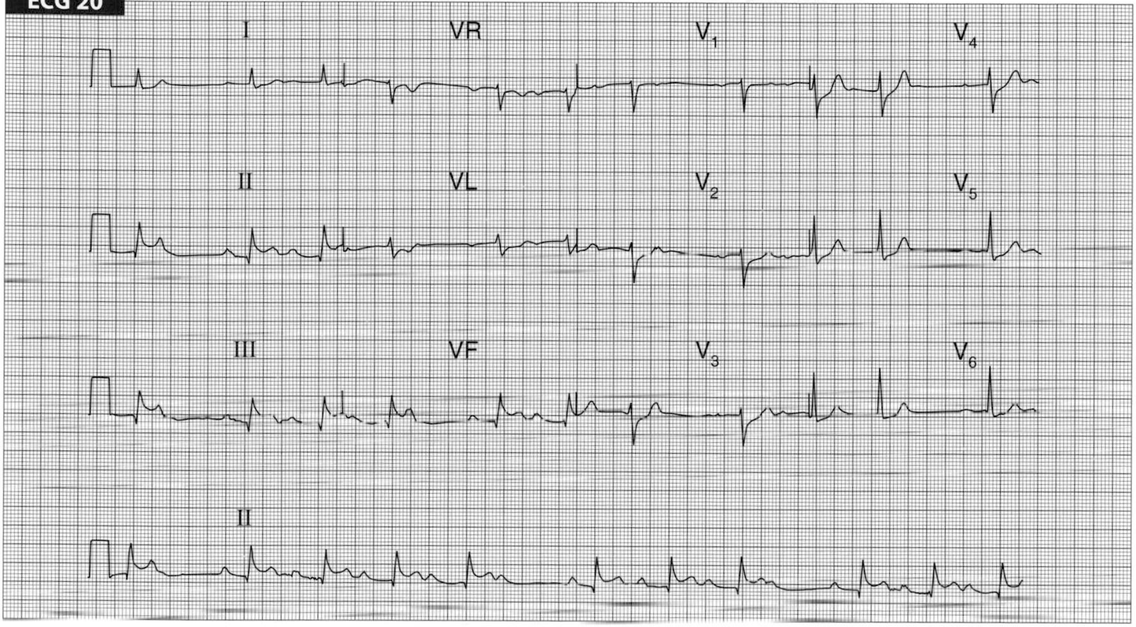

A 70-year-old man is admitted to hospital following the onset of severe central chest pain. This is his ECG. What does it show and what treatment is needed?

ANSWER 20

The ECG shows:

- Sinus rhythm, rate of sinus beats 75/min
- Second degree (Wenckebach) heart block (most obvious in the rhythm strip, recorded from lead II)
- Ventricular rate 70/min
- Normal axis
- Small Q waves in leads II, III, VF
- Raised ST segments in leads II, III, VF
- Depressed ST segments in leads V_5–V_6

Clinical interpretation

This patient has second degree block of the Wenckebach type (progressive lengthening of the PR interval followed by a nonconducted P wave, and then a return to a short PR interval and repeat of the sequence). There is also clear evidence of a recent acute inferior ST segment elevation myocardial infarction (STEMI).

What to do

The patient should be treated in the usual way for his acute myocardial infarction, with pain relief and immediate percutaneous coronary intervention (PCI) or thrombolysis. Wenckebach second degree block is usually benign when it occurs with an inferior infarction, and although he must obviously be monitored until sinus rhythm with normal conduction returns, temporary pacing is not necessary.

Summary ★
Second degree (Wenckebach) atrioventricular block with acute inferior STEMI.

ECG ME See p. 38, 8E

ECG IP See p. 84, 6E

ECG 21

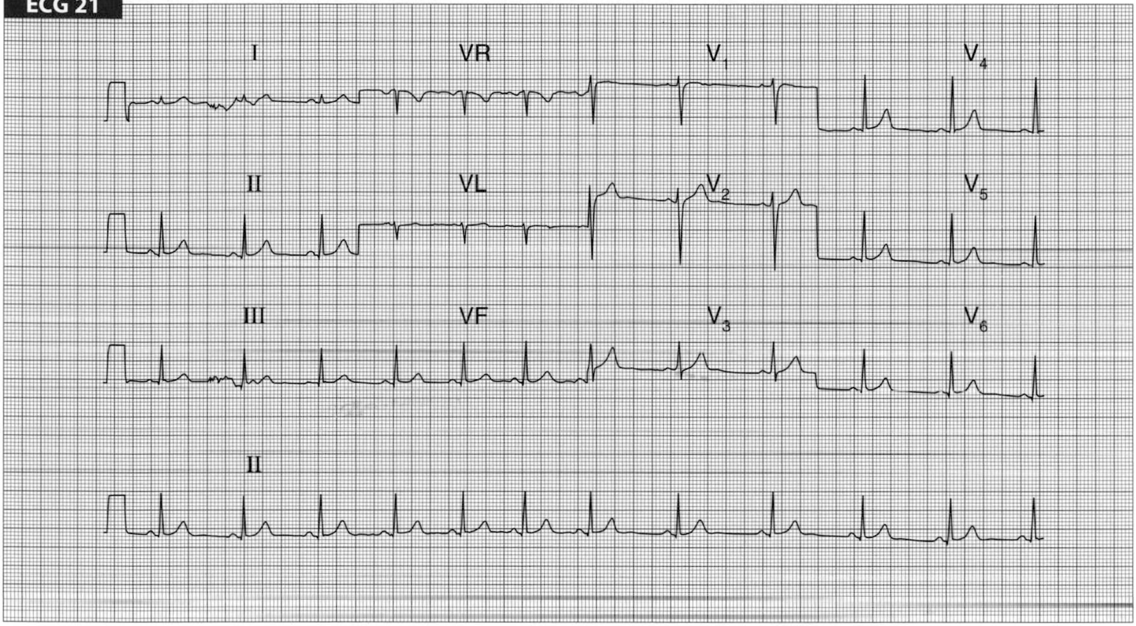

This ECG was recorded from a medical student during a practical class. What does it show?

ANSWER 21

The ECG shows:

- Sinus rhythm, rate 70/min
- Sinus arrhythmia
- Normal axis
- Normal QRS complexes
- Normal ST segments and T waves

Clinical interpretation

This is a perfectly normal ECG. There is a beat-to-beat variation in the interval between QRS complexes, with the heart rate speeding up and slowing down. Comparison of the rate recorded in lead VF with that recorded in lead V_3 may give a false impression of a change of rhythm, but the rhythm strip (lead II) clearly shows the progressive alteration of the R–R interval. This variation in heart rate relates to respiration and is called sinus arrhythmia, which is normal in young people. Sinus arrhythmia can be distinguished from atrial extrasystoles because in sinus arrhythmia the morphology of the P waves is unchanged.

What to do

Nothing!

Summary ★

Normal ECG with sinus arrhythmia.

ECG ME See p. 57, 8E

ECG IP See p. 113, 6E

ECG 22

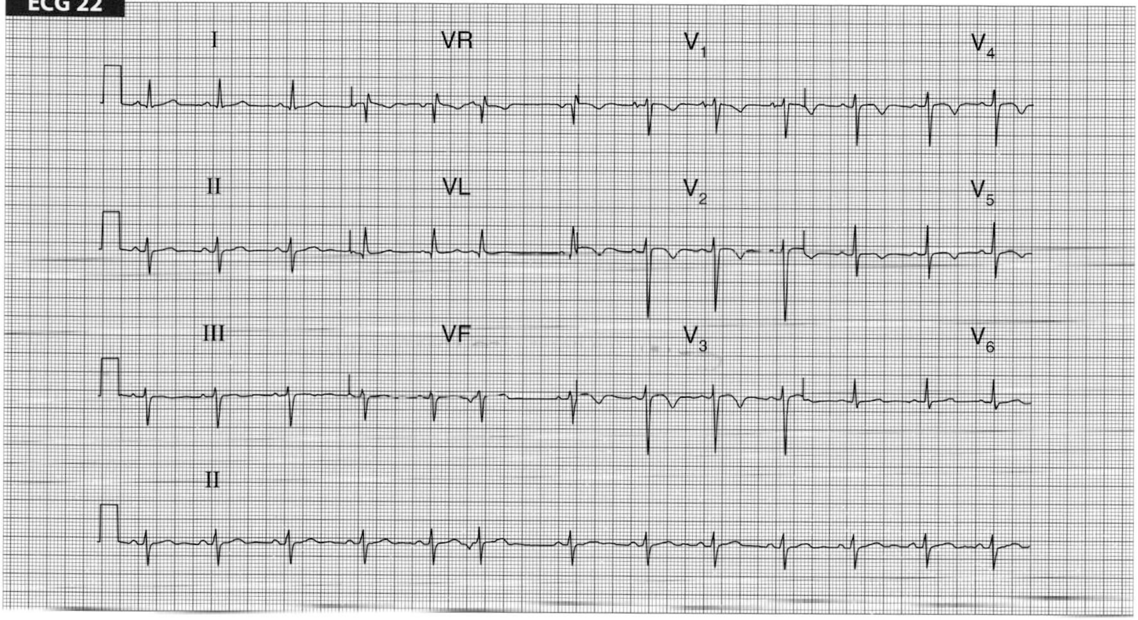

This ECG was recorded from a 48-year-old man who had had severe central chest pain for 1 h. What does it show and what would you do?

ANSWER 22

The ECG shows:

- Sinus rhythm, rate 75/min
- Left axis deviation (left anterior hemiblock)
- Normal QRS complexes, with a small Q wave (probably septal) in lead VL
- Inverted T waves in leads V_1–V_5

Clinical interpretation

This is a classic acute anterior non-ST segment elevation myocardial infarction (NSTEMI).

What to do

This ECG does not meet the conventional criteria for immediate percutaneous coronary intervention (PCI) or thrombolysis, which are raised ST segments or new left bundle branch block. The treatment is pain relief, aspirin, heparin, a beta-blocker and a statin – with PCI as soon as possible. The immediate outlook is good but the patient should be monitored and the ECG repeated after 1 h to see if ST segment elevation is appearing.

Summary ★
Acute anterior NSTEMI.

ECG ME See p. 142, 8E

ECG IP See p. 241, 6E

ECG 23

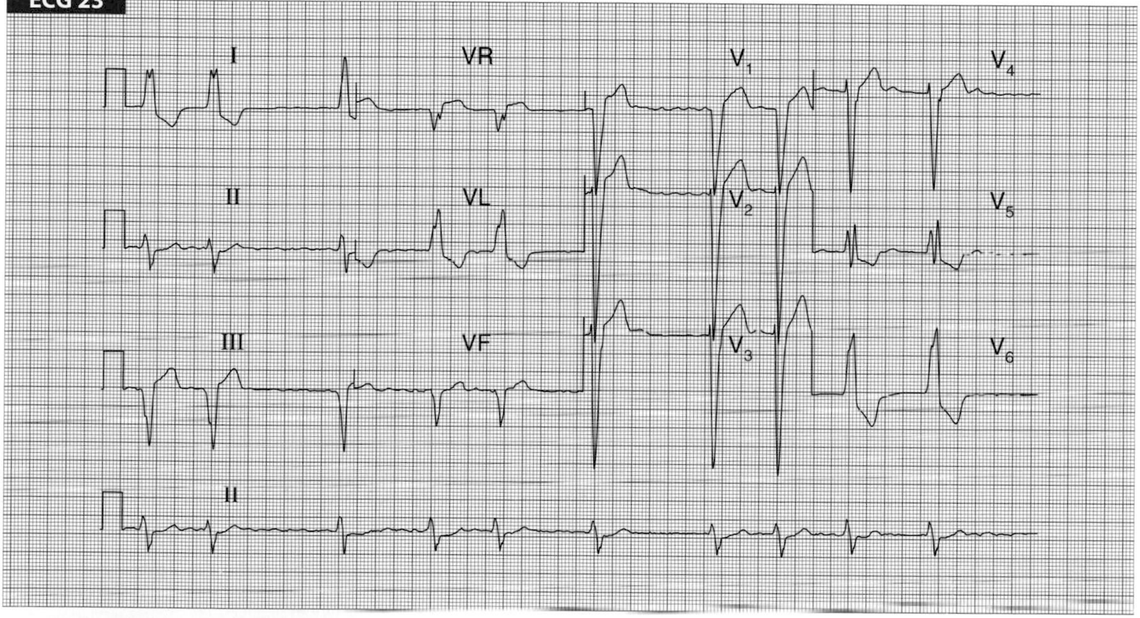

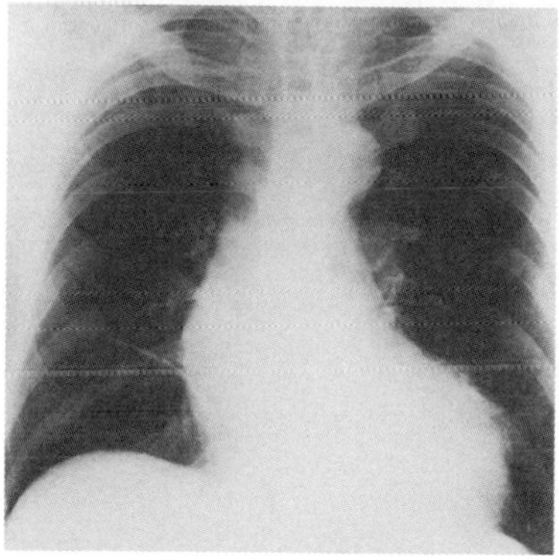

This ECG and chest X-ray are from a 70-year-old man who had had angina for some time and was being treated with a beta-blocker. He came to the A & E department complaining of pain similar to his angina, but much more severe and persistent for 4 h. He had a heart murmur. What do the ECG and chest X-ray show and what treatment would be appropriate?

ANSWER 23

The ECG shows:

- Atrial fibrillation; ventricular rate 62/min
- Left axis deviation (left anterior hemiblock)
- Broad QRS complexes (160 ms)
- 'M' pattern of QRS complexes in leads V_5–V_6
- Inverted T waves in leads I, VL, V_5–V_6

The chest X-ray shows an enlarged left ventricle and a dilated ascending aorta.

Clinical interpretation

This ECG shows atrial fibrillation and left bundle branch block (LBBB). No further interpretation is possible.

What to do

This patient has angina, and the chest X-ray suggests aortic stenosis. LBBB is characteristic of severe aortic stenosis. The problem is deciding whether his episode of severe pain is due to a bad attack of angina or to a myocardial infarction. An aortic dissection is also a possibility. Percutaneous coronary intervention (PCI) or thrombolytic agents should not be given unless there is evidence from previous records that the LBBB is new, and treatment will depend on whether the plasma troponin level is elevated. The patient urgently needs an echocardiogram, and probably needs early cardiac catheterization with a view to aortic valve replacement. He will need long-term anticoagulants because of the atrial fibrillation.

Summary ★
Atrial fibrillation and LBBB.

ECG ME See p. 43, 76, 8E

ECG IP See p. 127, 6E

ECG 24

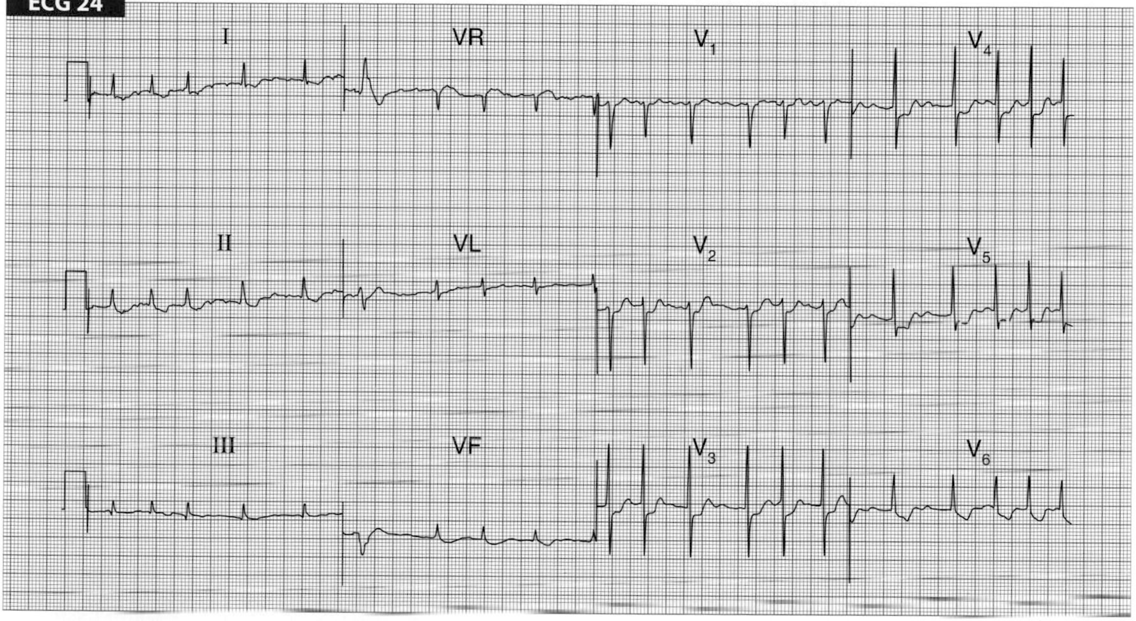

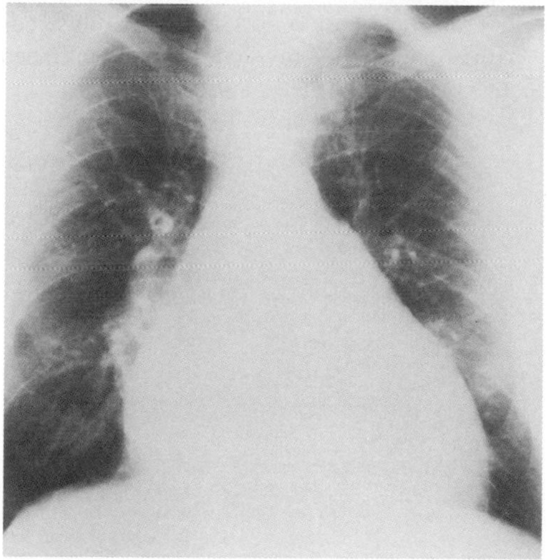

This ECG and chest X-ray are from a 60-year-old man being treated as an outpatient for severe congestive cardiac failure. What might be the diagnosis of the underlying heart condition and what would you do?

ANSWER 24

The ECG shows:

- Atrial fibrillation
- Average ventricular rate 120/min
- Normal axis
- Normal QRS complexes
- Horizontal ST segment depression in leads V_3–V_4
- Downward-sloping ST segment depression in leads I, II, V_5–V_6

The chest X-ray shows a generally enlarged heart, but especially an enlarged left ventricle and left atrium.

Clinical interpretation

The ventricular rate is not adequately controlled, though the downward-sloping ST segment depression suggests that he is taking digoxin. The horizontal ST segment depression suggests ischaemia.

What to do

Despite the ECG evidence of ischaemia, possible diagnoses include rheumatic heart disease, thyrotoxicosis, alcoholic heart disease, and other forms of cardiomyopathy. The chest X-ray suggests severe mitral regurgitation. Echocardiography is necessary. The serum digoxin level must be checked and the digoxin dose increased if appropriate. In addition to digoxin, the patient will need an angiotensin-converting enzyme inhibitor, a diuretic and, unless contraindicated, anticoagulants. Beta-blockers must be considered once his cardiac failure is controlled.

Summary ★★

Atrial fibrillation with an uncontrolled ventricular rate, probable ischaemia and digoxin effect.

ECG ME See p. 76, 101, 8E

ECG IP See p. 290, 6E

ECG 25

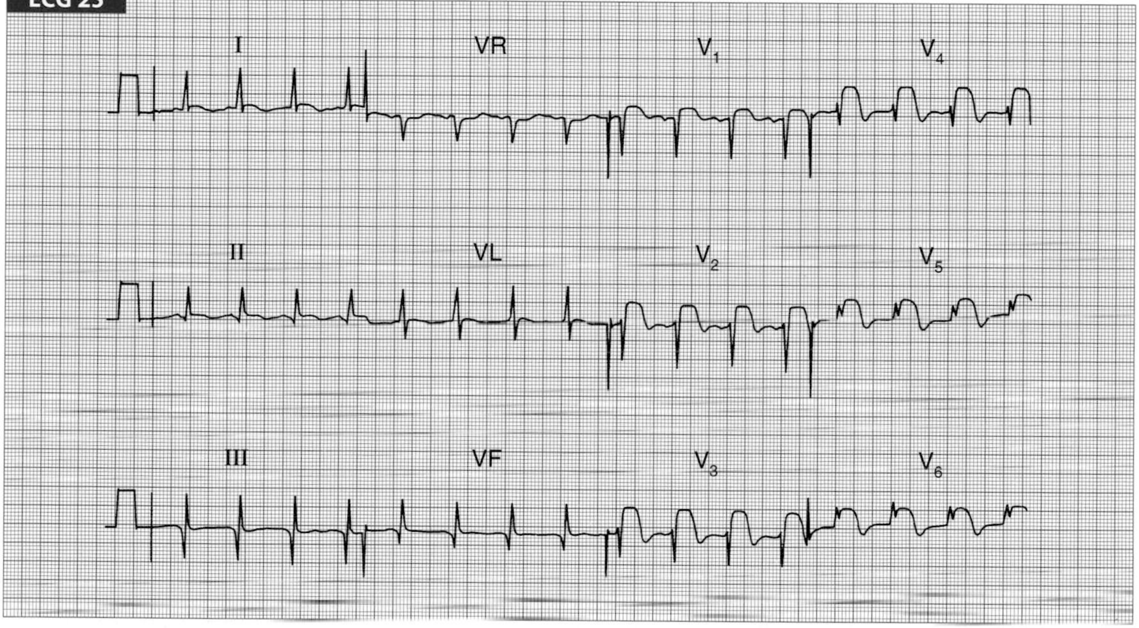

A 60-year-old man, who 3 years earlier had had a myocardial infarction followed by mild angina, was admitted to hospital with central chest pain that had been present for 1 h and had not responded to sublingual nitrates. What does his ECG show, and what would you do?

ANSWER 25

The ECG shows:

- Sinus rhythm, rate 103/min
- Normal axis
- Q waves in leads II, III, VF
- Normal QRS complexes in the anterior leads
- Marked ST segment elevation in leads V_1–V_6

Clinical interpretation

The Q waves in leads III and VF suggest an old inferior infarction, while the elevated ST segments in leads V_1–V_6 indicate an acute anterior ST segment elevation infarction.

What to do

The patient should be given pain relief, and in the absence of the usual contraindications should immediately be treated with aspirin, immediate percutaneous coronary intervention (PCI) or a thrombolytic agent. If he was treated with streptokinase for his previous infarction, he should be given alteplase or reteplase on this occasion.

Summary ★★

Old inferior and acute anterior myocardial infarctions.

ECG ME See p. 91, 8E

ECG IP See p. 231, 6E

ECG 26

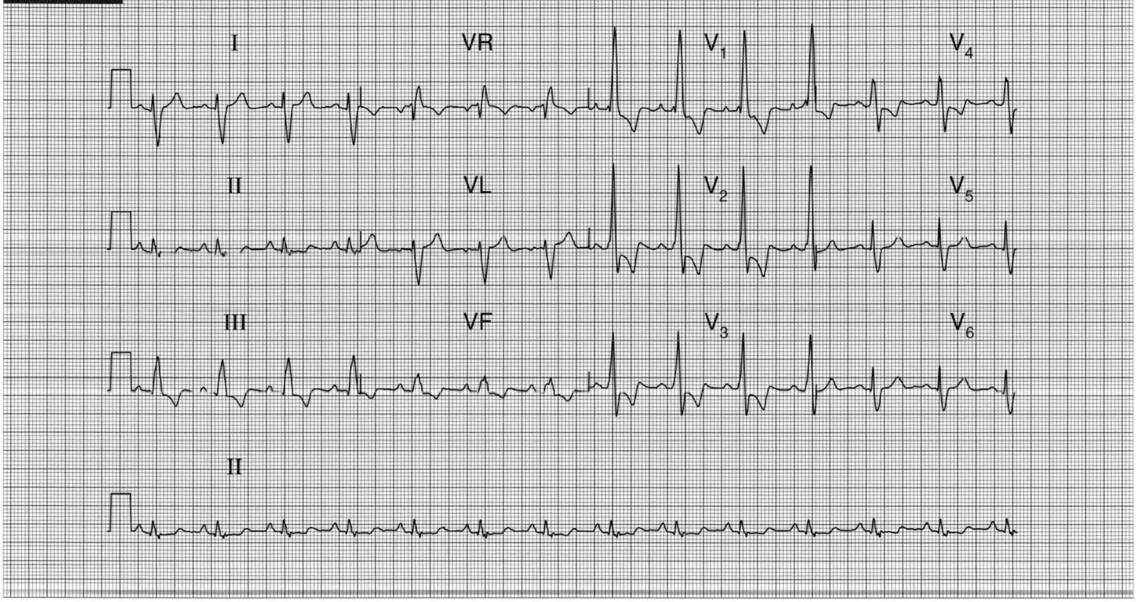

A 15-year-old boy was referred to the outpatient department because of a heart murmur. He had no symptoms. What does this ECG show and what physical signs would you look for?

ANSWER 26

The ECG shows:

- Sinus rhythm, rate 83/min
- Right axis deviation
- Broad QRS complexes (140 ms)
- RSR[1] pattern in leads V_1–V_3
- Wide and slurred S waves in lead V_6
- Normal ST segments
- T wave inversion in leads III, VF and V_1–V_4

Clinical interpretation

Right bundle branch block (RBBB). The right axis deviation suggests left posterior hemiblock.

What to do

RBBB is seen in a small proportion of people with otherwise perfectly normal hearts. In the presence of a heart murmur, however, the possibility of an atrial septal defect should be considered. This is what this patient had. The physical signs were a widely split pulmonary second sound which did not vary with inspiration (this is typical of RBBB), and an ejection systolic murmur best heard at the left sternal edge. On deep inspiration a soft diastolic murmur could be heard at the lower left sternal edge. The systolic murmur is a pulmonary flow murmur due to the extra flow through the right side of the heart, and the diastolic murmur that occurs on inspiration is a tricuspid flow murmur. The diagnosis was confirmed by echocardiography, and the defect was closed with a percutaneous 'umbrella' device. Following operation, the RBBB persisted.

Summary ★★
Sinus rhythm with RBBB.

ECG ME See p. 44, 8E

ECG IP See p. 327, 6E

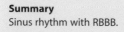

ECG 27

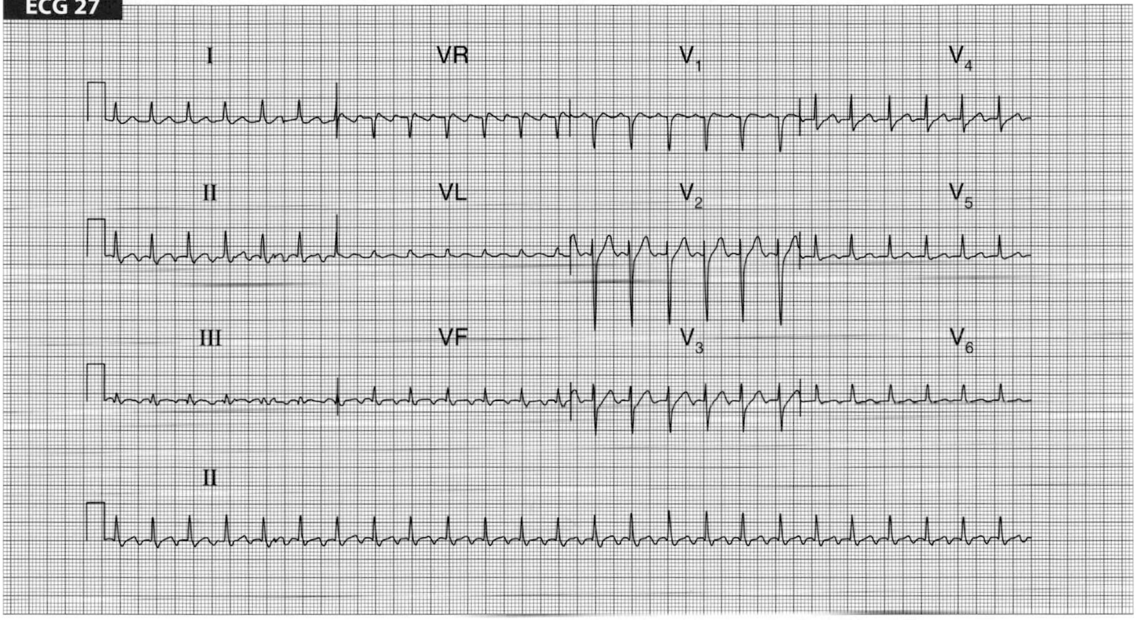

This ECG was recorded from a 40-year-old man who complained of breathlessness on climbing stairs. He was not aware of a fast heart rate and had had no chest pain. Apart from a rapid rate there were no cardiovascular abnormalities, but he looked a little jaundiced and had an enlarged spleen. What would you do?

ANSWER 27

The ECG shows:

- Atrial flutter
- Ventricular rate 148/min
- Normal axis
- Normal QRS complexes, ST segments and T waves

Clinical interpretation

Atrial flutter with 2:1 block.

What to do

Provided the patient is not in heart failure, it is always a good idea to identify the cause of an arrhythmia before treating it. The combination of an atrial arrhythmia, jaundice and splenomegaly suggests alcoholism. The patient needs anticoagulants, but his INR (international normalized ratio) may already be high. An echocardiogram is needed to assess left ventricular function. Carotid sinus massage will probably increase the degree of atrioventricular block, but is unlikely to correct the arrhythmia. Digoxin, a beta-blocker or verapamil could be given in an attempt to control the ventricular rate. After anticoagulation, cardioversion – either electrical or with flecainide – will be necessary.

Summary ★
Atrial flutter with 2:1 conduction.

ECG ME See p. 67, 8E

ECG IP See p. 117, 6E

ECG 28

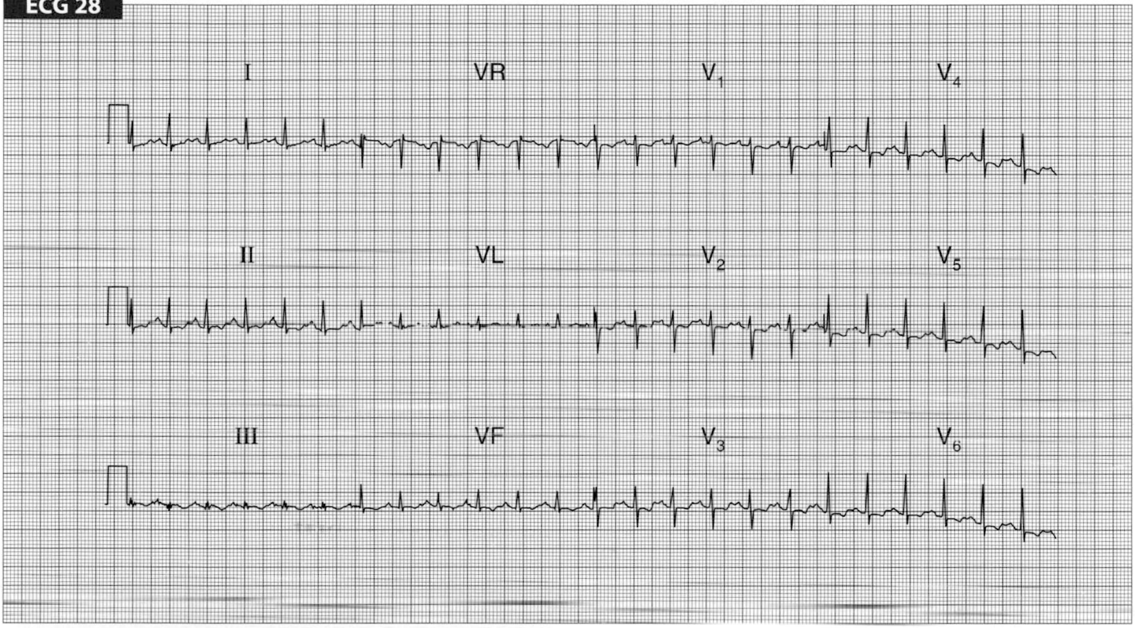

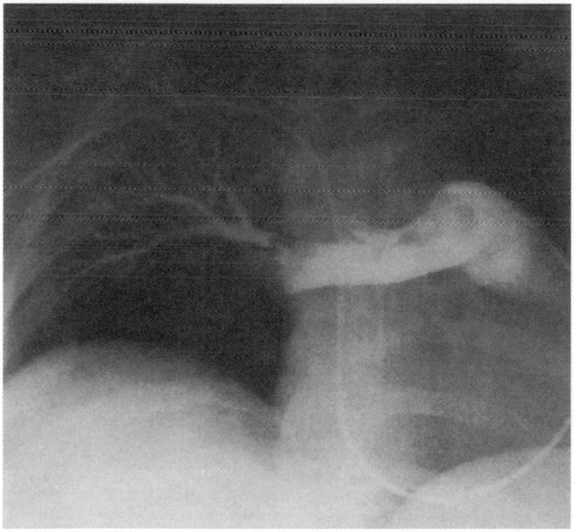

This ECG and pulmonary angiogram are from a 39-year-old woman who complained of a recent sudden onset of breathlessness. She had no previous history of breathlessness, and no chest pain. Examination revealed nothing, other than a rapid heart rate. A pulmonary angiogram was carried out as part of a series of investigations immediately after admission. What is the diagnosis?

ANSWER 28

The ECG shows:

- Sinus rhythm, rate 140/min
- Normal conduction
- Normal axis
- Normal QRS complexes
- Slightly depressed ST segments in leads V_1–V_4
- Biphasic or inverted T waves in the inferior leads and all the chest leads

Clinical interpretation

The ECG shows a marked sinus tachycardia, with no change in the cardiac axis and normal QRS complexes. The widespread ST segment/T wave changes are clearly very abnormal, but are not specific for any particular disease. However, the fact that leads V_1–V_3 are affected suggests a right ventricular problem.

The pulmonary angiogram shows a large central pulmonary embolus and occlusion of the arteries to the right lower lung.

What to do

This is a case where the ECG must be considered in the light of the patient's history and physical signs (if any). Clearly something has happened: the sudden onset of breathlessness without pain suggests a central pulmonary embolus – with pulmonary emboli that do not reach the pleural surface of the lung there may be little pain. In this patient, an echocardiogram and then a pulmonary angiogram demonstrated a large pulmonary embolus. Remember that sudden breathlessness with clear lung fields on a routine chest X-ray is always assumed to be due to a pulmonary embolus until proved otherwise. Heparin is essential; thrombolysis should be considered.

Summary ★★

Sinus tachycardia with widespread ST segment/T wave changes, suggesting pulmonary embolism.

ECG ME See p. 89, 8E

ECG IP See p. 247, 6E

ECG 29

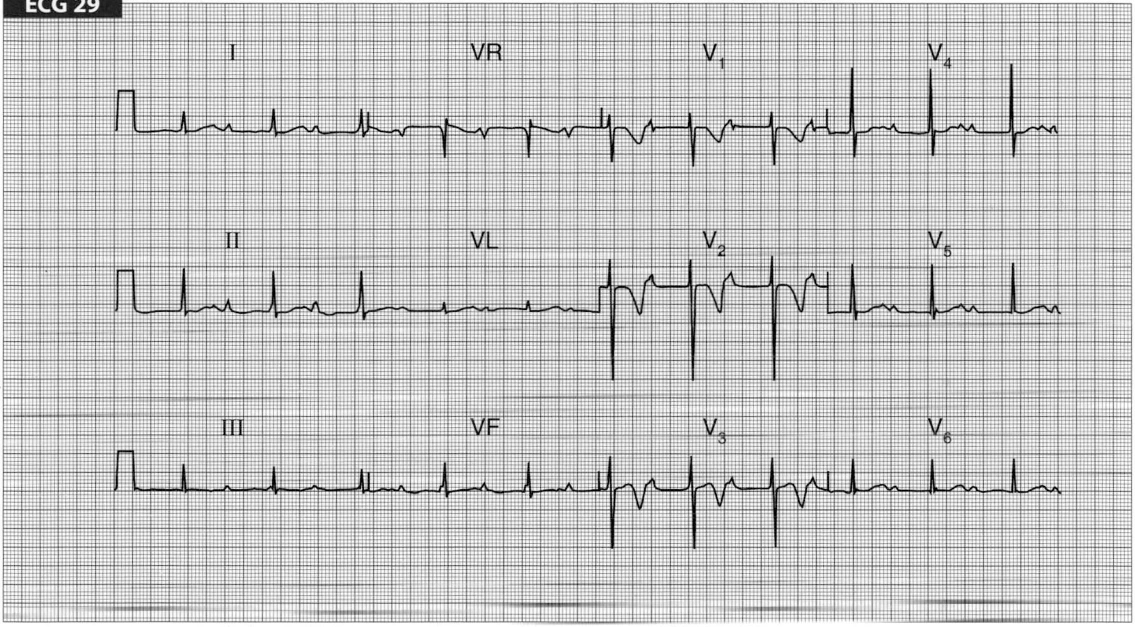

This ECG was recorded from a 50-year-old man who was admitted to hospital as an emergency, having had chest pain characteristic of a myocardial infarction for 3 h. What does the ECG show and how should the patient be treated?

ANSWER 29

The ECG shows:

- Sinus rhythm, rate 65/min
- PR interval markedly prolonged (480 ms)
- Normal axis
- Normal QRS complexes
- T wave inversion in leads V_1–V_3

Clinical interpretation

First degree block associated with a non-ST segment elevation anterior myocardial infarction (NSTEMI). Since the T wave inversion is in leads V_1–V_3 but not V_4, the possibility of a pulmonary embolus must be considered.

What to do

The ECG changes do not meet the conventional criteria for percutaneous coronary intervention (PCI) or thrombolysis for myocardial infarction (raised ST segments or new left bundle branch block), but the patient does need the full range of treatment for an NSTEMI – heparin, aspirin, clopidogrel, a beta-blocker, possibly a nitrate, and a statin. Early angiography must be considered. First degree block is not an indication for temporary pacing, but the patient must be monitored in case higher degrees of block develop.

Summary ★★

First degree block and anterior NSTEMI.

ECG ME See p. 98, 8E

ECG IP See p. 184, 6E

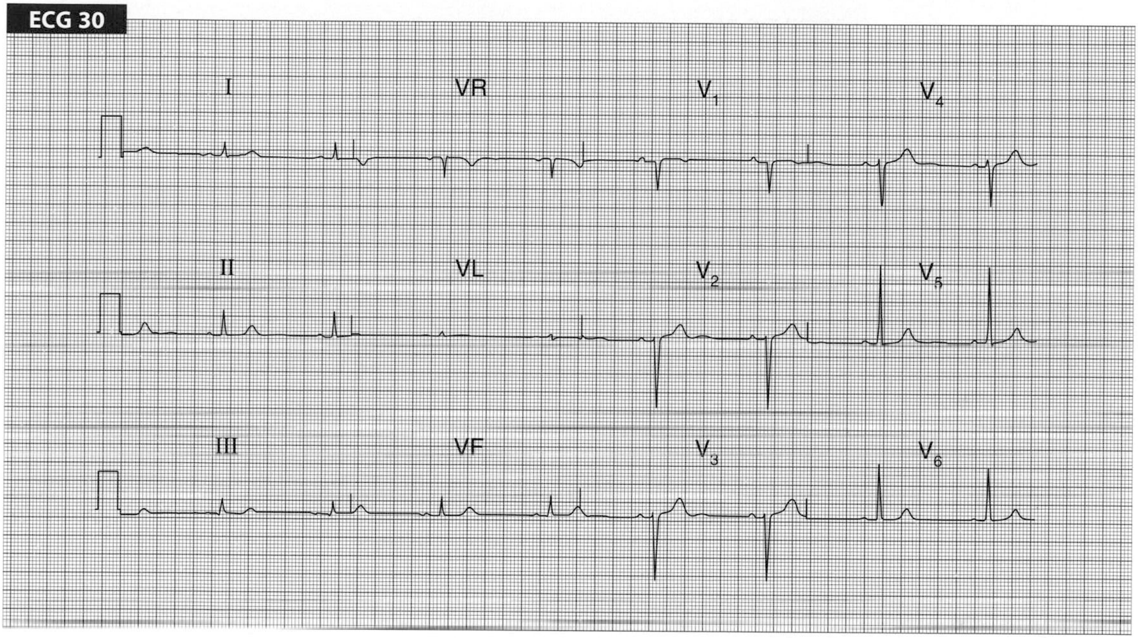

A 65-year-old man is seen in the outpatient department complaining of breathlessness and chest pain that has the characteristics of angina. He is untreated. Does his ECG help with his diagnosis and management?

ANSWER 30

The ECG shows:

- Sinus rhythm, rate 48/min
- Normal axis
- Small R waves in leads V_2–V_4 and a normal (tall) R wave in lead V_5

Clinical interpretation

The small R waves in leads V_2–V_4 and the 'sudden' appearance of a normal R wave in lead V_5 is called 'poor R wave progression', and despite the absence of Q waves this probably indicates an old anterior infarction. An alternative explanation might be poor lead positioning.

What to do

The ECG should be repeated, to ensure proper positioning of the chest leads. An echocardiogram and a chest X-ray are needed, to see if left ventricular impairment is responsible for the breathlessness, and stress echocardiography or perfusion imaging are needed, to investigate the chest pain.

Summary ★★

Poor R wave progression, suggesting an old anterior myocardial infarction.

ECG ME See p. 130, 8E

ECG IP See p. 225, 6E

ECG 31

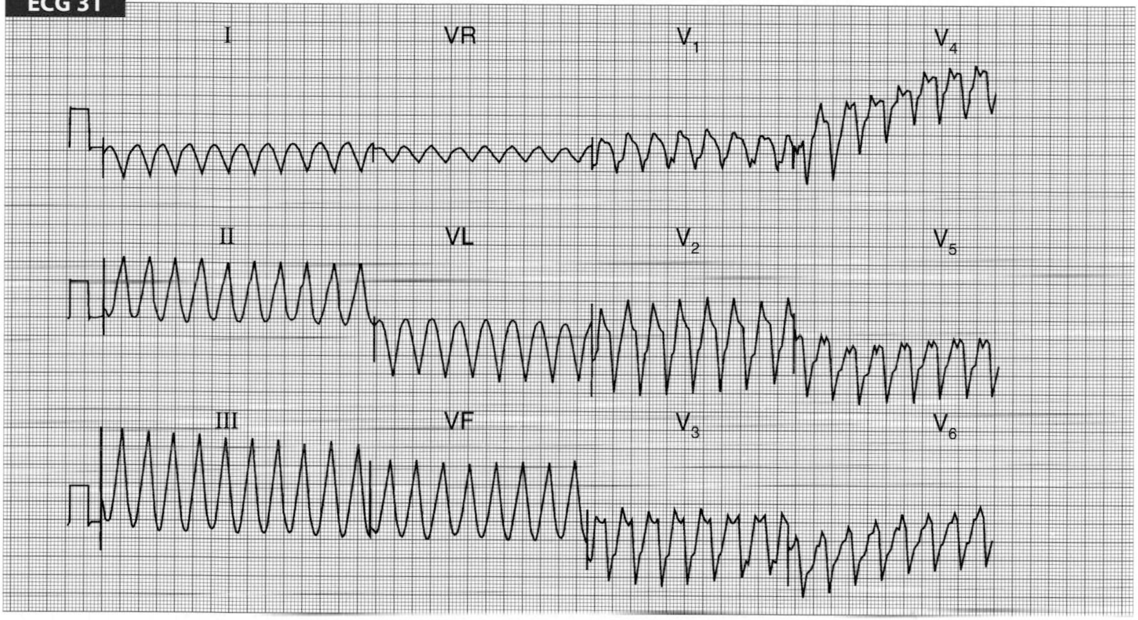

This ECG was recorded in a coronary care unit from a patient admitted 2 h previously with an acute anterior myocardial infarction. The patient was cold, clammy and confused, and his blood pressure was unrecordable. What does the ECG show and what would you do?

ANSWER 31

The ECG shows:

- Broad complex tachycardia, rate about 215/min
- Regular QRS complexes
- QRS complex duration uncertain: probably about 280 ms
- Indeterminate axis and QRS complex configuration

Clinical interpretation

In the context of acute myocardial infarction, broad complex tachycardias should be considered to be ventricular in origin – unless the patient is known to have bundle branch block when in sinus rhythm. Here the regularity of the rhythm and the very broad complexes of bizarre configuration leave no room for doubt that this is ventricular tachycardia.

What to do

In cases of severe circulatory failure, immediate DC cardioversion is needed.

Summary ★★★

Ventricular tachycardia.

ECG ME See p. 73, 8E

ECG IP See p. 126, 6E

ECG 32

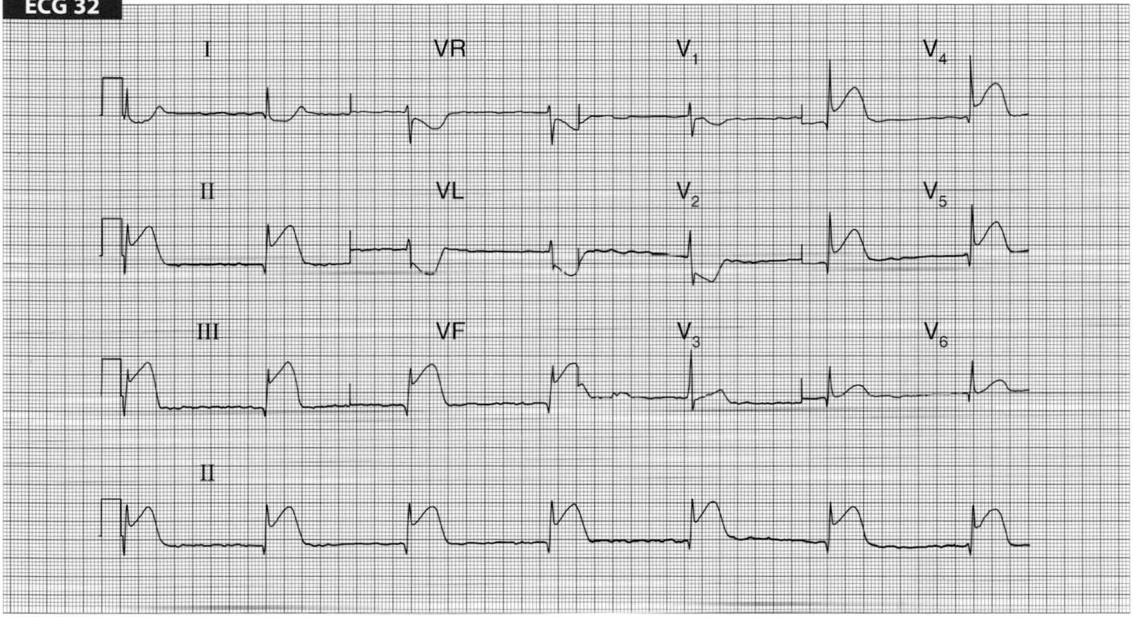

A 50-year-old man is admitted to hospital as an emergency, having had chest pain for 4 h. The pain is characteristic of a myocardial infarction. Apart from signs due to pain, the examination is normal. What does this ECG show and what would you do?

ANSWER 32

The ECG shows:

- Sinus rhythm, rate 38/min
- Normal axis
- Small Q waves in leads II, III, VF, V_4–V_6
- Normal QRS complexes in the chest leads
- Raised ST segments in leads II, III, VF and to a lesser extent in V_4 and V_5
- Downward-sloping ST segments in leads VL and V_2

Clinical interpretation

This is an acute ST segment elevation inferior myocardial infarction (STEMI). The rapidity of Q wave development is extremely variable, but the trace is certainly consistent with a 4 h history. The depressed and downward-sloping ST segment in lead V_2 suggests involvement of the posterior wall of the left ventricle.

What to do

Pain relief is the most important part of the treatment. In the absence of contra-indications, the patient should be given aspirin immediately, and then percutaneous coronary intervention (PCI) or thrombolysis as soon as possible.

Summary ★
Acute inferior STEMI.

ECG ME See p. 91, 138, 8E

ECG IP See p. 215, 6E

ECG 33

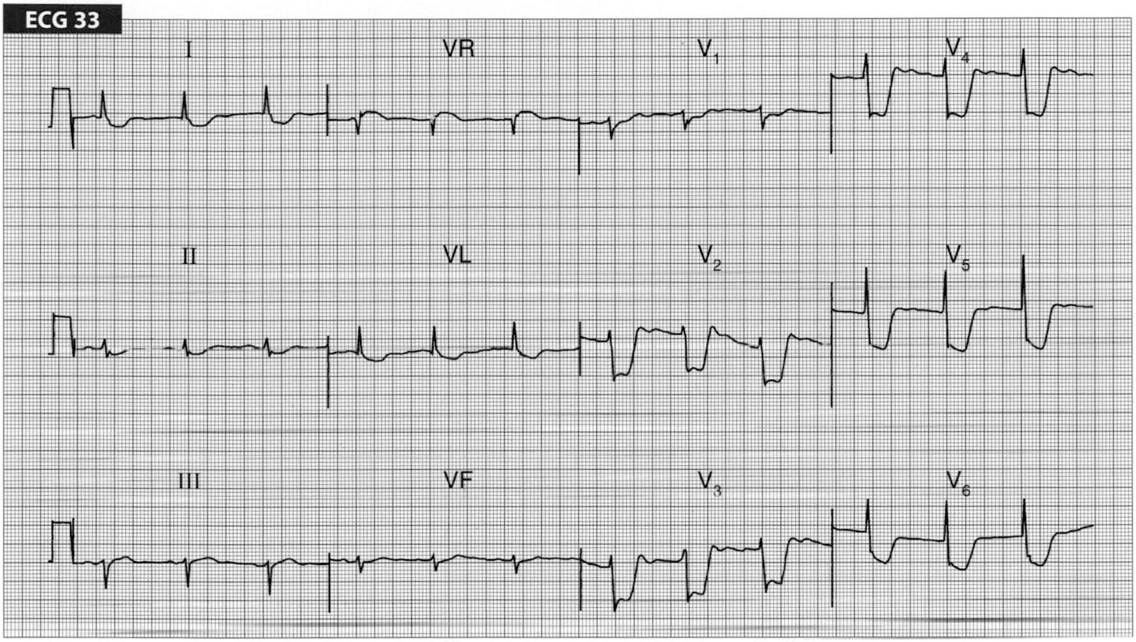

An 80-year-old man being observed in the recovery room following a femoral–popliteal bypass operation was noted to have this abnormal ECG. What does it show and what would you do?

ANSWER 33

The ECG shows:

- Sinus rhythm, rate 68/min
- Normal axis
- Normal QRS complexes
- Marked horizontal ST segment depression (about 8 mm) in leads V_2–V_4, and downward-sloping ST segment depression in the lateral leads

Clinical interpretation

The patient is elderly and has peripheral vascular disease, so coronary disease is likely to be present. The appearance of the ECG is characteristic of severe cardiac ischaemia. The lack of a tachycardia is surprising.

What to do

This is not an easy situation to deal with because the patient's postoperative condition dictates management. He needs anticoagulation with aspirin and heparin, though his postoperative state may prevent this, and intravenous nitrates should be given cautiously.

Summary ★★

Severe anterolateral ischaemia.

ECG ME See p. 144, 8E

ECG IP See p. 243, 6E

ECG 34

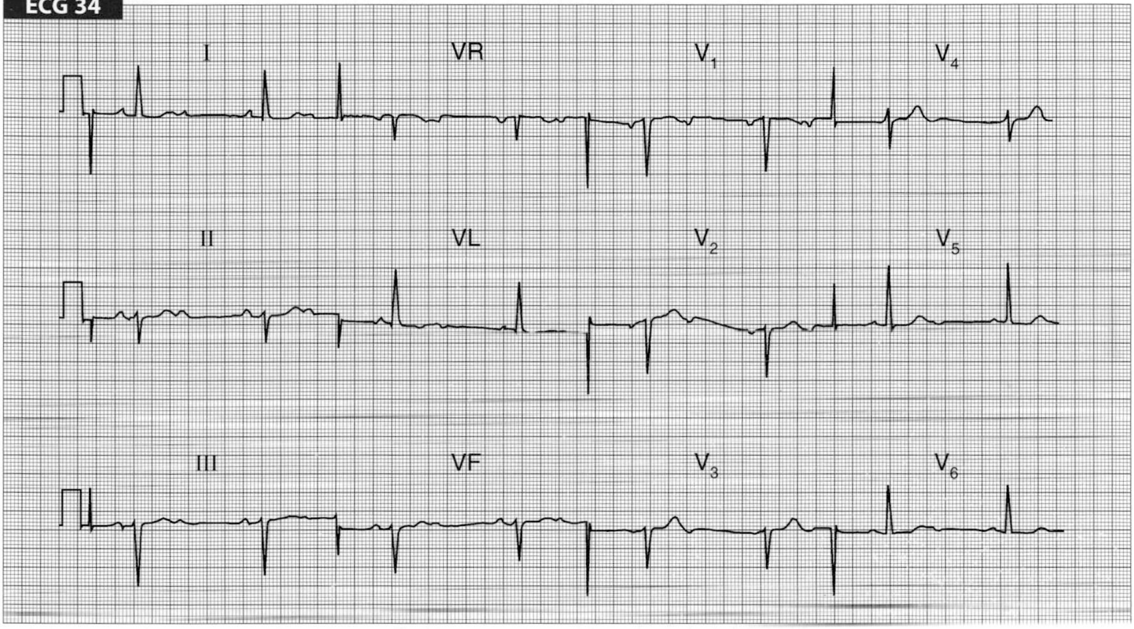

This ECG was recorded from a 75-year-old man who complained of breathlessness. He had not had any chest pain or dizziness. Apart from a slow pulse, there were no abnormalities on examination. What three abnormalities are present in this record and how would you treat the patient?

ANSWER 34

The ECG shows:

- Sinus rhythm; ventricular rate 45/min
- Second degree (2 : 1) block
- Left axis deviation
- Poor R wave progression in the anterior leads
- Normal T waves

Clinical interpretation

The second degree block is associated with a ventricular rate of 45/min, which may well be the cause of his breathlessness. The left axis deviation indicates left anterior hemiblock. The poor R wave progression (virtually no R wave in lead V_3, a small R wave in lead V_4, and a normal R wave in lead V_5) suggests an old anterior infarction.

What to do

This patient needs a permanent pacemaker.

Summary ★★★

Second degree (2 : 1) block, left anterior hemiblock, and probable old anterior infarction.

ECG ME See p. 38, 8E

ECG IP See p. 89, 6E

ECG 35

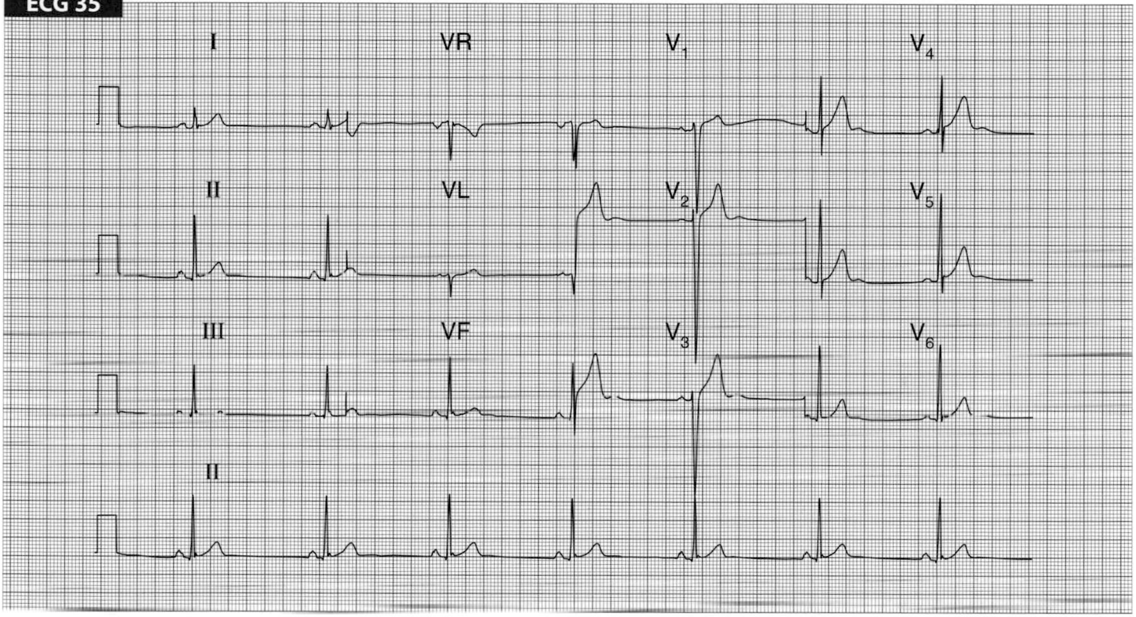

This ECG was recorded from a fit 22-year-old male medical student. He was worried – should he have been?

ANSWER 35

The ECG shows:

- Sinus rhythm, rate 44/min
- Normal axis
- Tall R waves (23 mm in lead V_5) and deep S waves (41 mm in lead V_2)
- Normal ST segments and T waves
- Prominent U waves in leads V_2–V_5

Clinical interpretation

This record shows left ventricular hypertrophy by 'voltage criteria' (R waves greater than 25 mm in lead V_5 or V_6, or the sum of the R wave in lead V_5 or V_6 plus the S wave in lead V_1 or V_2 is greater than 35 mm). There are, however, no T wave changes. 'Voltage criteria' on their own are unreliable, and in a fit young man this may well be a normal variant. The U waves are perfectly normal, and this pattern is common in athletes.

What to do

Tell the student to buy a good book on ECG interpretation, but if reassurance is not enough, echocardiography could be used to measure the left ventricular thickness.

Summary ★★

Left ventricular hypertrophy on 'voltage criteria', but probably normal.

ECG ME See p. 90, 8E

ECG IP See p. 19, 6E

ECG 36

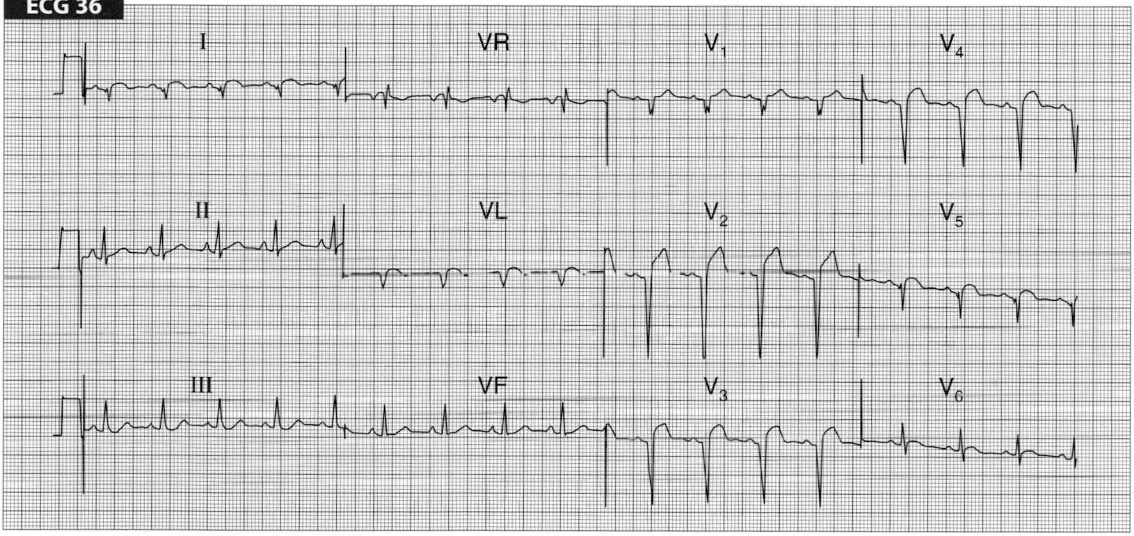

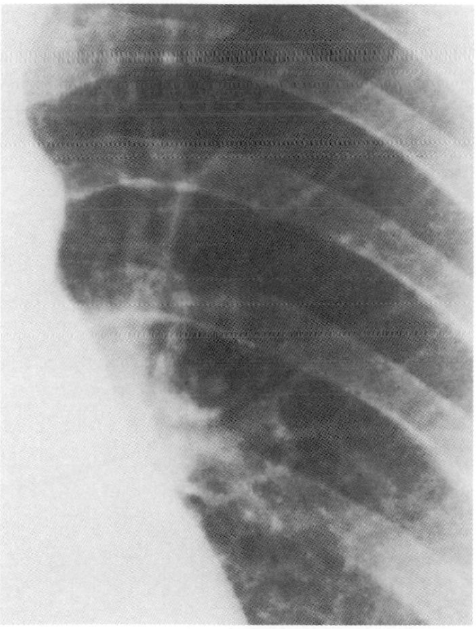

A 70-year-old man was seen as an outpatient with symptoms and signs of heart failure. His problem had begun quite suddenly a few weeks previously, when he had had a few hours of dull central chest discomfort. What do his ECG and the enlarged part of his chest X-ray show and what would you do?

ANSWER 36

The ECG shows:

- Sinus rhythm, rate 100/min
- Normal axis
- Q waves in leads I, VL, V_2–V_5
- Raised ST segments in leads I, VL, V_2–V_6

The chest X-ray shows diversion of blood flow to the upper zones of the lungs, which is an early radiological sign of heart failure.

Clinical interpretation

The raised ST segments suggest an acute infarction, but the deep Q waves suggest that the infarction occurred at least several hours previously. From the patient's story it seems clear that he had an infarction several weeks before he was seen, and there was nothing in the history to suggest a more recent episode. These ECG changes are therefore probably all old; the anterior changes might indicate a left ventricular aneurysm.

What to do

An ECG should always be interpreted in the light of the patient's clinical state. Since the ECG is compatible with an old infarction it should be assumed that this diagnosis is correct, and the patient should be treated for heart failure in the usual way with diuretics, angiotensin-converting enzyme inhibitors and beta-blockers. Since the heart failure is clearly due to ischaemia he also needs aspirin and a statin.

Summary ★

Anterolateral myocardial infarction of uncertain age.

ECG ME See p. 91, 8E

ECG IP See p. 225, 6E

ECG 37

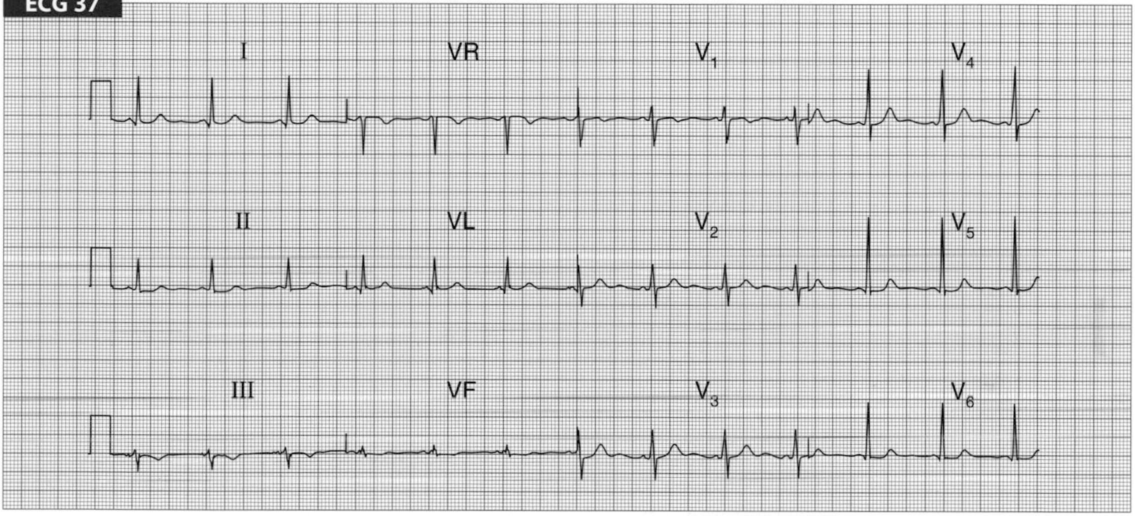

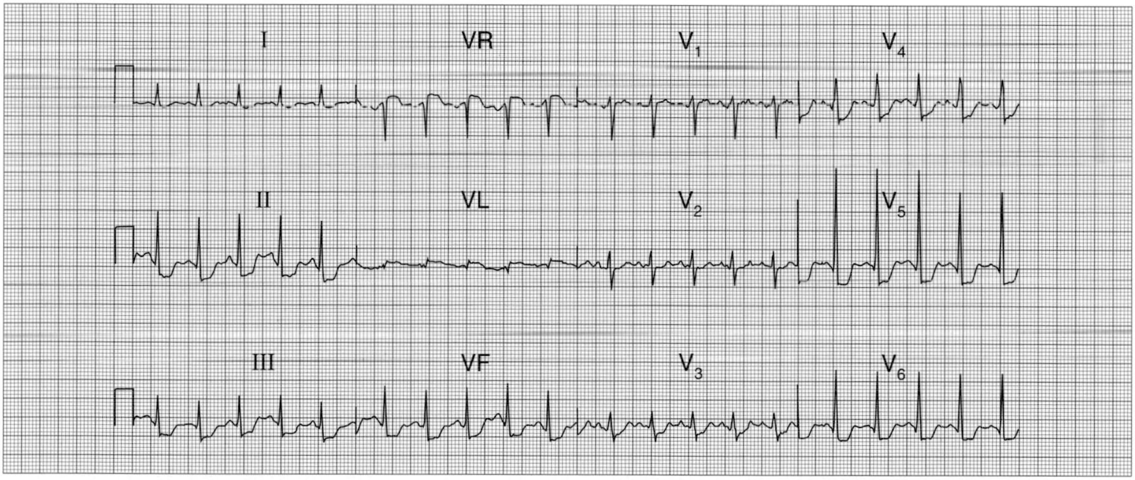

A 60-year-old man was referred to the outpatient department because of exercise-induced chest pain. The upper ECG is his record at rest, and the lower one was taken during stage 1 of the Bruce exercise protocol (1.7 mph and 10% grade on the treadmill). What do these ECGs show and what would you do?

ANSWER 37

Upper ECG

The ECG shows:

- Sinus rhythm, rate 75/min
- Normal axis
- Normal QRS complexes
- Slight ST segment depression in leads II, VF, V_6
- T wave inversion in lead III

Clinical interpretation

The ST segment changes in leads II, VF and V_6 are nonspecific, and the T wave inversion in lead III could well be a normal variant. Nevertheless, with the story of exercise-induced chest pain a diagnosis of angina seems likely, and an exercise test is the appropriate next step.

Lower ECG

The ECG shows:

- Sinus rhythm at 140/min
- Normal axis
- Normal QRS complexes
- ST segment depression in most leads, the maximum being 4 mm in lead V_5

Clinical interpretation

The resting ECG shows only nonspecific changes, but the ECG on exercise shows the classic changes of ischaemia – appearing during the first stage of the Bruce protocol. Even this light exercise level markedly increased the heart rate. Both the inferior and the anterior chest leads show definite ischaemia, so widespread coronary disease is likely, possibly including the main stem of the left coronary artery.

What to do

This patient can be treated immediately with short- and long-acting nitrates, beta-blockers and calcium antagonists, but he also needs urgent coronary angiography with a view to percutaneous coronary intervention (PCI) or coronary artery bypass graft surgery. Risk factors such as smoking, weight and hypercholesterolaemia must also be addressed.

See p. 144, 8E ECG ME

Summary ★

Nonspecific ECG changes at rest; strongly positive exercise test.

See p. 270, 6E ECG IP

ECG 38

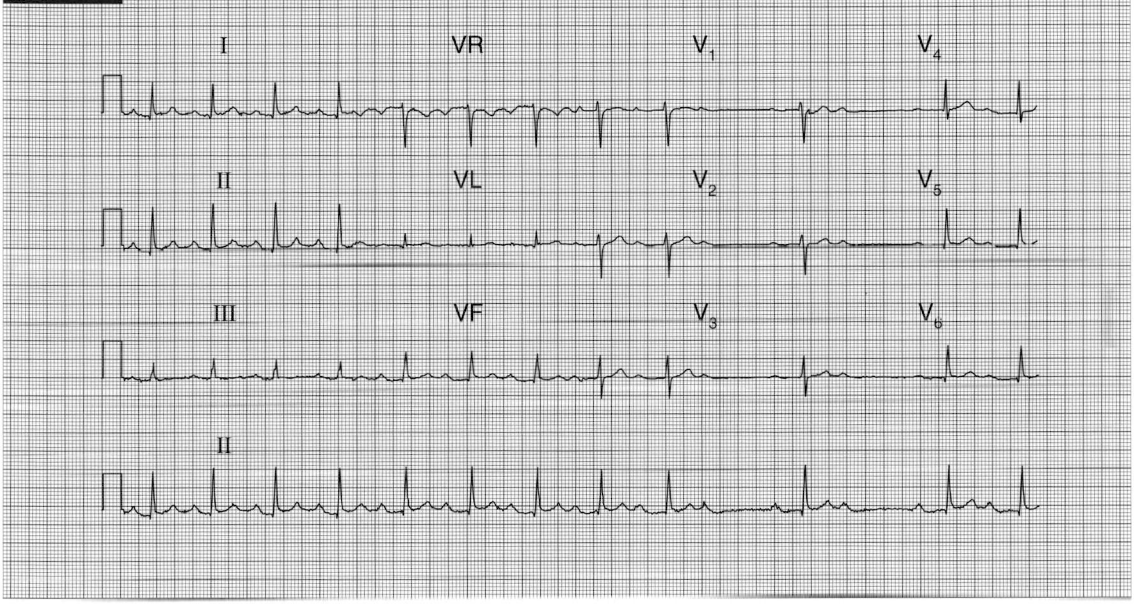

A 70-year-old man with long-standing high blood pressure has had attacks of dizziness over several weeks. His pulse feels irregular but there are no other abnormal signs. This was his ECG. What does it show and what would you do?

ANSWER 38

The ECG shows:

- The first nine beats with sinus rhythm and a ventricular rate of about 80/min
- The PR interval in these nine beats slowly increases, from 240 ms to 360 ms
- There is then a nonconducted P wave, followed by a conducted P wave with a PR interval of 360 ms
- There is then a second nonconducted P wave, followed by two conducted P waves, again with a PR interval of 360 ms
- Normal axis
- Normal QRS complexes, ST segments and T waves

Clinical interpretation

This ECG shows a mixture of different types of heart block. The progressively increasing PR intervals followed by a nonconducted P wave represent second degree block of the Wenckebach (Mobitz type 1) type. The next nonconducted P wave followed by a conducted P wave with a long PR interval is second degree block of Mobitz type 2. The final beat, with the same prolonged PR interval, shows first degree block. The changing heart rate is presumably the cause of his attacks of dizziness.

What to do

Since this man has had no pain, and there is no evidence of ischaemia on the ECG, it is perhaps unlikely that coronary disease is responsible for the conduction problem. You should always think about myocarditis, and about infiltrative diseases that might affect the bundle of His, but in a hypertensive patient the most likely cause of this sort of heart block is medication. He may well be taking either a beta-blocker or a calcium-blocker, and the first thing to do would be to discontinue these.

Summary ★★★

Second degree block of both the Wenckebach type and Mobitz type 2, and also first degree block.

ECG ME See p. 38, 8E

ECG IP See p. 179, 6E

ECG 39

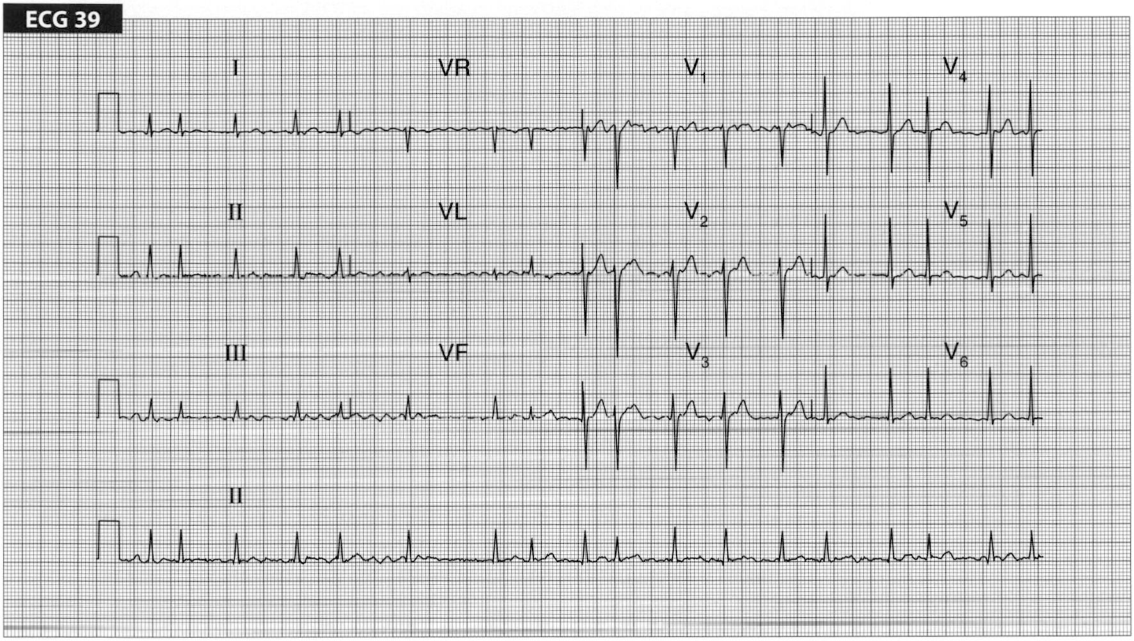

A 70-year-old woman, from whom this ECG was recorded, was admitted to hospital with increasing congestive cardiac failure. What does the ECG show and what would you do?

ANSWER 39

The ECG shows:

- Atrial fibrillation, rate about 110/min
- Normal axis
- Normal QRS complexes
- Normal ST segments

Clinical interpretation

The rhythm could be interpreted as atrial flutter, particularly in lead VL. However, the flutter-like activity is variable, and the QRS complexes are completely irregular, so this is atrial fibrillation. The ST segments are normal, with no suggestion of digoxin effect, and the ventricular rate is not controlled, so the patient is probably not taking digoxin.

What to do

The ventricular rate in this case is rapid, and the uncontrolled rate may be contributing to the patient's heart failure. Her thyroid function tests should be checked, and she needs an echocardiogram to assess heart size and left ventricular function. The heart rate needs to be controlled, and digoxin is the first drug to use. Her heart failure must be treated with a diuretic and probably an angiotensin-converting enzyme inhibitor, and then a decision has to be taken regarding cardioversion. This is unlikely to be successful unless some remediable cause of the atrial fibrillation, such as thyrotoxicosis, is detected. At this age, she will need life-long anticoagulation with warfarin, whatever her echocardiogram shows.

Summary ★

Atrial fibrillation with an uncontrolled ventricular rate.

ECG ME See p. 76, 8E

ECG IP See p. 290, 6E

ECG 40

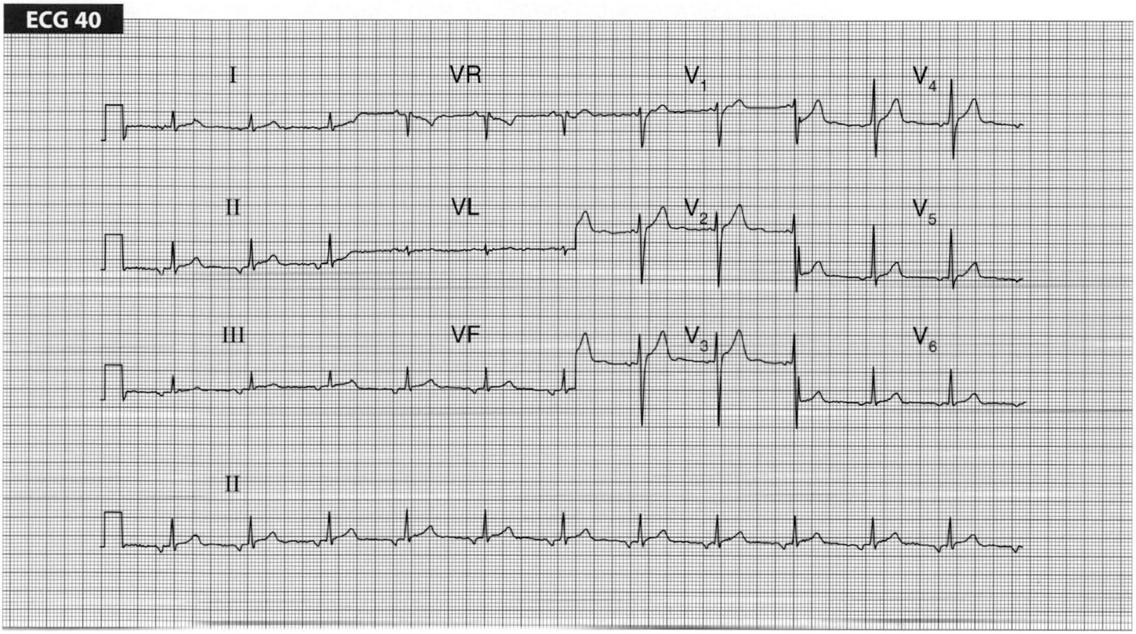

This ECG was recorded from a 30-year-old woman who complained of palpitations. Does it help in making a diagnosis?

ANSWER 40

The ECG shows:

- Ectopic atrial rhythm, with inverted P waves in leads II, III, VF, V_3–V_6; ventricular rate 69/min
- Normal axis
- Normal QRS complexes and T waves

Clinical interpretation

This appears to be a stable rhythm originating in the atrial muscle rather than the SA node – hence the abnormal P wave and the slightly short PR interval (130 ms). This rhythm is not uncommon, and is usually of no clinical significance. It is unlikely to be the cause of her symptoms unless at times she has a paroxysmal atrial tachycardia.

What to do

Take a careful history and attempt to determine whether her symptoms sound like a paroxysmal tachycardia – ask about any sudden onset and ending of the palpitations; associated symptoms like breathlessness; precipitating and terminating factors; and so on. If in doubt, some sort of ambulatory recording will be needed.

Summary ★★
Ectopic atrial rhythm.

ECG ME See p. 111, 8E

ECG IP See p. 7, 6E

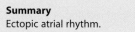

ECG 41

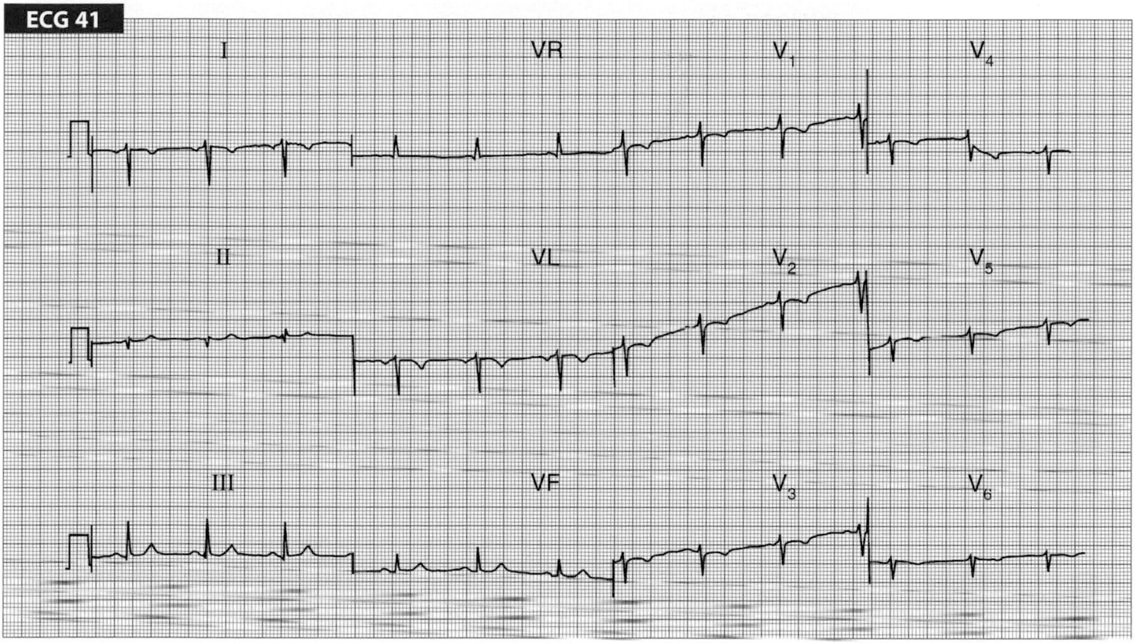

This ECG was recorded from a healthy 25-year-old man during a routine medical examination. Any comments?

ANSWER 41

The ECG shows:

- A very odd appearance
- Sinus rhythm, rate 70/min
- Inverted P waves in lead I
- Right axis deviation
- Dominant R waves in lead VR
- No R wave development in the chest leads, with lead V_6 still showing a right ventricular pattern
- Normal-width QRS complexes

Clinical interpretation

This is dextrocardia. A normal trace would be obtained with the limb leads reversed and the chest leads attached in the usual rib spaces but on the right side of the chest.

What to do

Ensure that the leads are properly attached – for example, inverted P waves in lead I will be seen if the right and left arm attachments are reversed. Of course, this would not affect the appearance of the ECG in the chest leads.

Summary ★★★
Dextrocardia.

ECG ME See p. 19, 8E

ECG IP See p. 10, 6E

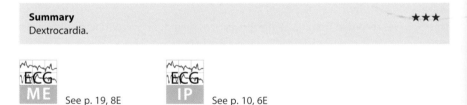

ECG 42

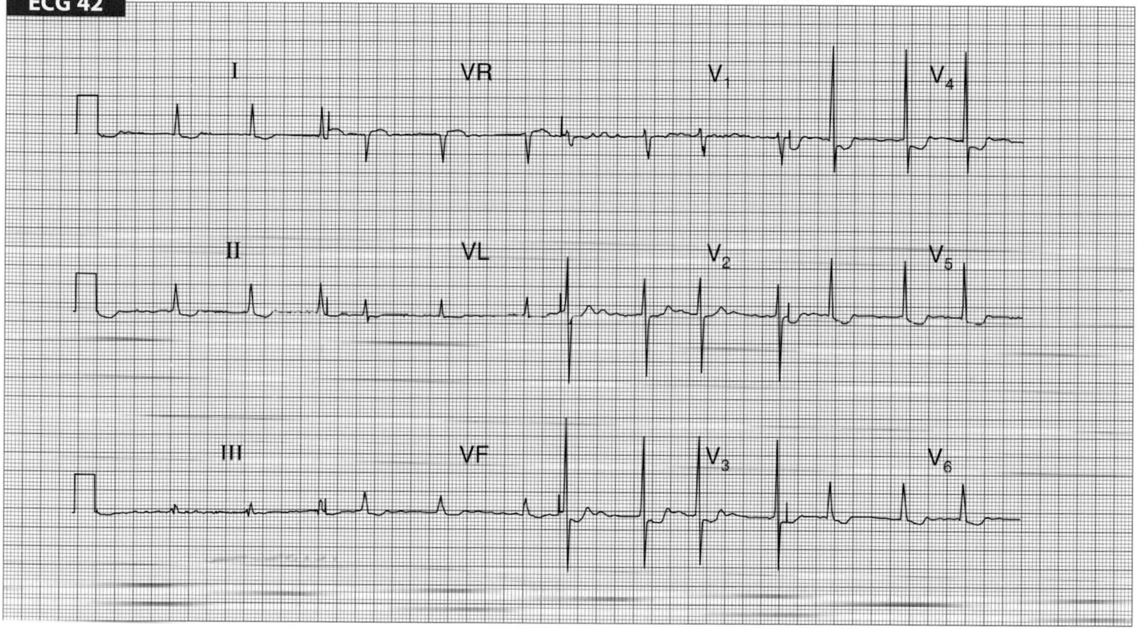

An 80-year-old woman, who has apparently been treated for heart failure for years, complains of nausea and vomiting. No previous records are available. Does her ECG help her management?

ANSWER 42

The ECG shows:

- Atrial fibrillation, ventricular rate 80/min
- Normal axis
- Normal QRS complexes
- Downward-sloping ST segment depression, especially in leads V_4–V_6
- T waves probably upright
- Prominent U waves in leads V_2–V_3

Clinical interpretation

The ECG shows atrial fibrillation with a controlled ventricular rate. There is nothing on the ECG to suggest a cause for the arrhythmia or the patient's heart failure. The 'reversed tick' ST segment depression suggests that she is being treated with digoxin. The ECG does not suggest digoxin toxicity, but nevertheless this is the most likely cause of her nausea. The U waves may be normal, but raise the possibility of hypokalaemia.

What to do

Digoxin therapy should be temporarily discontinued, and her plasma potassium and digoxin levels should be checked.

Summary ★

Atrial fibrillation and digoxin effect.

ECG ME See p. 101, 8E

ECG IP See p. 335, 6E

ECG 43

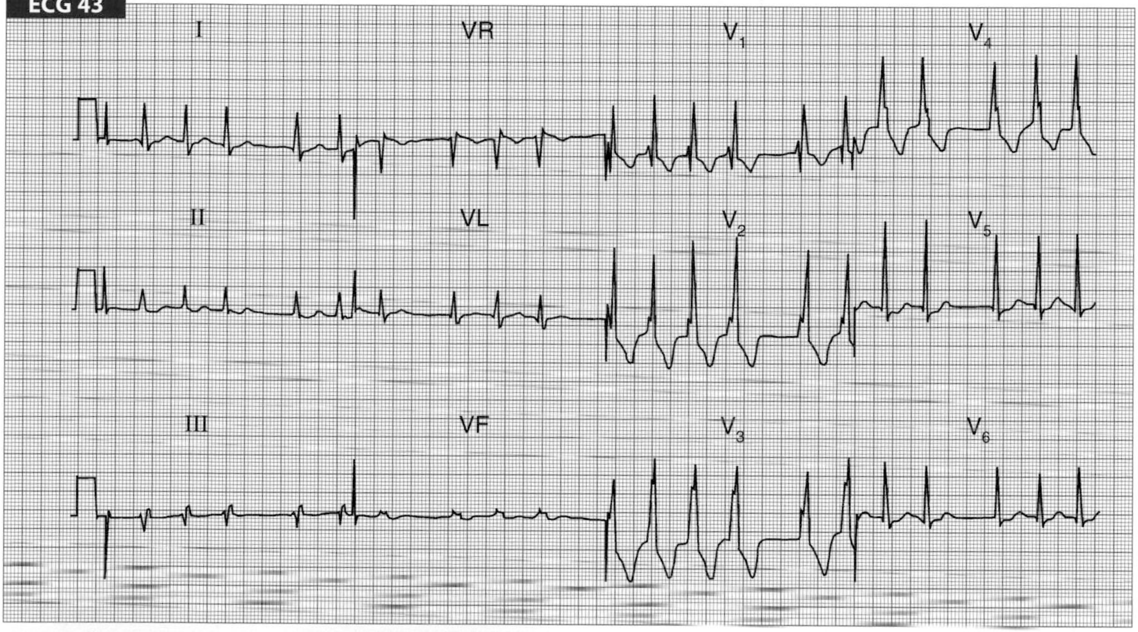

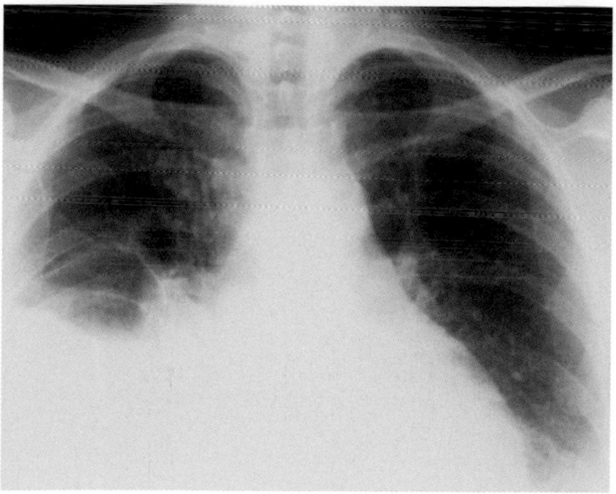

A 60-year-old man, whose heart and preoperative ECG had been normal, developed a cough with pleuritic chest pain a few days after a cholecystectomy. These are his ECG and chest X-ray: what do they show and what might be the problem?

ANSWER 43

The ECG shows:

- Atrial fibrillation
- Normal axis
- RSR^1 pattern in leads V_1–V_3, indicating right bundle branch block (RBBB)

The chest X-ray shows a large pleural effusion on the right side with some atelectasis above it, and also a small left-sided effusion. There is upper-zone blood diversion, indicating heart failure.

Clinical interpretation

In this ECG the usual 'irregular baseline' of atrial fibrillation is not apparent, but the QRS complexes are so irregular that this must be the rhythm. The rhythm change, together with the development of RBBB, could be due to a chest infection but is more likely to have been caused by a pulmonary embolus. The right-sided pleural effusion could also be due to either infection or embolism, but the patient clearly has heart failure because the effusions are bilateral (although asymmetrical) and there is diversion of blood flow to the upper zones of the lungs.

What to do

In a postoperative patient, anticoagulation can always cause haemorrhage. Nevertheless, the risk of death from a pulmonary embolus is so high that the patient should immediately be given heparin while steps are taken (white blood cell count, sputum culture, CT scan) to differentiate between a chest infection and a pulmonary embolus.

Summary ★★★

Atrial fibrillation with RBBB.

ECG ME See p. 43, 76, 8E

ECG IP See p. 125, 6E

ECG 44

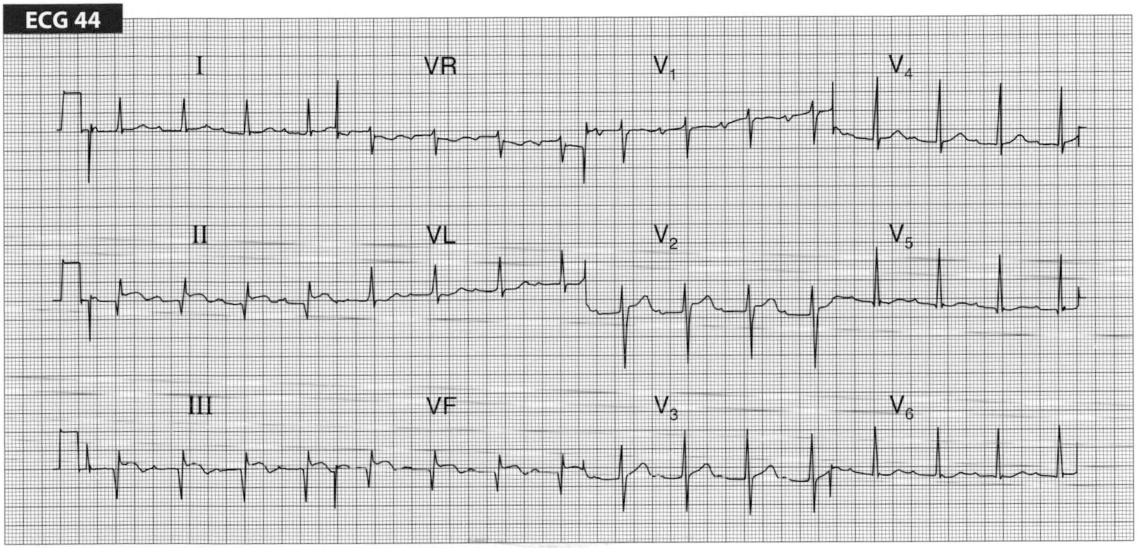

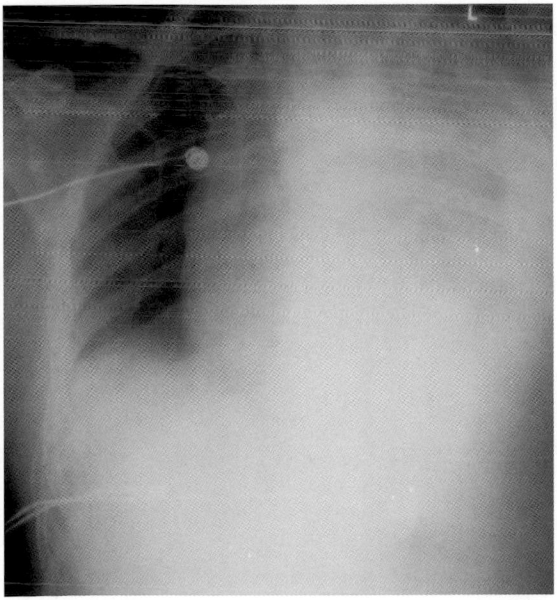

This ECG and chest X-ray were recorded in the A & E department from a 50-year-old man with severe central chest pain that radiated into his back. The pain had been present for 6 h. What do the ECG and X-ray show and what would you do?

ANSWER 44

The ECG shows:

- Sinus rhythm, rate 88/min
- PR interval 320 ms – first degree block
- Q waves in leads II, III, VF
- Raised ST segments in leads II, III, VF
- Inverted T waves in leads III, VF

The chest X-ray shows opacification of the left side of the chest, with probable shift of the mediastinum to the right.

Clinical interpretation

This ECG shows an acute inferior myocardial infarction, which often causes first degree block. The Q waves and raised ST segments are consistent with the story of 6 h of chest pain, and the first degree block is not important.

What to do

Chest pain radiating through to the back has to raise the possibility of aortic dissection, which can occlude the opening of the coronary arteries and so cause a myocardial infarction. However, this is relatively rare compared with back pain associated with myocardial infarction, which is common. In this case, the chest X-ray suggests that blood has leaked into the left pleural cavity from a dissection of the aorta. Thrombolysis for the myocardial infarction is obviously contraindicated, and the patient needs immediate investigation by CT or MR scanning to see if surgical repair of the dissection is possible.

Summary ★★

Acute inferior myocardial infarction with first degree block, due to dissection of the aorta.

ECG ME See p. 91, 8E

ECG IP See p. 215, 6E

ECG 45

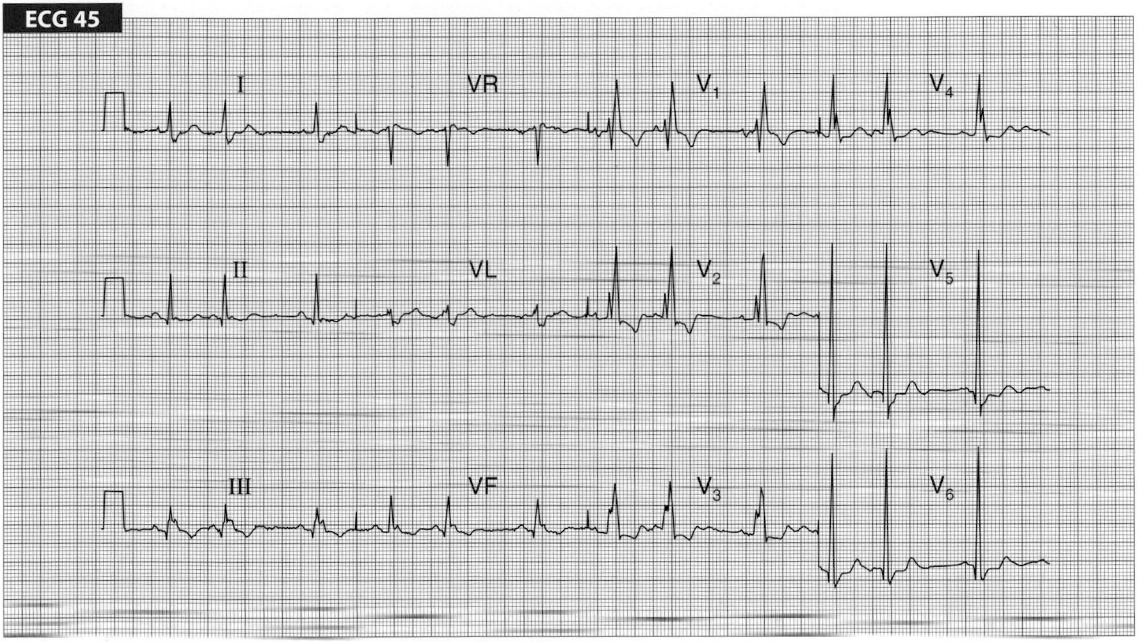

This ECG was recorded from a 23-year-old pregnant woman who had complained of palpitations, and who had been found to have a heart murmur. What does it show and what might be the problem?

ANSWER 45

The ECG shows:

- Sinus rhythm, underlying rate 61/min
- Supraventricular (atrial) extrasystoles
- Normal PR interval
- Normal axis
- Wide QRS complex (160 ms)
- RSR^1 pattern in lead V_1
- Broad slurred S wave in lead V_6
- Inverted T waves in leads V_1–V_3

Clinical interpretation

The broad QRS complex with an RSR^1 pattern in lead V_1 and a slurred S wave in lead V_6, together with the inverted T waves in leads V_1–V_3, indicate right bundle branch block (RBBB). The extrasystoles are supraventricular because they have the same (abnormal) QRS pattern as the sinus beats; they are atrial in origin because each is preceded by a T wave of slightly different shape from the sinus beats.

What to do

The palpitations of which the patient complains may well be due to the extrasystoles: it is important to ensure that they correspond to her symptoms. RBBB in a young person may indicate an atrial septal defect, and she should have an echocardiogram. The heart murmur could be due to a septal defect, but could well be a 'flow murmur' due to the increased cardiac output associated with pregnancy.

Summary ★

RBBB and atrial extrasystoles.

ECG ME See p. 43, 8E

ECG IP See p. 115, 6E

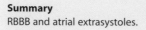

ECG 46

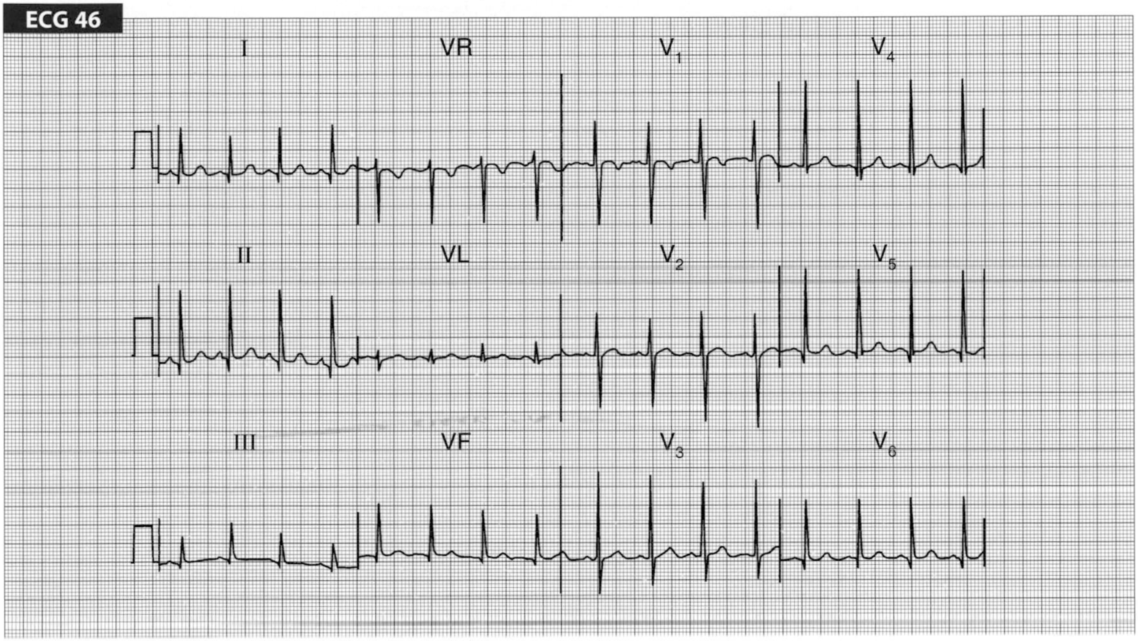

This ECG was recorded from a 9-year-old girl who was asymptomatic but who had been found to have a heart murmur at a school medical examination. What does it tell you about the murmur?

ANSWER 46

The ECG shows:

- Sinus rhythm, rate 107/min
- Normal axis
- Normal QRS complexes, but narrow, deep Q waves in leads I, II, V_4–V_6
- Inverted T waves in lead V_1

Clinical interpretation

A sinus tachycardia with normal QRS complexes, showing prominent 'septal' Q waves, is characteristic of ECGs of children. The inverted T wave in lead V_1 is normal at any age. A normal ECG helps to exclude serious causes of heart murmurs, but the record has not been very helpful in this case.

What to do

If in doubt, an echocardiogram will show whether there is any important structural abnormality of the heart.

Summary ★★

Normal ECG in a 9-year-old child.

ECG IP See p. 53, 6E

ECG 47

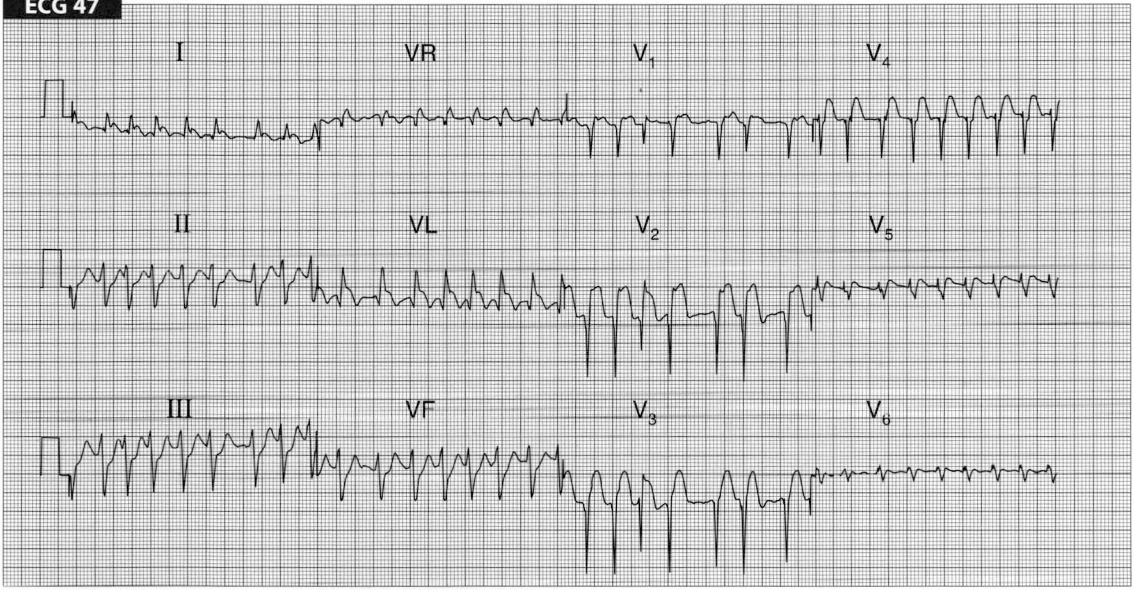

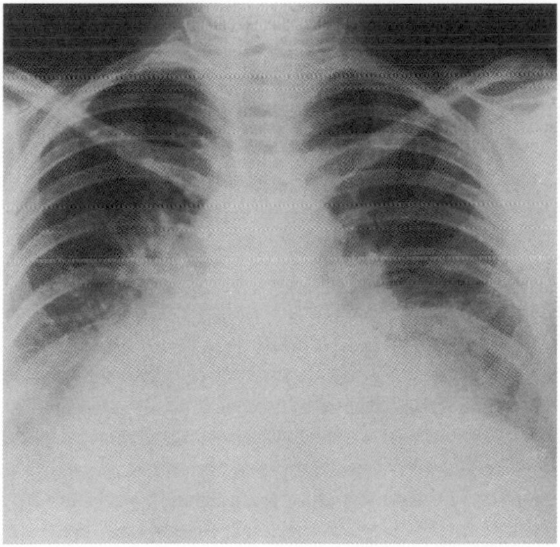

This ECG and chest X-ray were recorded from a diabetic man who was admitted to hospital because of the sudden onset of pulmonary oedema. What do you think has happened?

ANSWER 47

The ECG shows:

- Atrial fibrillation with a ventricular rate of about 180/min
- Left axis deviation
- Probable Q waves in leads V_2–V_4
- QRS complexes of normal width and height
- Raised ST segments in leads I, VL, V_2–V_4

The chest X-ray shows pulmonary oedema; it is difficult to see the heart borders.

Clinical interpretation

This ECG shows uncontrolled atrial fibrillation with left anterior hemiblock and an acute anterolateral ST segment elevation myocardial infarction (STEMI). The onset of atrial fibrillation may have been the cause or the consequence of the myocardial infarction, and the rapid ventricular rate will at least in part explain the pulmonary oedema. The left anterior hemiblock is probably a consequence of the infarction. The patient may not have experienced pain because of his diabetes.

What to do

The most important thing is to relieve the patient's distress and the pulmonary oedema. He needs diamorphine, an intravenous diuretic, intravenous nitrates, and intravenous digoxin to control the ventricular rate – all with careful monitoring. Attention can then be turned to the treatment of his myocardial infarction. He will need anticoagulation with heparin.

Summary ★★

Atrial fibrillation, left anterior hemiblock and acute anterolateral STEMI.

ECG ME See p. 49, 76, 91, 8E

ECG IP See p. 217, 6E

ECG 48

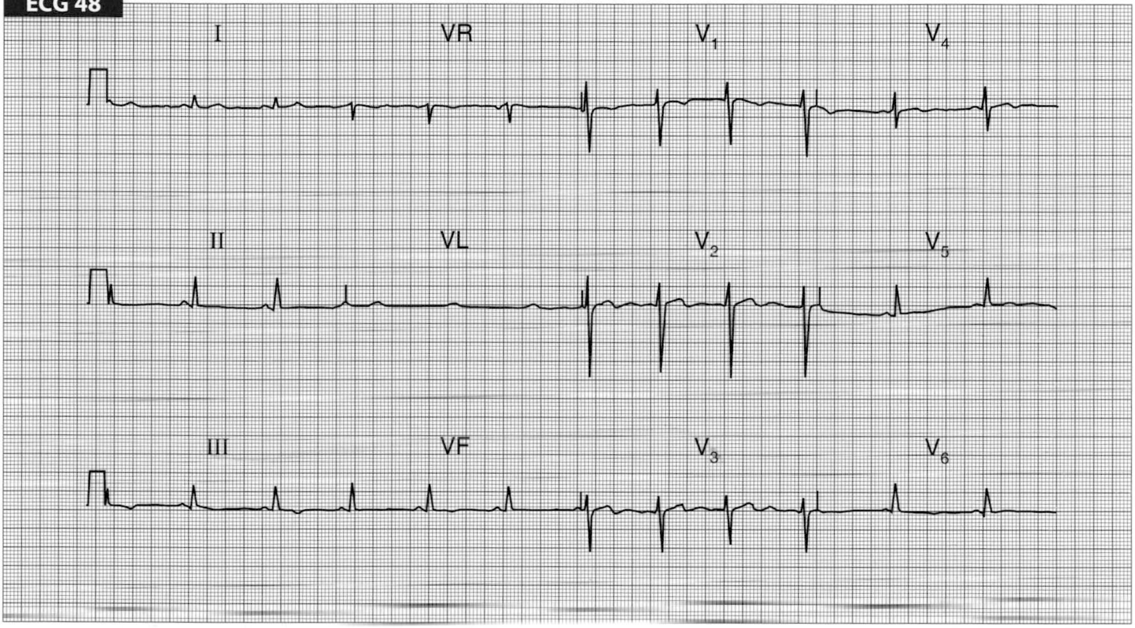

This ECG was recorded from a young man seen in the outpatient department because of chest pain which appeared to be nonspecific. How would you interpret the ECG and what action would you take?

ANSWER 48

The ECG shows:

- Sinus rhythm, rate 71/min
- Normal axis
- Normal QRS complexes
- Inverted T waves in leads III, VF; biphasic T waves in lead V_4; flattened T waves in leads V_5–V_6
- U waves in leads V_2–V_3 (normal)

Clinical interpretation

These T wave changes, particularly those in the inferior leads, could well be caused by ischaemia. The flattened T waves in the lateral leads can only be described as 'nonspecific'.

What to do

When confronted with an ECG showing this sort of 'nonspecific' abnormality, action depends primarily on the clinical diagnosis. If the patient is asymptomatic it is fair to report the ECG as showing 'nonspecific changes'; if the patient has symptoms at all – as in this case – it is probably worth proceeding to an exercise test. In this patient, the exercise test was perfectly normal, and his symptoms cleared without any intervention. A repeat ECG, recorded purely out of interest a month later, showed similar changes.

Summary ★★★
Nonspecific ST segment and T wave changes.

ECG ME See p. 123, 8E

ECG IP See p. 34, 6E

ECG 49

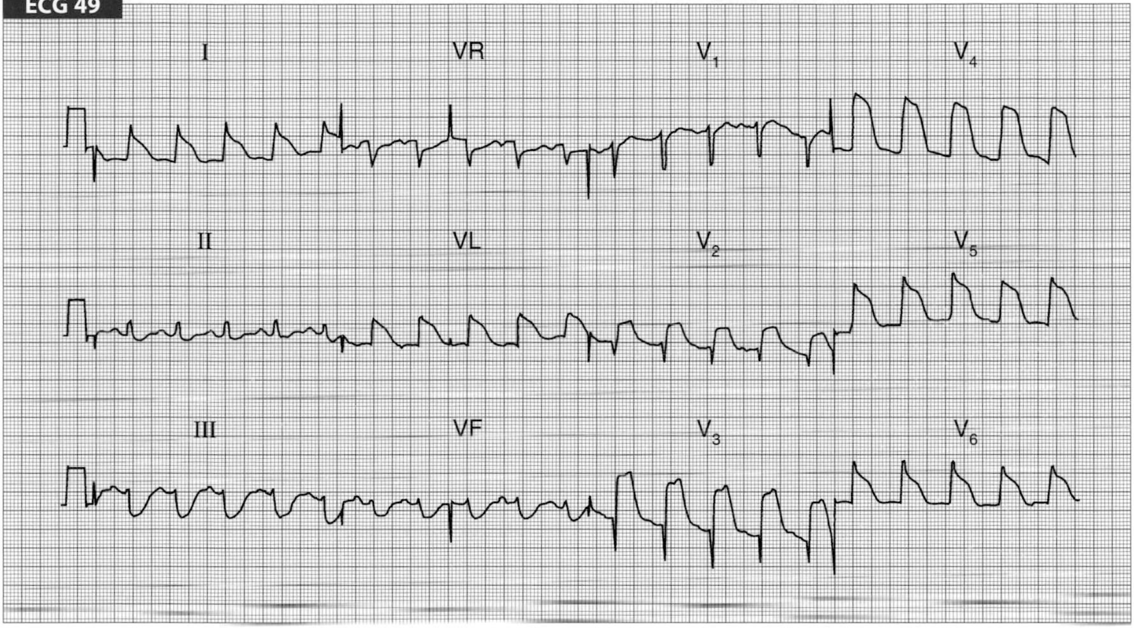

This ECG was recorded from a 65-year-old woman admitted to hospital as an emergency because of severe chest pain for 1 h. What does the ECG show? What other investigations would you order?

ANSWER 49

The ECG shows:

- Sinus rhythm, rate 111/min
- Normal axis
- Probably normal QRS complexes
- Gross elevation of ST segments in anterior and lateral leads
- Depressed ST segments in the inferior leads (III, VF)

Clinical interpretation

Acute ST segment elevation anterolateral myocardial infarction (STEMI). In the lateral leads I, VL and V_4–V_6, it is difficult to see where the QRS complexes end and the ST segments begin, but in lead II it is clear that the QRS complex is of normal width.

What to do

If the patient gives a history suggestive of a myocardial infarction and has this ECG, no further investigations are needed in the acute phase of the illness, and in particular there is no place for a chest X-ray. Routine treatment for a myocardial infarction – pain relief, aspirin and percutaneous coronary intervention (PCI) or thrombolysis – should be commenced immediately.

Summary ★
Acute anterolateral STEMI.

ECG ME See p. 91, 8E

ECG IP See p. 217, 6E

ECG 50

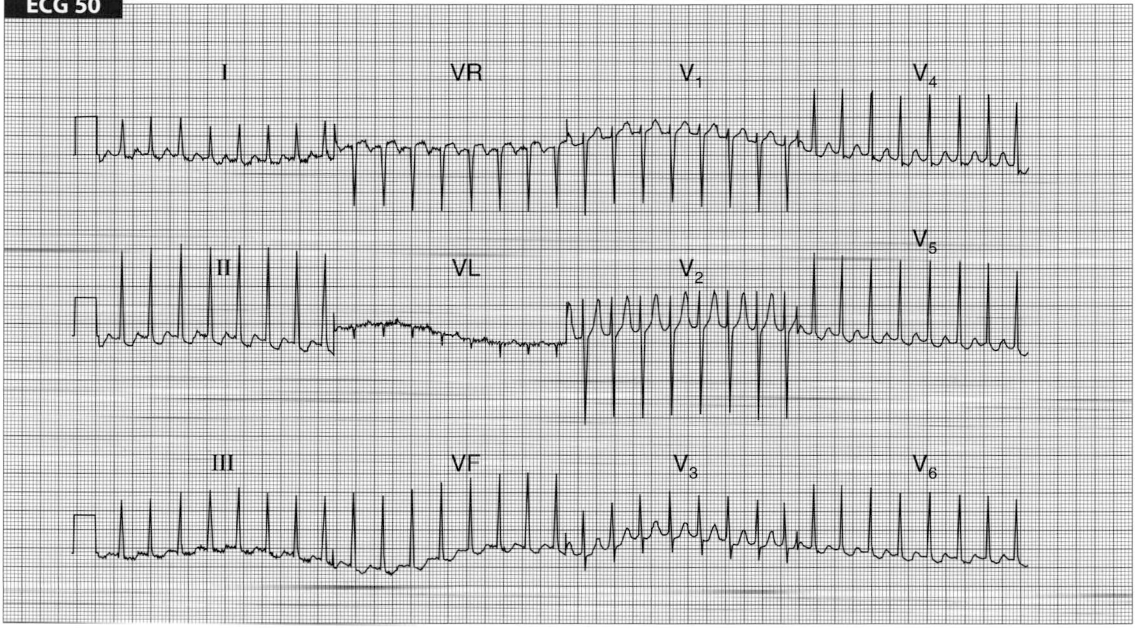

A 45-year-old woman had complained of occasional attacks of palpitations for 20 years, and eventually this ECG was recorded during an attack. What are the palpitations due to, and what would you do?

ANSWER 50

The ECG shows:

- Narrow complex tachycardia at 188/min
- No P waves visible
- Normal axis
- QRS complexes normal
- Some ST segment depression

Clinical interpretation

This ECG shows supraventricular tachycardia. This rhythm is usually due to a re-entry pathway within, or near to, the atrioventricular node, so the rhythm is properly called AV nodal re-entry tachycardia (AVNRT), although the term ‘supraventricular tachycardia’ is often (inappropriately) used. The ST segment depression could indicate ischaemia, but the ST segments are not horizontally depressed, nor is the depression greater than 2 mm, so it is probably of no significance.

What to do

The first action is carotid sinus pressure, which may terminate the attack. If this fails it will almost certainly respond to adenosine. As with any tachycardia, electrical cardioversion must be considered if there is haemodynamic compromise. Once sinus rhythm has been restored, the patient must be taught the various methods (e.g. the Valsalva manoeuvre) with which she might try to terminate an attack. Prophylactic medication may not be needed if attacks are infrequent, but most patients with this problem should have an electrophysiological study to try to identify a re-entry pathway that can be ablated.

Summary ★

AV nodal re-entry (junctional) tachycardia (AVNRT).

ECG ME See p. 81, 8E

ECG IP See p. 109, 6E

ECG 51

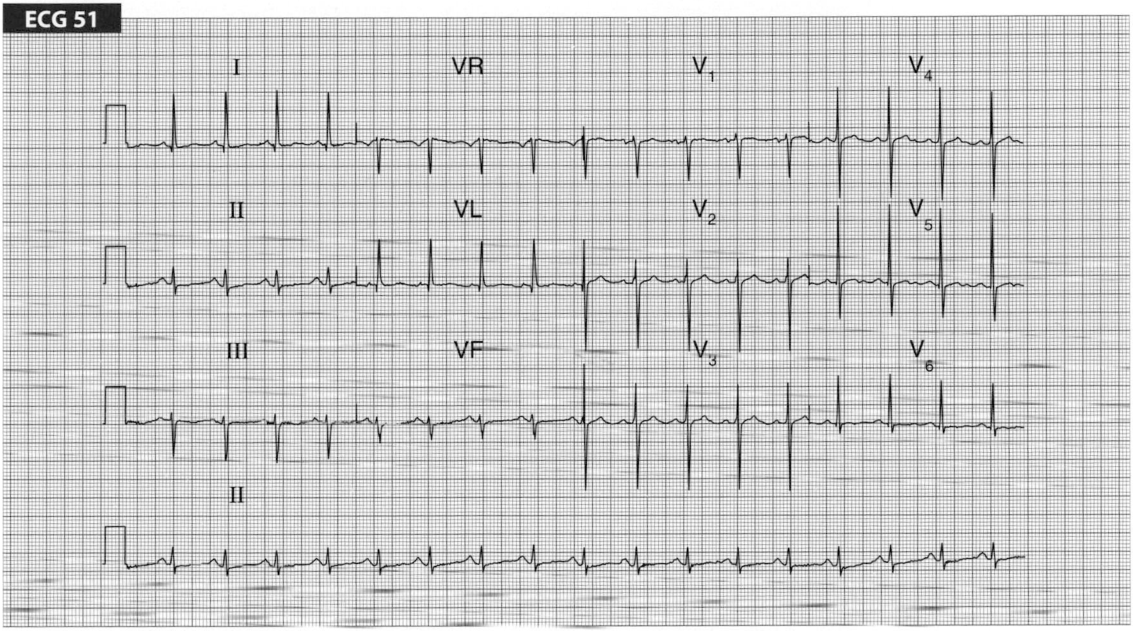

This ECG was recorded from a 35-year-old woman who complained of breathlessness but not of pain. She was anxious, but there were no abnormalities on examination. Does this ECG help with her diagnosis and management?

ANSWER 51

The ECG shows:

- Sinus rhythm, rate 106/min
- Normal axis
- Normal QRS complexes (septal Q waves in leads I and VL)
- Slight ST segment depression, especially in leads II and V_6
- T wave flattening in leads II, III, VF, V_6
- T wave inversion in lead III

Clinical interpretation

A sinus rate of over 100/min would be compatible with anxiety, though other causes of 'high output' (e.g. pregnancy, thyrotoxicosis, anaemia, volume loss, CO_2 retention, beri-beri) have to be considered. The widespread ST segment and T wave changes have to be described as 'nonspecific'; in an anxious patient they could be due to hyperventilation. The ECG does not help with the diagnosis and management.

What to do

If a full history and examination fail to suggest any underlying physical disease, further investigations are unlikely to be helpful.

Summary ★★

Nonspecific ST segment and T wave changes.

ECG ME See p. 101, 8E

ECG IP See p. 35, 6E

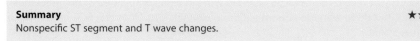

ECG 52

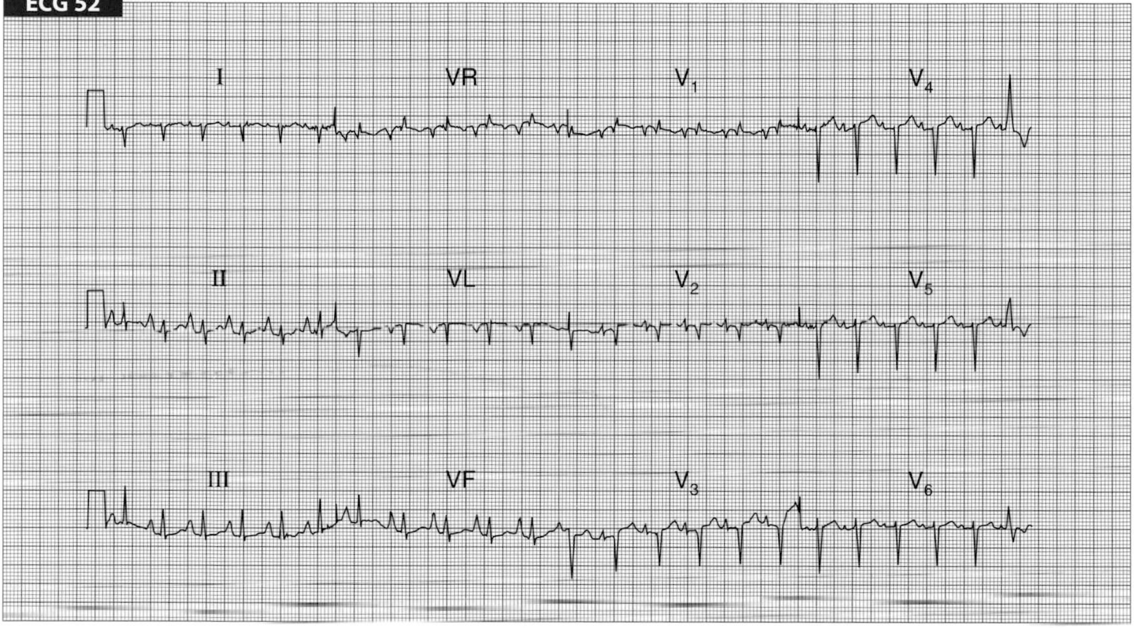

This ECG was recorded from a 60-year-old man seen in the clinic because of severe breathlessness, which had developed over several years. His jugular venous pressure is raised. What do you think the problem is?

ANSWER 52

The ECG shows:

- Sinus rhythm, rate 140/min
- One ventricular extrasystole
- Peaked P waves (best seen in leads II, III, VF)
- Normal PR interval
- Right axis deviation
- Dominant R wave in lead V_1
- Deep S wave in lead V_6
- Normal ST segments and T waves

Clinical interpretation

The sinus tachycardia suggests a major problem. The peaked P waves indicate right atrial hypertrophy. The right axis deviation and dominant R wave in lead V_1 suggest right ventricular hypertrophy. The deep S wave in lead V_6, with no 'left ventricular' complexes in the chest leads, indicates 'clockwise rotation' of the heart, with the right ventricle occupying the precordium. These changes suggest lung disease.

What to do

Since the ECG is entirely 'right-sided', one can assume that the problem is due to chronic lung disease or recurrent pulmonary embolism. The story sounds more in keeping with a lung problem. The raised jugular venous pressure is presumably due to cor pulmonale. The sinus tachycardia is worrying, and suggests respiratory failure.

Summary ★★

Sinus tachycardia and one ventricular extrasystole; right atrial and right ventricular hypertrophy; and clockwise rotation – suggesting chronic lung disease.

ECG ME See p. 19, 8E

ECG IP See p. 305, 6E

ECG 53

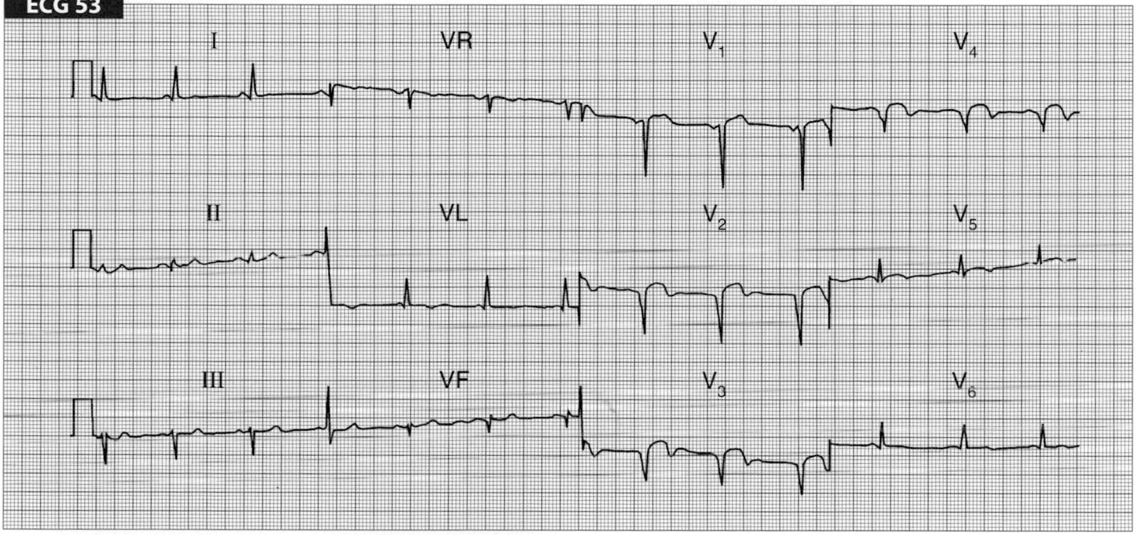

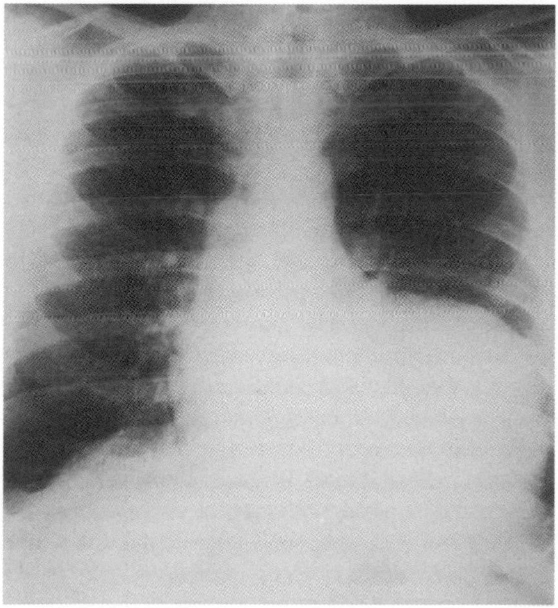

A 60-year-old man is seen in the outpatient department complaining of breathlessness which began quite suddenly 2 months previously. He had had no chest pain. Examination revealed a raised jugular venous pressure, basal crackles in the lungs and a third sound at the cardiac apex. These are his ECG and chest X-ray. What do they show and how does this fit the clinical picture? What would you do?

ANSWER 53

The ECG shows:

- Sinus rhythm, rate 72/min
- Normal axis
- Large Q waves in leads V_1–V_4 and small Q waves in leads I, VL
- Elevated ST segments and inverted T waves in leads V_2–V_5
- Flattened T waves in leads I and V_6; inverted T waves in lead VL

The chest X-ray shows a left ventricular aneurysm.

Clinical interpretation

This ECG would be compatible with an acute anterior myocardial infarction, but this does not fit the clinical picture: it appears that an event occurred 2 months previously. This pattern of ST segment elevation in the anterior leads can persist following a large infarction, and is often seen in the presence of a ventricular aneurysm. This is confirmed by the chest X-ray.

What to do

An echocardiogram will show the extent of the aneurysm and whether the remaining left ventricular function is impaired, which it almost certainly will be. The patient should be treated with diuretics and an angiotensin-converting enzyme inhibitor, and surgical resection of the aneurysm might be considered.

Summary ★★★

Old anterior myocardial infarction with a left ventricular aneurysm.

ECG ME See p. 130, 8E

ECG IP See p. 225, 6E

ECG 54

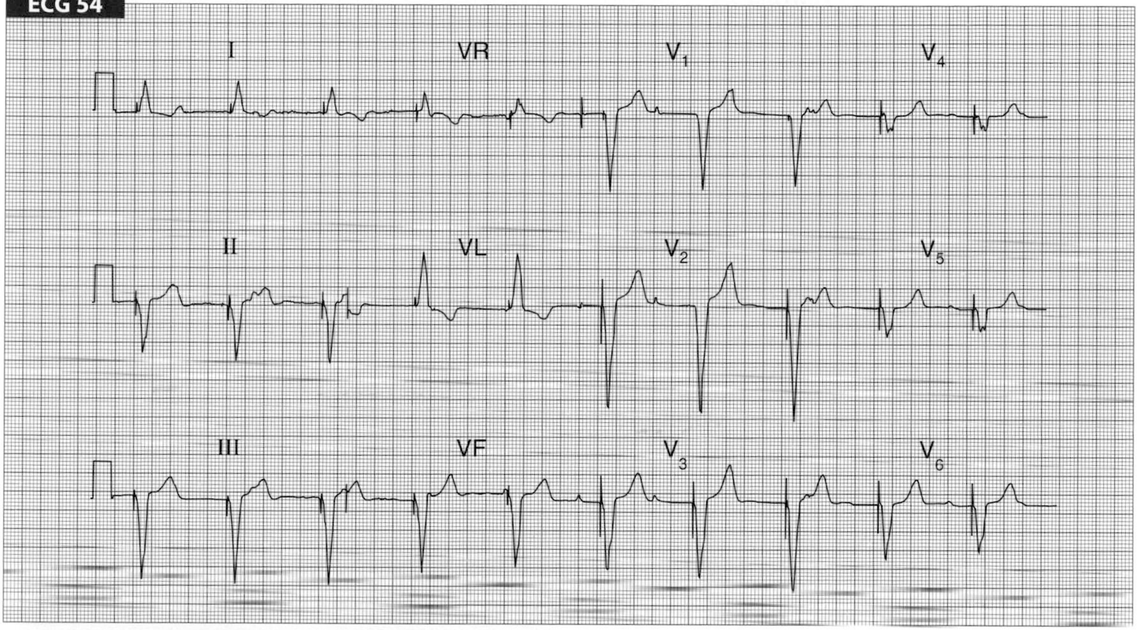

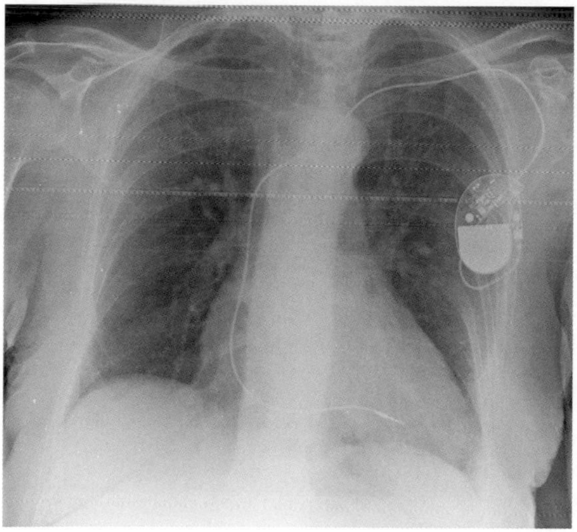

The senior house officer in the A & E department is puzzled by this ECG which was recorded from an 80-year-old admitted unconscious with a stroke. What has the house officer missed? Perhaps he did not make a proper examination and did not look at the chest X-ray?

ANSWER 54

The ECG shows:

- Regular rhythm at 60/min
- Occasional P waves, not related to QRS complexes (e.g. in lead I)
- Left axis deviation
- QRS complexes preceded by a sharp 'spike'
- Broad QRS complexes (160 ms)
- Deep S wave in lead V_6
- Inverted T waves in leads I, VL

The chest X-ray shows a permanent pacemaker, with a single lead in the right ventricle.

Clinical interpretation

The broad QRS complexes show that this is either a supraventricular rhythm with bundle branch block, or a ventricular rhythm. This rhythm is ventricular. The sharp spikes preceding each QRS complex are due to the pacemaker. The P waves that can occasionally be seen indicate that the underlying rhythm is complete heart block – presumably the reason why the pacemaker was inserted.

What to do

The house officer has missed the pacemaker, which is usually buried below the left clavicle. There is no particular reason why the pacemaker should be related to the stroke, except that patients with vascular disease in one territory usually have it in others – this man probably has both coronary and cerebrovascular disease.

Summary ★
Permanent pacemaker and underlying complete block.

ECG ME See p. 169, 8E

ECG IP See p. 187, 6E

ECG 55

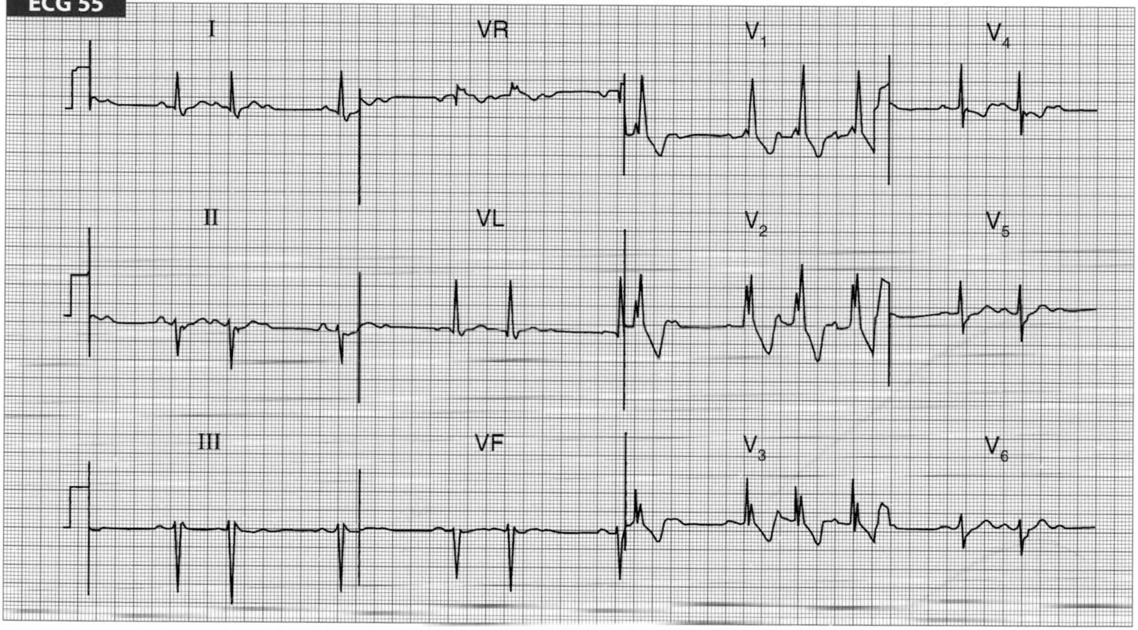

A 70-year-old woman who complained of 'dizzy turns' was found to have an irregular pulse, and this ECG was recorded. There are three abnormalities. What advice would you give her?

ANSWER 55

The ECG shows:

- Sinus rhythm; sinus rate 100/min
- Normal and constant PR intervals in the conducted beats
- Occasional nonconducted P waves (best seen in lead I)
- Left axis deviation
- Right bundle branch block (RBBB)

Clinical interpretation

This ECG shows second degree block (Mobitz type 2) and bifascicular block – left axis deviation (left anterior hemiblock) and RBBB. This combination of conduction abnormalities indicates disease throughout the conduction system, and is sometimes called 'trifascicular' block.

What to do

The 'dizzy turns' may represent intermittent complete block. Permanent pacing is essential.

Summary ★★

Second degree block (Mobitz type 2) and bifascicular block.

ECG ME See p. 39, 8E

ECG IP See p. 89, 6E

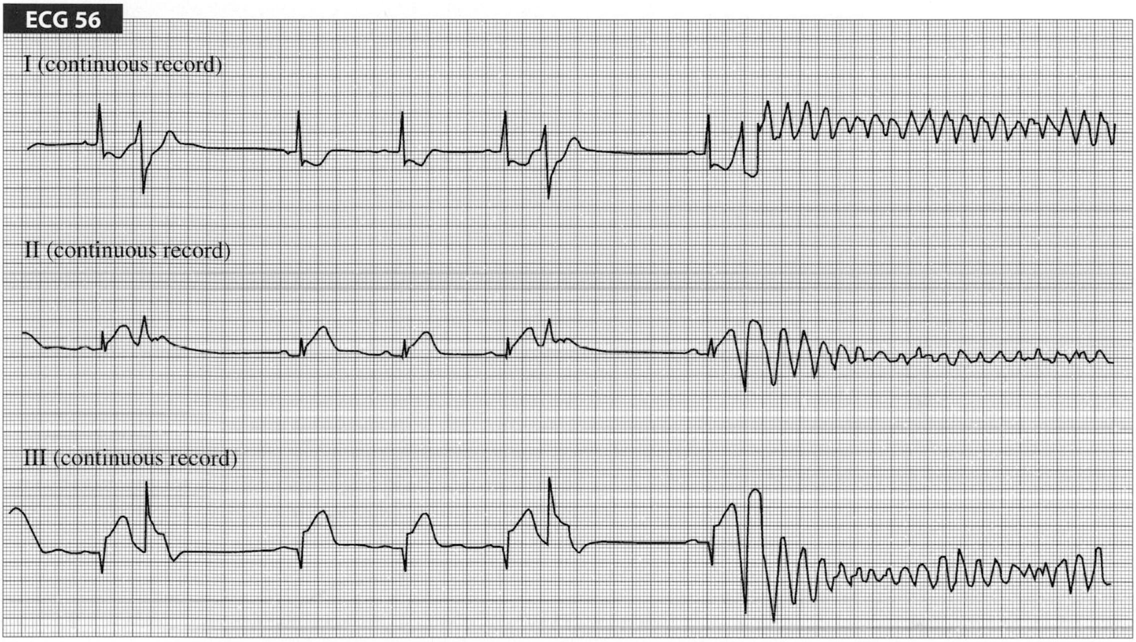

A 50-year-old man, who had come to the A & E department with chest pain, collapsed while his ECG was being recorded. What happened and what would you do?

ANSWER 56

The ECG shows:

- Sinus rhythm initially 55/min, with ventricular extrasystoles
- The third extrasystole occurs on the peak of the T wave of the preceding sinus beat
- After three or four beats of ventricular tachycardia, ventricular fibrillation develops
- In the sinus beats there is a Q wave in lead III; and there are raised ST segments in leads II and III, and ST segment depression and T wave inversion in lead I

Clinical interpretation

Although only leads I, II and III are available, it looks as if the chest pain was due to an inferior myocardial infarction. This was probably the cause of the ventricular extrasystoles, and an 'R on T' extrasystole caused ventricular tachycardia, which rapidly decayed into ventricular fibrillation. It might be argued that in lead III, and perhaps also in lead I, 'torsade de pointes' ventricular tachycardia is present, but this is not apparent in lead II.

What to do

Precordial thump and immediate defibrillation, but if no defibrillator is at hand then cardiopulmonary resuscitation should be performed, and the usual procedure for the management of cardiac arrest instituted.

Summary ★
Probable inferior myocardial infarction; R on T ventricular extrasystole, causing ventricular fibrillation.

ECG ME See p. 79, 8E

ECG IP See p. 115, 6E

ECG 57

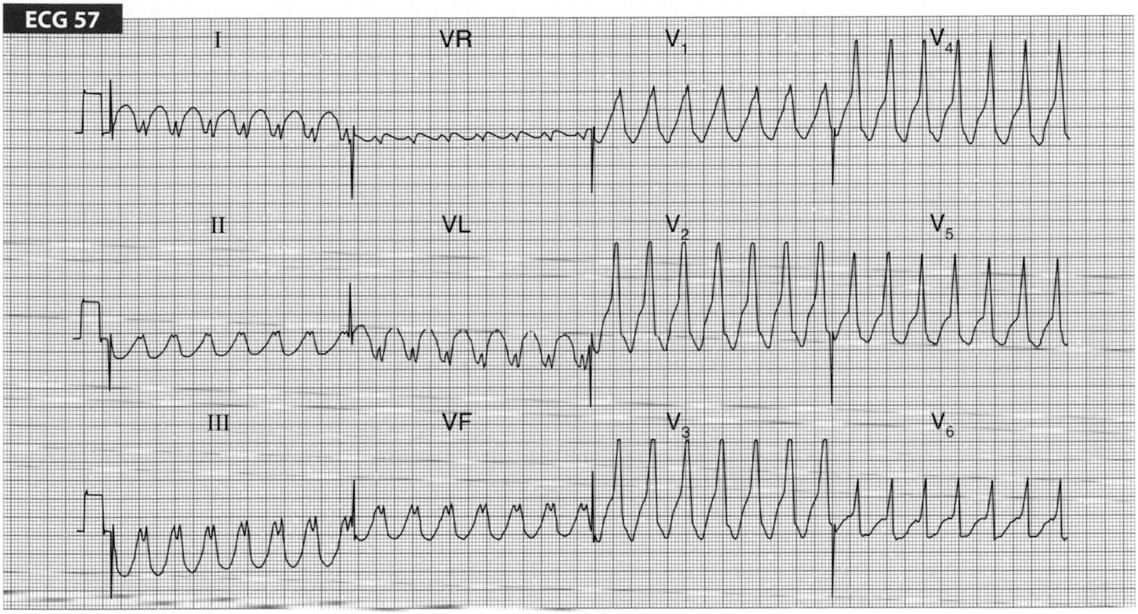

A 60-year-old man complained of severe central chest pain, and a few minutes later became extremely breathless and collapsed. He was brought to the A & E department, where his heart rate was found to be 165/min, his blood pressure was unrecordable and he had signs of left ventricular failure. This is his ECG. What has happened and what would you do?

ANSWER 57

The ECG shows:

- Broad complex tachycardia at 165/min
- No P waves visible
- QRS complex duration about 200 ms
- Concordance of QRS complexes (i.e. all point upwards) in the chest leads

Clinical interpretation

A broad complex tachycardia can be ventricular in origin, or can be due to a supraventricular tachycardia with aberrant conduction (i.e. bundle branch block). Here the very broad complexes and the QRS complex concordance suggest a ventricular tachycardia. In a patient with a myocardial infarction it is always safe to assume that such a rhythm is ventricular. From the story, one would guess that this patient had a myocardial infarction and then developed ventricular tachycardia, but it is possible that the chest pain was due to the arrhythmia.

What to do

This patient has haemodynamic compromise – low blood pressure and heart failure – and needs immediate cardioversion. While preparations are being made it would be reasonable to try intravenous lidocaine or amiodarone.

Summary ★
Ventricular tachycardia.

ECG ME See p. 73, 8E

ECG IP See p. 126, 6E

ECG 58

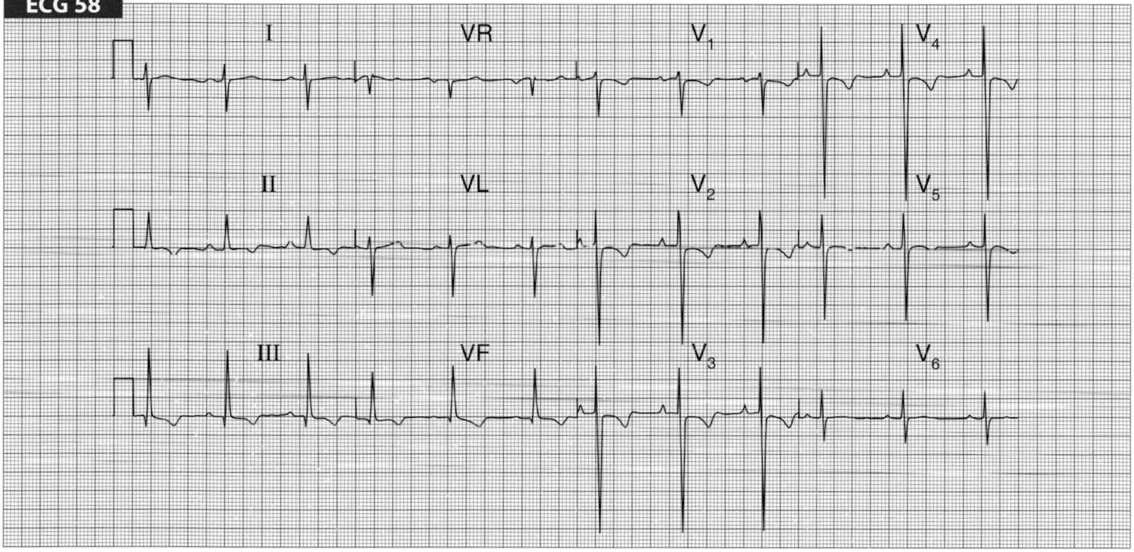

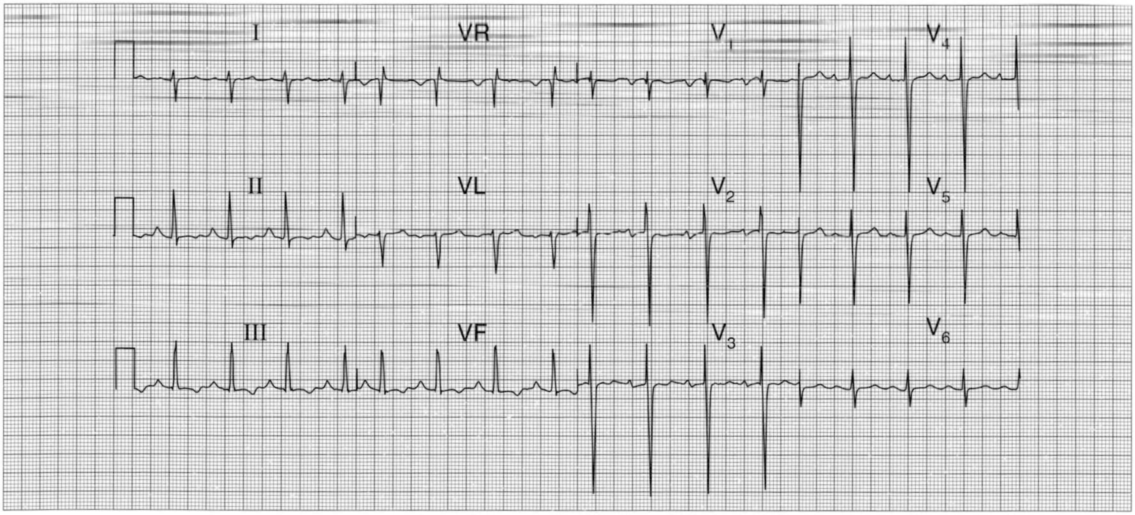

A 70-year-old man gave a history of several years of chest pain on exertion. These are his ECGs at rest (upper trace) and on exercise (lower trace). What do they show?

ANSWER 58

The upper ECG shows:

- Sinus rhythm, rate 68/min
- Right axis deviation
- Small Q waves in leads III, VF
- Persistent S wave in leads V_5–V_6
- Inverted T waves in leads II, III, VF, V_1–V_5

The lower record was taken during stage 2 of the Bruce protocol. It shows:

- Sinus rhythm at 100/min
- T wave inversion persists in leads II, III, VF; but the T waves are now upright in the chest leads

Clinical interpretation

The widespread T wave inversion suggests a non-ST segment elevation myocardial infarction, although there is nothing in the history to suggest when this occurred. The S wave in lead V_6 suggests the possibility of chronic lung disease. The change in the T waves in the anterior leads, from inverted at rest to normal on exercise, is an example of 'pseudonormalization', which is an indication of ischaemia.

What to do

'Pseudonormalization' must be regarded in the same way as the usual ST segment response to ischaemia, which is depression. This patient's exercise test was positive (i.e. indicates ischaemia) at a relatively low level – so although his symptoms can be treated medically in the usual way, a coronary angiogram with a view to intervention is indicated. The risk factors for coronary disease must be assessed and treated, whatever course of action is chosen.

Summary ★★★

Ischaemia with 'pseudonormalization' of the ECG on exercise.

ECG IP

See p. 275, 6E

ECG 59

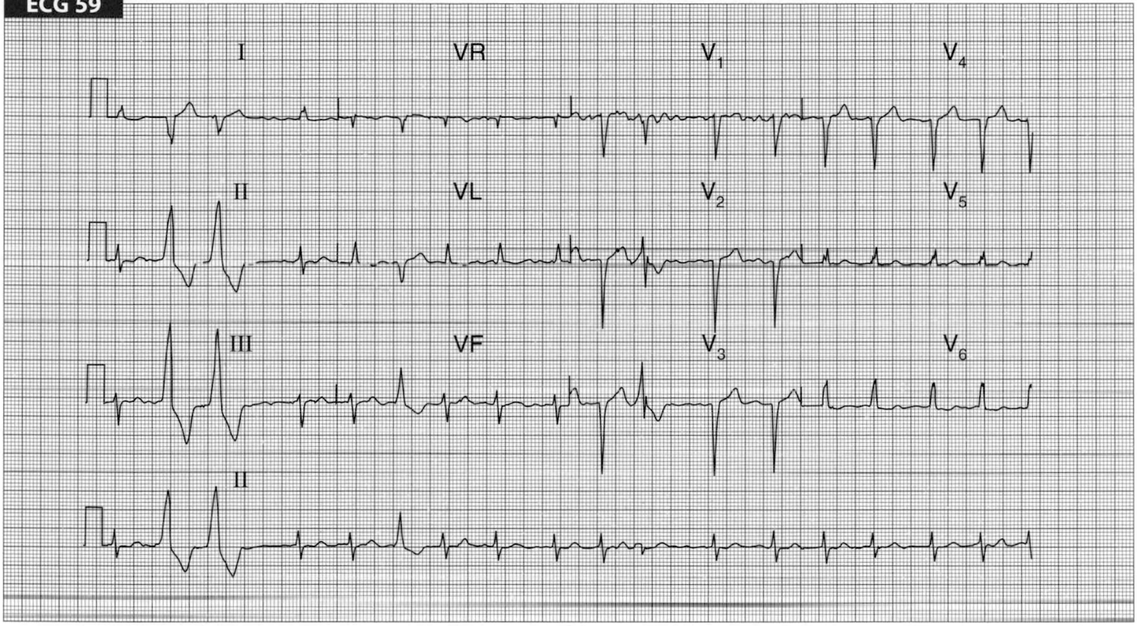

This ECG was recorded from a 70-year-old woman who complained of an irregular heartbeat. What does it show and what would you do?

ANSWER 59

The ECG shows:

- Atrial fibrillation, rate about 110/min
- Frequent multifocal ventricular extrasystoles
- Normal axis in the sinus beats
- Loss of R waves in leads V_3–V_4
- There is downward-sloping ST segment depression in lead V_6

Clinical interpretation

This ECG shows an old anterior myocardial infarction, so ischaemia is probably (but not certainly) the cause of the patient's atrial fibrillation and extrasystoles. The ventricular rate is not well controlled. The ST segment depression suggests that she is taking digoxin.

What to do

It would be prudent to check the patient's serum potassium and digoxin levels to make sure that the extrasystoles are not a manifestation of digoxin toxicity. An echocardiogram should be recorded to check her heart size and left ventricular function; remember that atrial fibrillation may be the only indication of thyrotoxicosis in the elderly. Her complaint of palpitations may be due to her atrial fibrillation or to the extrasystoles (or both). The extrasystoles themselves are not important, but she should avoid smoking, alcohol and caffeine. A beta-blocker may reduce the extrasystoles as well as control her ventricular rate. It is unlikely that cardioversion would be successful, and she will need long-term treatment with digoxin, possibly a beta-blocker, probably an angiotensin-converting enzyme inhibitor, and certainly anticoagulants.

Summary ★★

Atrial fibrillation, multifocal ventricular extrasystoles, and an old anterior myocardial infarction.

ECG ME See p. 64, 8E

ECG IP See p. 225, 6E

ECG 60

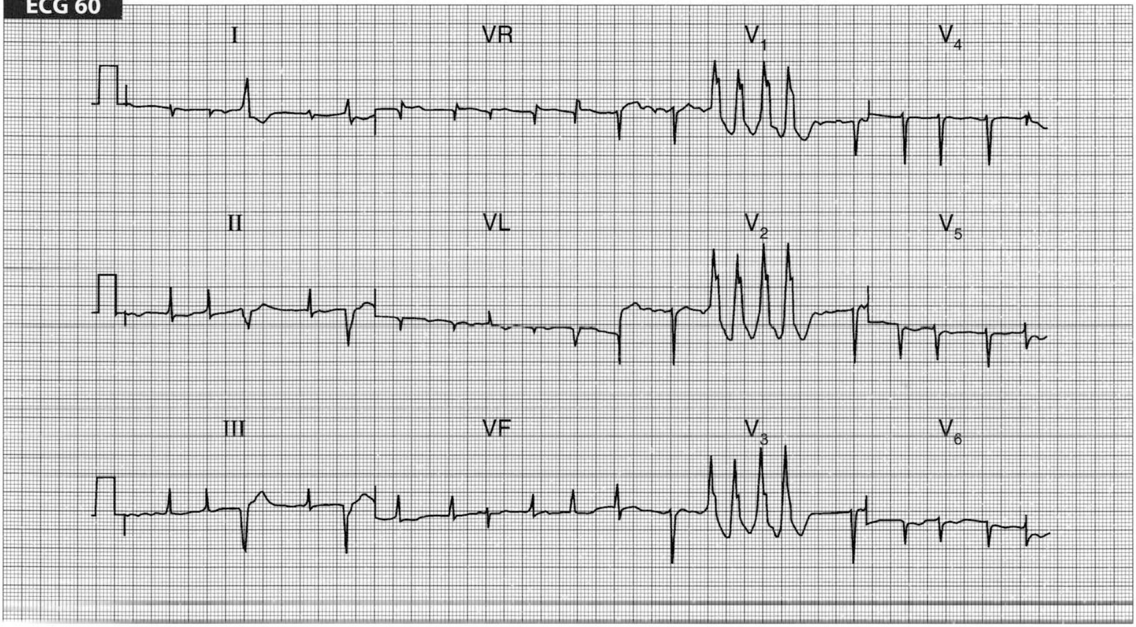

A 60-year-old man who was being treated in hospital complained of palpitations, and this ECG was recorded. What do you think the underlying disease was, and what were the palpitations due to?

ANSWER 60

The ECG shows:

- Atrial fibrillation
- Ventricular extrasystoles with two distinct morphologies (best seen in lead II)
- A four-beat run of ventricular tachycardia
- Right axis deviation
- Small QRS complexes
- No R wave development in the chest leads; lead V_6 shows a dominant S wave
- T wave inversion in leads V_5–V_6

Clinical interpretation

This ECG suggests chronic lung disease – small complexes, right axis deviation, and marked 'clockwise rotation', with lead V_6 still showing a right ventricular type of complex (i.e. a complex with a small R wave and a deeper S wave, as normally seen in lead V_1). The atrial fibrillation is probably secondary to the lung disease, though the other possibilities must be considered. The patient's lung condition is probably being treated with a beta-agonist, such as salbutamol, and this could be the cause of the extrasystoles and ventricular tachycardia.

What to do

Stop the beta-agonist but do not give a beta-blocker. Check the electrolyte levels; consider the possibility of digoxin toxicity.

Summary ★★★

Atrial fibrillation with ventricular extrasystoles and ventricular tachycardia; changes suggesting chronic lung disease.

ECG ME See p. 19, 73, 8E

ECG IP See p. 307, 6E

ECG 61

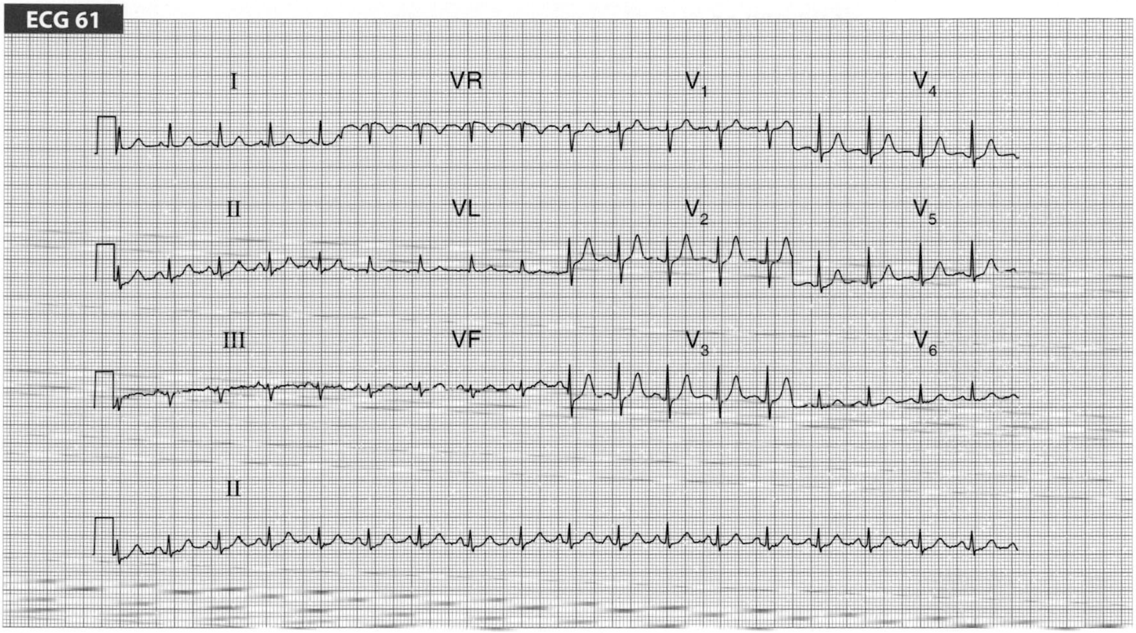

A 45-year-old man complained of palpitations, weight loss and anxiety. His blood pressure was 180/110, and his heart seemed normal. This is his ECG. His thyroid function tests, measured several times, were normal. What might be going on?

ANSWER 61

The ECG shows:

- Narrow complex rhythm at 110/minute
- One P wave per QRS complex – sinus tachycardia
- Normal PR interval
- Normal axis
- Normal QRS complexes

Clinical interpretation

The most common causes of a sinus tachycardia are exercise and anxiety, but this patient was losing weight, and although he was anxious it is necessary to think about other diagnoses. His diastolic blood pressure was high, which should not happen with anxiety. He was not thyrotoxic but there must have been some other physical cause of his problems – it turned out he had a phaeochromocytoma.

Summary ★★

Sinus tachycardia.

ECG ME See p. 57, 8E

ECG IP See p. 3, 6E

ECG 62

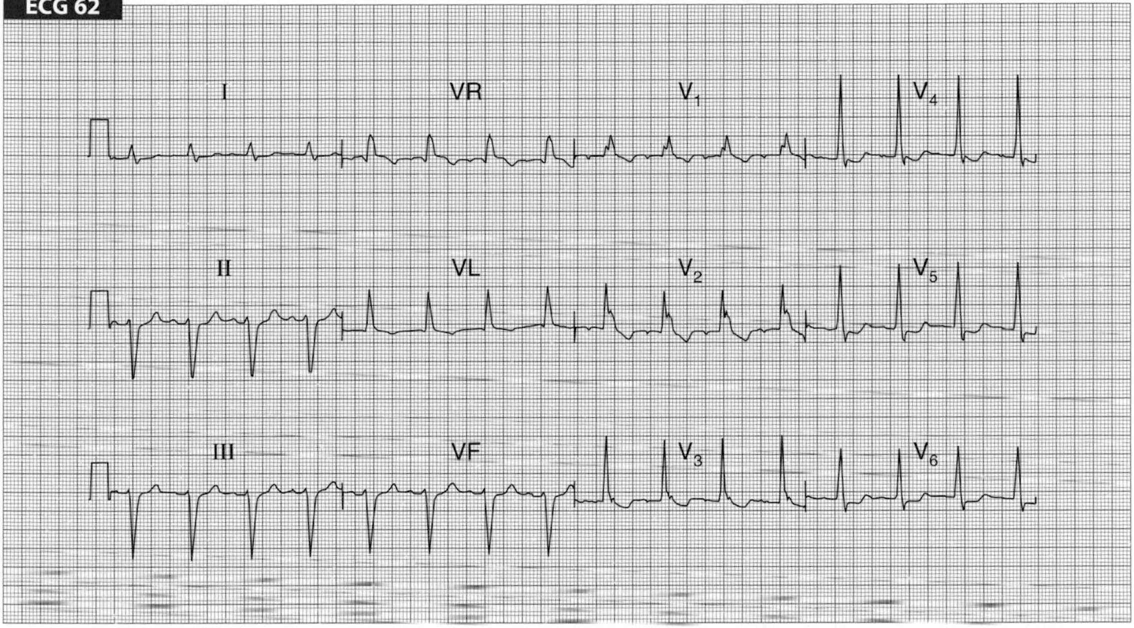

A 70-year-old man is sent to the clinic because of rather vague attacks of dizziness, which occur approximately once per week. Otherwise he is well, and there are no abnormalities on examination. Does this ECG help with his management?

ANSWER 62

The ECG shows:

- Sinus rhythm, rate 94/min
- PR interval at the upper limit of normal (200 ms)
- Left axis deviation
- QRS complex duration prolonged (160 ms)
- RSR^{1} pattern in leads V_1–V_2; wide S wave in lead V_6
- Inverted T waves in leads VL, V_1–V_4

Clinical interpretation

The left axis deviation is characteristic of left anterior hemiblock. There is also right bundle branch block (RBBB), so two of the main conducting pathways are blocked, resulting in 'bifascicular block'. The fact that the PR interval is at the upper limit of normal raises the possibility of delayed conduction in the remaining pathway; if the PR interval were definitely prolonged, this would indicate 'trifascicular block'.

What to do

Bifascicular block is not an indication for pacing if the patient is asymptomatic. The problem here is to decide if the attacks of dizziness are due to intermittent complete heart block. Ideally an ECG would be recorded during an attack – since they occur only every week or so, ambulatory ECG recording may not be helpful, but an event recorder would be worth trying. In the absence of clear evidence, the decision whether or not to insert a permanent pacemaker is a matter of judgement, but in a patient with this story and ECG it would be a perfectly reasonable thing to do.

Summary ★★
Left anterior hemiblock and RBBB – bifascicular block.

ECG ME See p. 51, 8E

ECG IP See p. 89, 6E

ECG 63

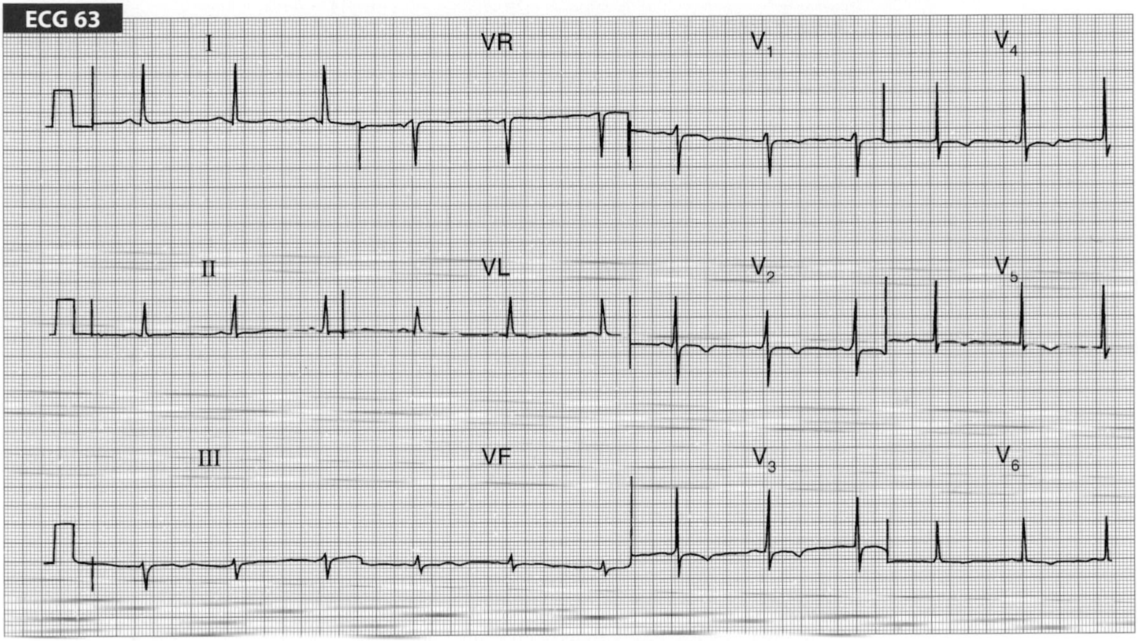

This ECG was recorded from a 25-year-old black professional footballer. What does it show, and what would you do?

ANSWER 63

The ECG shows:

- Sinus rhythm, rate 61/min
- Normal axis
- Normal QRS complexes
- Widespread T wave inversion, particularly in leads V_2–V_5

Clinical interpretation

Repolarization (T wave) abnormalities are quite common in black people, but alternative explanations for this ECG appearance would be a non-ST segment elevation myocardial infarction, or a cardiomyopathy.

What to do

This man is a professional football player, so it is important to exclude hypertrophic cardiomyopathy, and this can be done by echocardiography. Because his career depended upon coronary disease being excluded, a coronary angiogram was performed and was entirely normal.

Summary ★★

Widespread T wave inversion, probably normal in a black man.

ECG ME See p. 124, 8E

ECG IP See p. 39, 6E

ECG 64

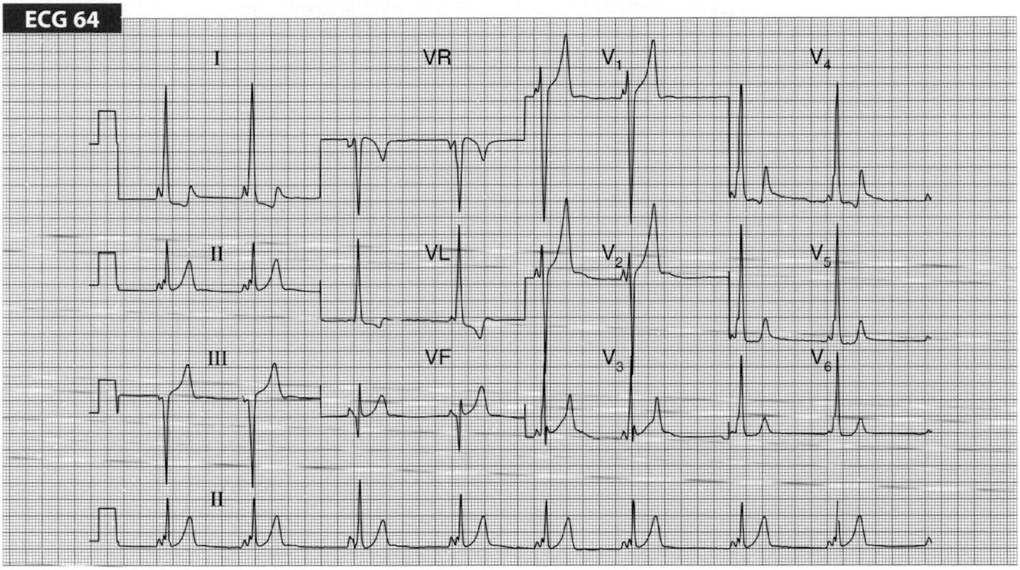

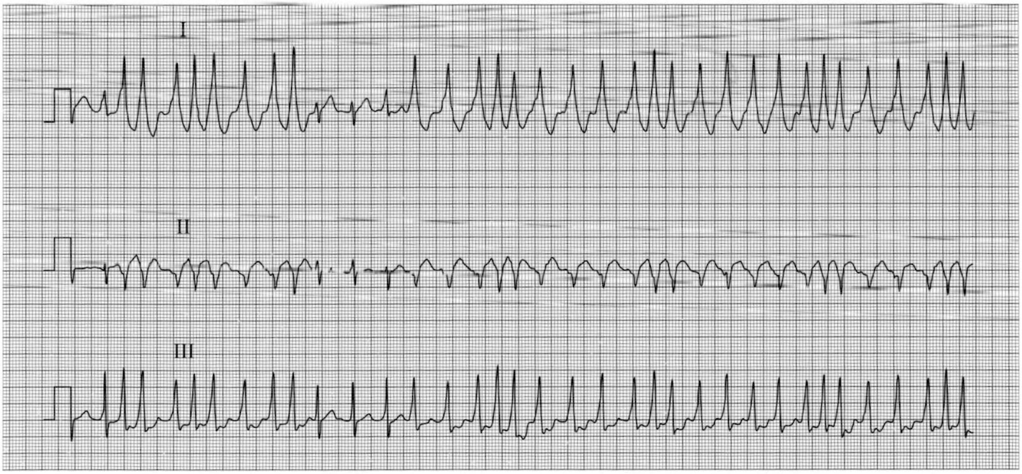

These ECGs were recorded from a 20-year-old man who had had attacks of a fast and irregular heartbeat for several years. The upper trace was recorded when he was asymptomatic; the lower trace (rhythm strips only) was recorded during one of his attacks. What is the diagnosis and what would you do next?

ANSWER 64

The upper ECG shows:

- Sinus rhythm, rate 51/min
- Very short PR interval
- Normal axis
- Bizarre and widened QRS complexes with a slurred upstroke (delta wave), best seen in leads I and V_4–V_6

The lower ECG shows:

- A very irregular tachycardia with a ventricular rate of up to 200/min
- No visible P waves
- A few normal complexes, but the majority are wide and have a slurred upstroke

Clinical interpretation

This is the Wolff–Parkinson–White (WPW) syndrome: the accessory pathway is on the right side, and this is sometimes called 'type B'. The irregular tachycardia is due to atrial fibrillation.

What to do

Atrial fibrillation in the WPW syndrome can lead to sudden death due to ventricular fibrillation, so ablation of the abnormal pathway is needed urgently. Immediate treatment of the atrial fibrillation should be by cardioversion if there is haemodynamic compromise; otherwise flecaidine can be used. Digoxin, verapamil and diltiazem should be avoided because these block the atrioventricular node and encourage conduction through the accessory pathway.

Summary ★★

The WPW syndrome type B.

ECG ME See p. 154, 8E

ECG IP See p. 69, 6E

ECG 65

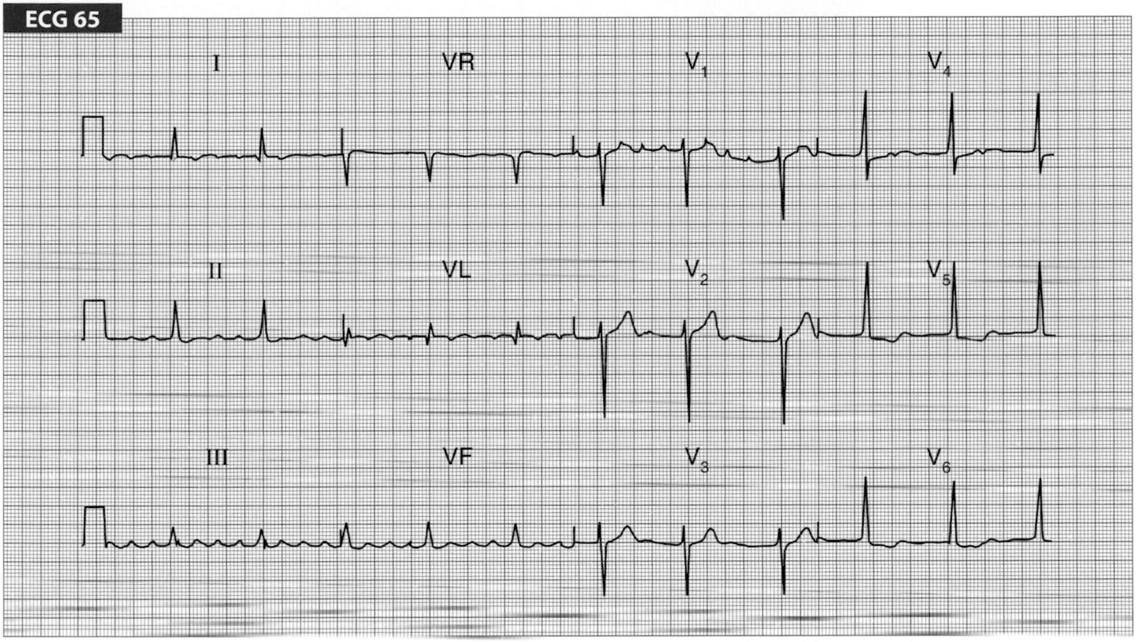

A 60-year-old woman is seen in the outpatient department, complaining of breathlessness. There are no abnormal physical findings. What does this ECG show, what might be the underlying problem, and how would you treat her?

ANSWER 65

The ECG shows:

- Atrial flutter, best seen in lead III
- 4 : 1 block
- Normal axis
- Normal QRS complexes
- Sloping ST segment depression, best seen in leads V_5–V_6

Clinical interpretation

This shows atrial flutter with what appears to be a stable 4 : 1 block. The ST segment depression suggests digoxin effect.

What to do

The stable 4 : 1 block has caused a regular heartbeat, so the arrhythmia was not suspected at the time of the clinical examination. There is nothing in this ECG to indicate the underlying disease, which could be ischaemic, rheumatic or a cardiomyopathy: echocardiography is needed. The downward-sloping ST segments suggest digoxin treatment. Digoxin will tend to maintain a fairly high degree of block but will not affect the underlying rhythm. Intravenous flecainide may convert the heart to sinus rhythm, but DC cardioversion may be necessary.

Summary ★★

Atrial flutter with 4 : 1 block.

ECG ME See p. 67, 8E

ECG IP See p. 117, 6E

ECG 66

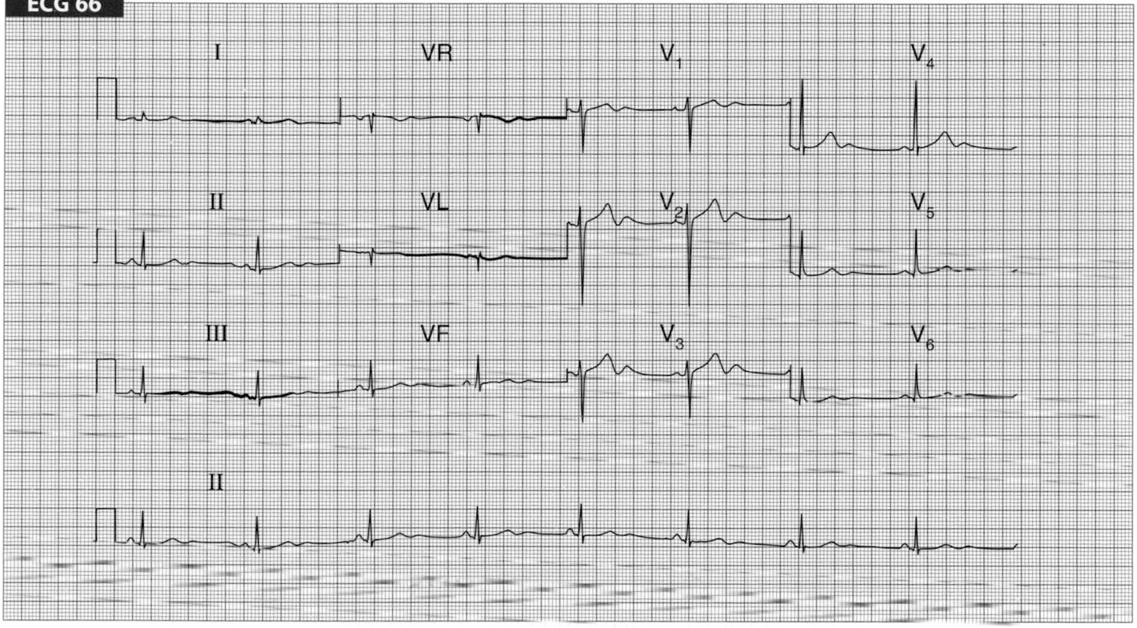

This ECG was recorded from a 30-year-old man at a medical examination required by the Civil Aviation Authority. Is it normal?

ANSWER 66

The ECG shows:

- Sinus rhythm, rate 52/min
- Prominent U waves, especially in leads V_2–V_4

Clinical interpretation

U waves can indicate hypokalaemia, but when associated with normal T waves (as here) they are a normal variant.

What to do

Provide reassurance – he is fit to fly.

Summary ★★
Normal ECG, with prominent U waves.

ECG ME See p. 5, 8E

ECG IP See p. 47, 6E

ECG 67

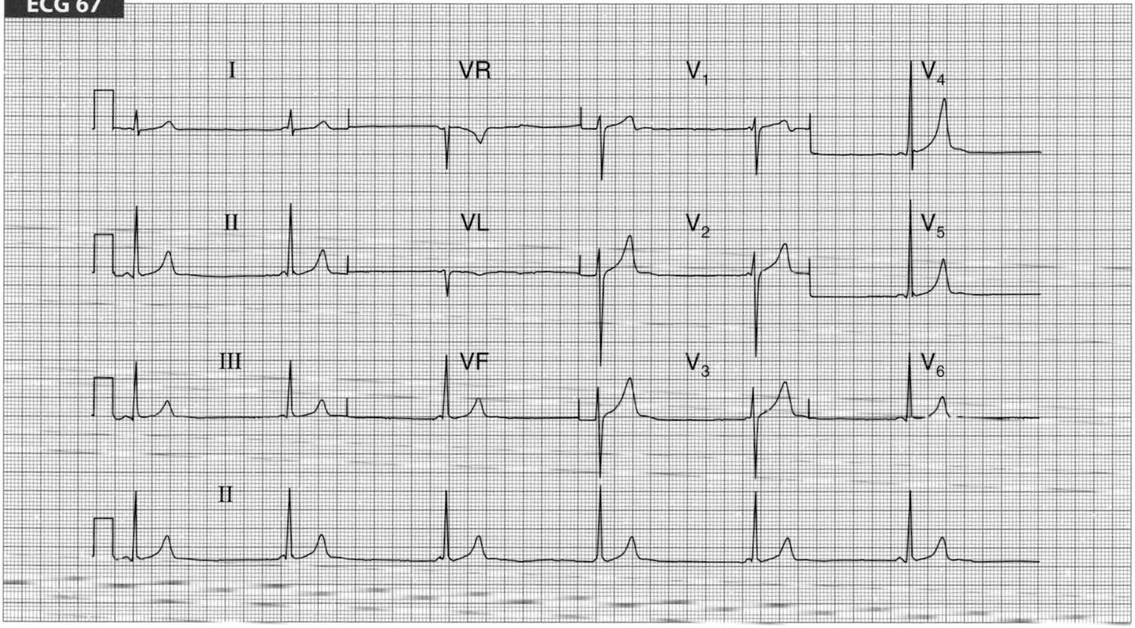

This ECG was recorded as part of the 'screening' examination of a young professional football player. Is it normal?

ANSWER 67

The ECG shows:

- Regular narrow complex rhythm at 35/min
- P waves sometimes, but not always, visible just before the QRS complexes
- PR interval, when measurable, is always short but varies
- Height of R wave in lead V_4 plus depth of S wave in lead V_2 = 49 mm
- Normal QRS complexes and ST segments
- Peaked T waves, especially in lead V_4

Clinical interpretation

The short PR interval raises the possibility of pre-excitation, but the interval varies, and in the first complex of leads V_1–V_3 no P wave can be seen. The slow, narrow complex rhythm suggests atrioventricular nodal escape. Here there is a pronounced slowing of the sinoatrial node, presumably due to athletic training, and an accelerated idionodal rhythm has taken over. This pattern used to be called a 'wandering atrial pacemaker'. The tall R waves are perfectly normal in young fit people, and so are the peaked T waves.

What to do

This is a normal variant in athletes, and no action is required.

Summary ★★

Accelerated idionodal rhythm.

ECG ME See p. 60, 8E

ECG IP See p. 102, 6E

ECG 68

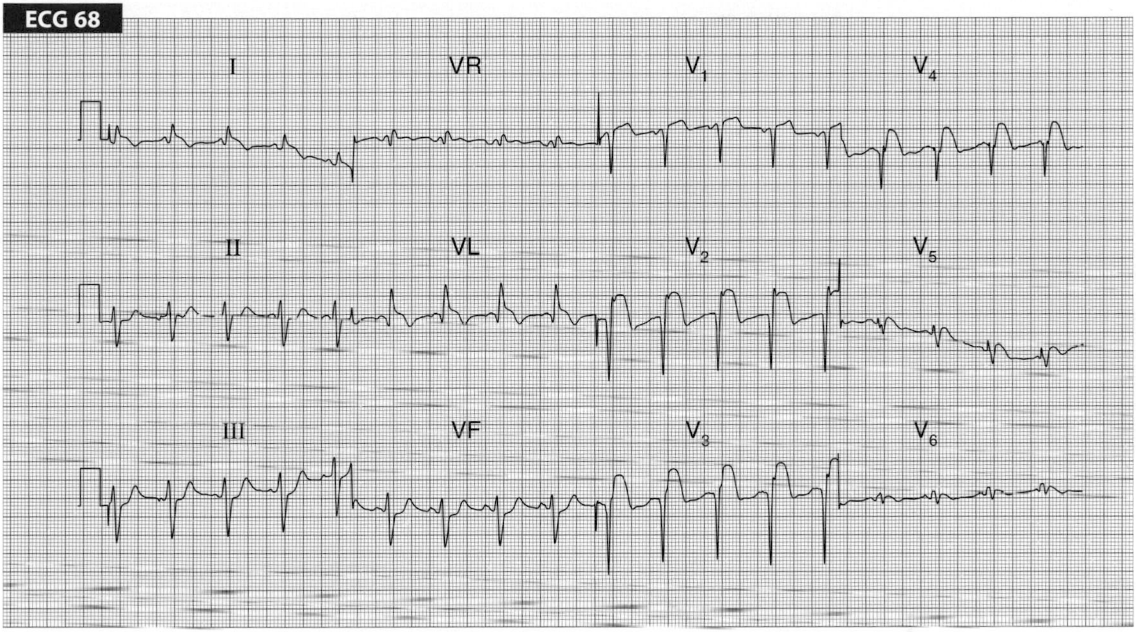

A 45-year-old patient is admitted to the A & E department having had severe central chest pain for 1 h. There are no signs of heart failure, and this is his ECG. What does the ECG show and what would you do?

ANSWER 68

The ECG shows:

- Sinus rhythm, rate 100/min
- Left axis deviation
- Q waves in leads V_2–V_4
- Raised ST segments in leads I, VL, V_2–V_5

Clinical interpretation

This ECG shows left anterior hemiblock, with an acute ST segment elevation antero-lateral myocardial infarction (STEMI).

What to do

Unless there are any potential risks of bleeding (previous stroke, peptic ulcer, diabetic retinopathy, etc.), this patient should be given aspirin, 300 mg to be chewed, and immediate percutaneous coronary intervention (PCI), or immediate thrombolysis if PCI is not available.

Summary ★
Acute antero-lateral STEMI and left anterior hemiblock.

ECG ME See p. 91, 8E

ECG IP See p. 85, 6E

ECG 69

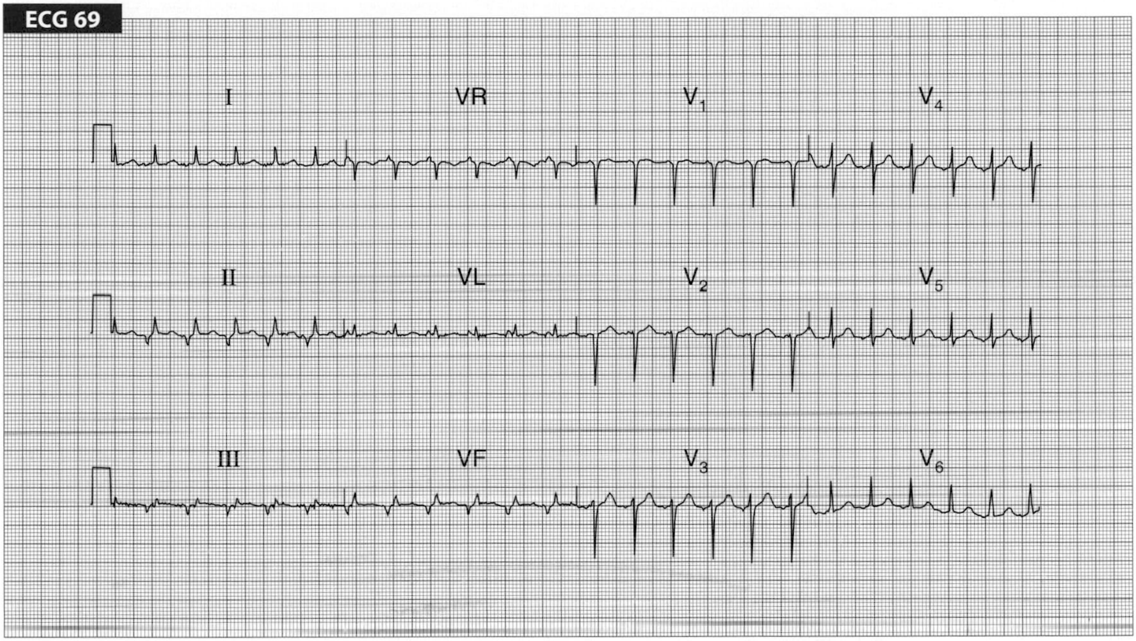

A 30-year-old man, who had complained of palpitations for many years without anything abnormal being found, came to the A & E department during an attack, and this ECG was recorded. Apart from signs of marked anxiety there were no unusual findings except a heart rate of 140/min. What does the ECG show?

ANSWER 69

The ECG shows:

- Narrow complex tachycardia at 140/min
- Inverted P waves, most obvious in leads II, III, VF
- Short PR interval (about 100 ms)
- Normal axis
- Normal QRS complexes, ST segments and T waves

Clinical interpretation

The story of attacks of palpitations could indicate episodes of sinus tachycardia due to anxiety, but the heart rate of 140/min suggests that a rhythm other than sinus rhythm is likely. This ECG clearly shows a supraventricular tachycardia of some sort, with one P wave per QRS complex. It could be sinus tachycardia, and the short PR interval could indicate pre-excitation, but the abnormal P waves in the inferior leads show that this is an atrial tachycardia.

What to do

Carotid sinus massage may terminate the attack, but if not it will almost certainly respond to adenosine. Further attacks may be prevented by a beta-blocker, but the patient should be referred for an electrophysiological study in the hope that a re-entry pathway can be identified and ablated.

Summary ★★

Atrial tachycardia.

ECG ME See p. 66, 8E

ECG IP See p. 107, 6E

ECG 70

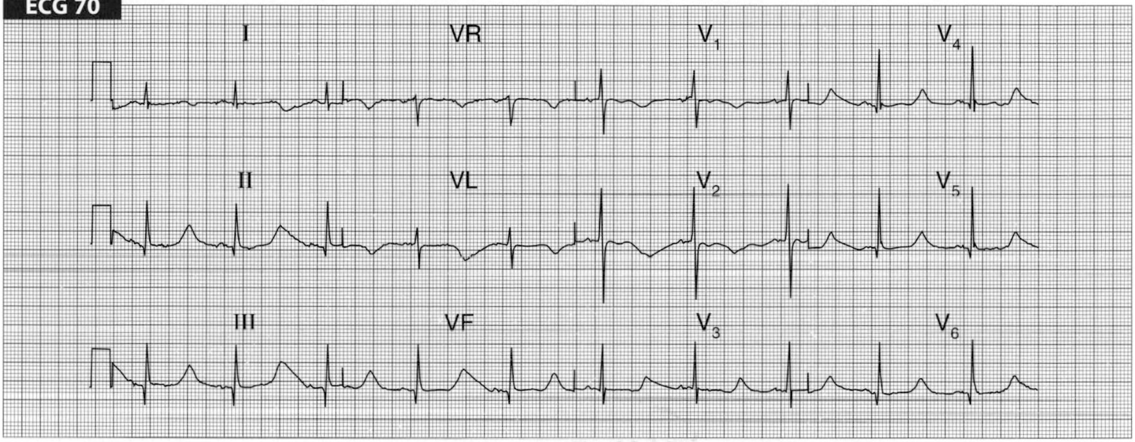

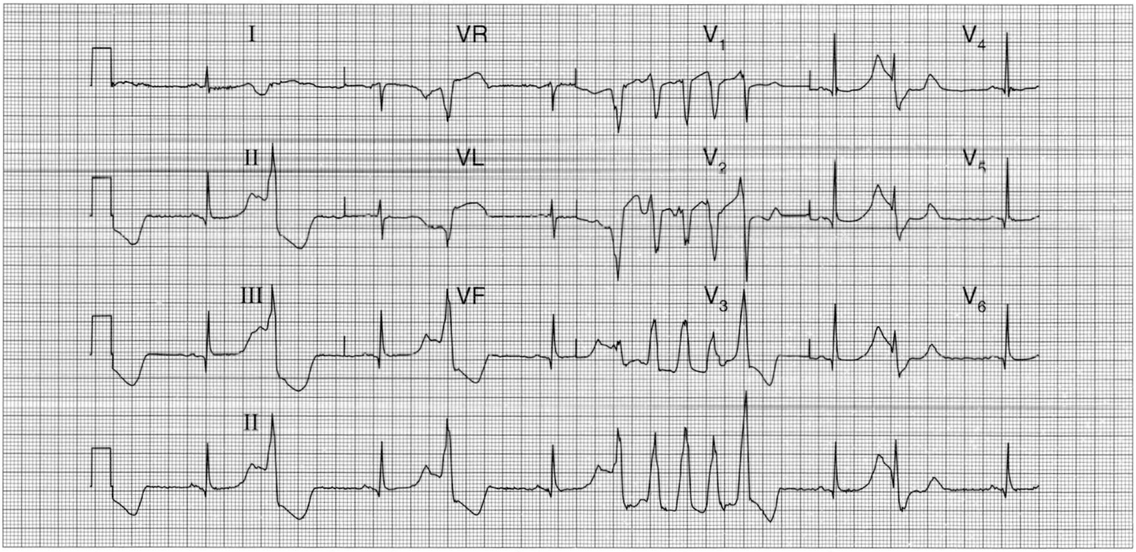

A confused 80-year-old woman was sent to hospital from a nursing home because of a collapse. No other history was available, except that she was said to be having treatment for her heart. There were no obvious physical signs. The upper ECG was recorded on admission, and the lower ECG was recorded shortly afterwards. What is going on?

ANSWER 70

The upper ECG shows:

- Sinus rhythm, with a rate of 60/min
- Narrow Q waves in leads II, III, VF, V_4–V_6
- Abnormally shaped T waves in most leads
- Prolonged QT interval (about 650 ms)

The lower ECG shows:

- Sinus rhythm with multifocal ventricular extrasystoles
- A run of polymorphic (i.e. changing shape) ventricular tachycardia

Clinical interpretation

In the upper trace the inferolateral Q waves could represent an old infarction, but they are narrow and are probably septal in origin. The prolonged QT interval and abnormal T waves suggest either an electrolyte abnormality or that the patient is being treated with one of the many drugs that have these effects. A collapse in a patient with an ECG with a long QT interval suggests episodes of torsade de pointes ventricular tachycardia.

What to do

The electrolyte levels, including magnesium, must be checked, and in this case were found to be normal. It is essential immediately to establish what medication the patient is taking, and pending that information it would be sensible to leave her untreated and simply to monitor her for arrhythmias. It turned out that this woman was taking sotalol – a beta-blocker with class III antiarrhythmic activity which is known to cause QT interval prolongation. When this drug was stopped, her ECG returned to normal.

Summary ★★★
Drug-induced QT interval prolongation and polymorphic ventricular tachycardia.

ECG ME See p. 157, 8E

ECG IP See p. 144, 6E

ECG 71

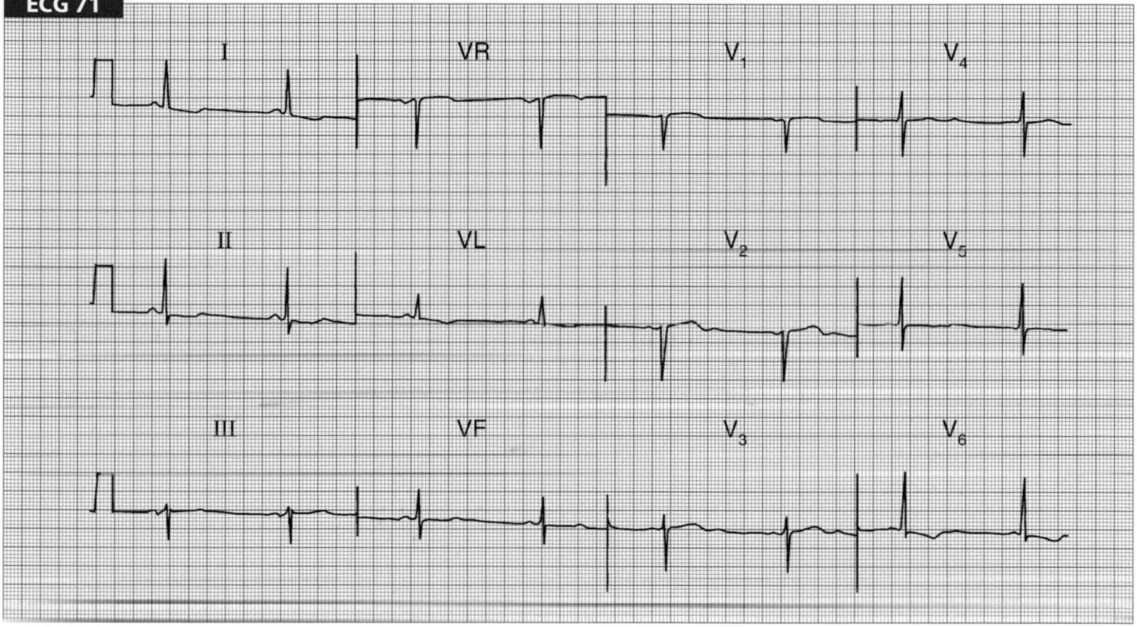

This ECG was recorded as part of a routine health check on a 50-year-old woman who said she was asymptomatic. The only abnormality detected in the other usual screening tests was a serum cholesterol level of 7.2 mmol/l. What would you do?

ANSWER 71

The ECG shows:

- Sinus rhythm, rate 45/min
- Normal axis
- Normal QRS complexes
- Widespread T wave flattening and inversion
- Prominent U waves, especially in leads V_2–V_5

Clinical interpretation

Flattened T waves with prominent U waves usually result from hypokalaemia. The serum potassium level is usually checked during health screening, but the same ECG changes can result from hypomagnesaemia; hypocalcaemia causes a long QT interval but not U waves. A high cholesterol level can be a marker for coronary disease, but elevated cholesterol levels can also be secondary to thyroid or renal disease.

What to do

Check the thyroid function. This woman had myxoedema, and her ECG became normal when it was treated.

Summary ★★★

Widespread T wave flattening with prominent U waves – classically due to hypokalaemia, but in this case due to myxoedema.

ECG ME See p. 101, 8E

ECG IP See p. 335, 6E

ECG 72

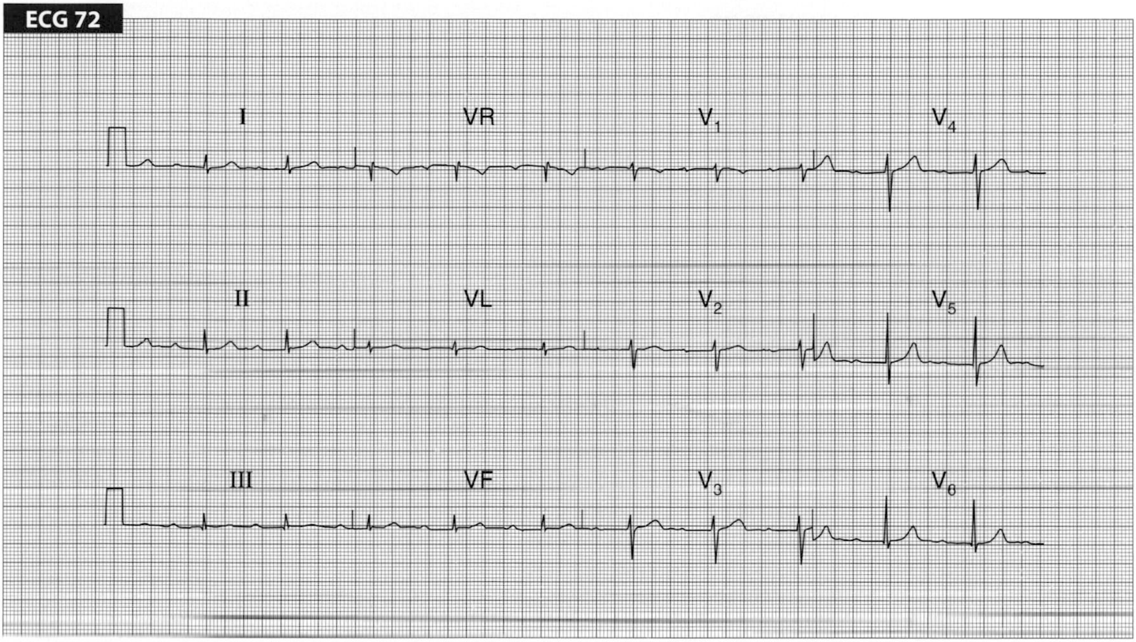

This ECG was recorded from an asymptomatic 45-year-old man at a 'health screening' examination. Is it normal, and what advice would you give him?

ANSWER 72

The ECG shows:

- Sinus rhythm, rate 64/min
- Prolonged PR interval (360 ms)
- Normal QRS complexes, ST segments, and T waves

Clinical interpretation

This ECG shows first degree atrioventricular block but is otherwise entirely normal.

What to do

Although the upper limit of the PR interval is usually taken to be 220 ms, longer durations (technically first degree block) are frequently seen in healthy people. Provided you can be sure that this patient has no symptoms, and provided the physical examination is normal, no further action is required. Some individuals in occupations that require a totally normal ECG may have to have an ambulatory ECG recording to demonstrate that there are no episodes of higher-degree block.

Summary ★
First degree atrioventricular block.

ECG ME See p. 37, 8E

ECG IP See p. 49, 6E

ECG 73

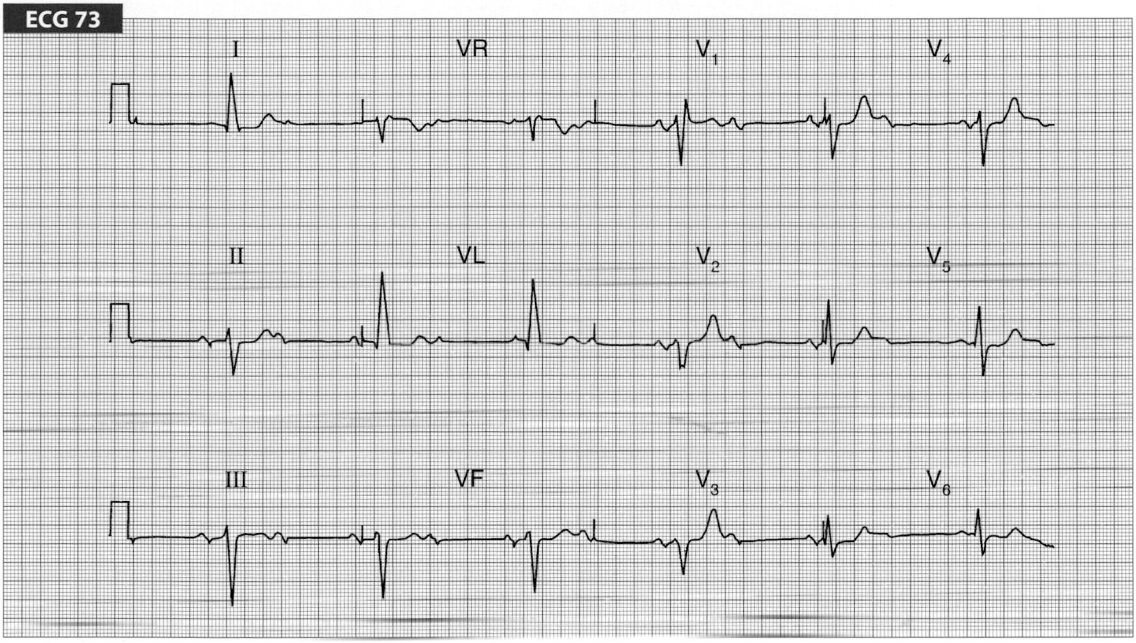

An 80-year-old man is found at routine examination to have a slow heart rate and a harsh systolic murmur. This is his ECG. What does it show, and what is the likely diagnosis? Is treatment necessary?

ANSWER 73

The ECG shows:

- Sinus rhythm, P wave rate 75/min
- Second degree (2:1) block
- Left axis deviation
- QRS complex duration 140 ms, with an RSR^1 pattern in lead V_1, indicating right bundle branch block (RBBB)

Clinical interpretation

This is second degree block and not complete (third degree) block because the PR interval in the conducted beats is normal: at times it appears to vary but in fact this variation is due to lead changes (shown by the small spikes). Left axis deviation (left anterior hemiblock) and RBBB constitute bifascicular block, but the 2:1 block shows that there is also disease in either the His bundle or the remaining posterior fascicle. This combination is sometimes called 'trifascicular' block.

What to do

The combination of a heart murmur and heart block suggests aortic stenosis. The severity of this can be assessed with echocardiography, though the slow rate (and thus high stroke volume) will accentuate the recorded valve gradient. Aortic valve replacement may or may not be needed, but the patient certainly needs a permanent pacemaker to prolong his survival.

Summary ★★

Second degree (2:1) block and trifascicular block.

ECG ME See p. 38, 8E

ECG IP See p. 89, 6E

ECG 74

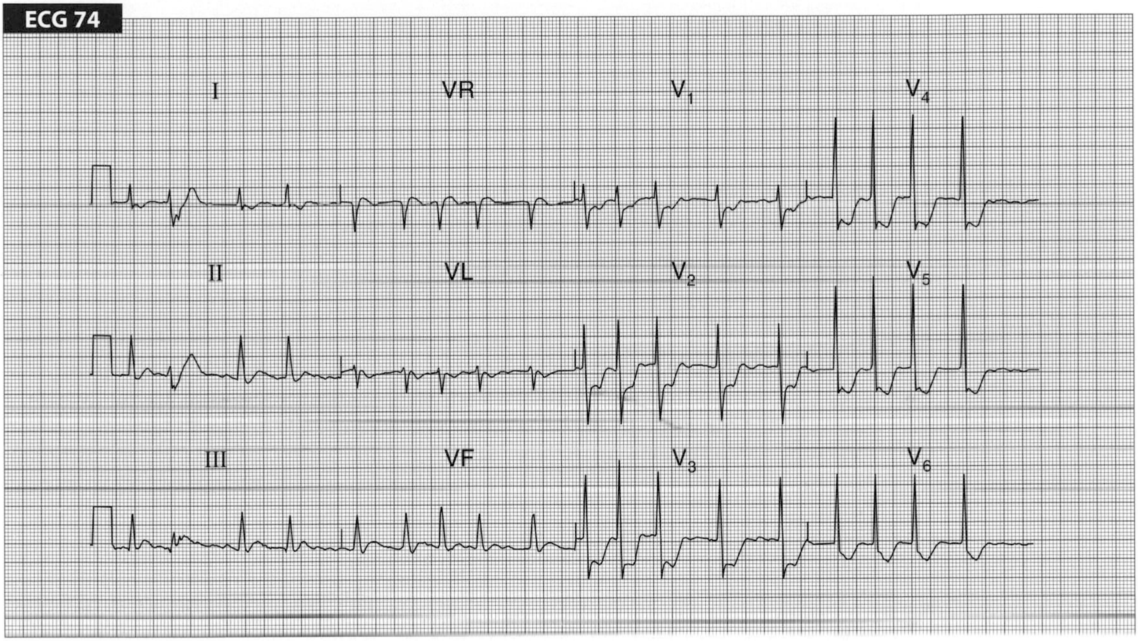

A 70-year-old woman, who had been breathless for several months, was admitted to hospital with chest pain, and this is her ECG. What does it show and what would you do?

ANSWER 74

The ECG shows:

- Atrial fibrillation, with one ventricular extrasystole
- Ventricular rate about 110/min
- Normal axis
- Normal QRS complexes
- Horizontal ST segment depression of 7 mm in lead V_2
- Downward-sloping ST segment depression in leads V_3–V_6
- Inverted T waves in leads I, VL, V_6; indeterminate T waves elsewhere

Clinical interpretation

The anterior horizontal ST segment depression indicates severe ischaemia, which is presumably the cause of the chest pain. The downward-sloping ST segment in lead V_6 could be due to digoxin therapy. The ventricular rate is not too fast, and although the heart rate may be contributing to the ischaemia it seems unlikely that it is the main problem.

What to do

The patient should be treated for an acute coronary syndrome with heparin, a beta-blocker and nitrates. If the pain does not settle, early angiography with a view to revascularization by a coronary artery bypass graft (CABG) or percutaneous coronary intervention (PCI) will have to be considered.

Summary ★★

Atrial fibrillation and anterior ischaemia.

ECG ME See p. 76, 8E

ECG IP See p. 243, 6E

ECG 75

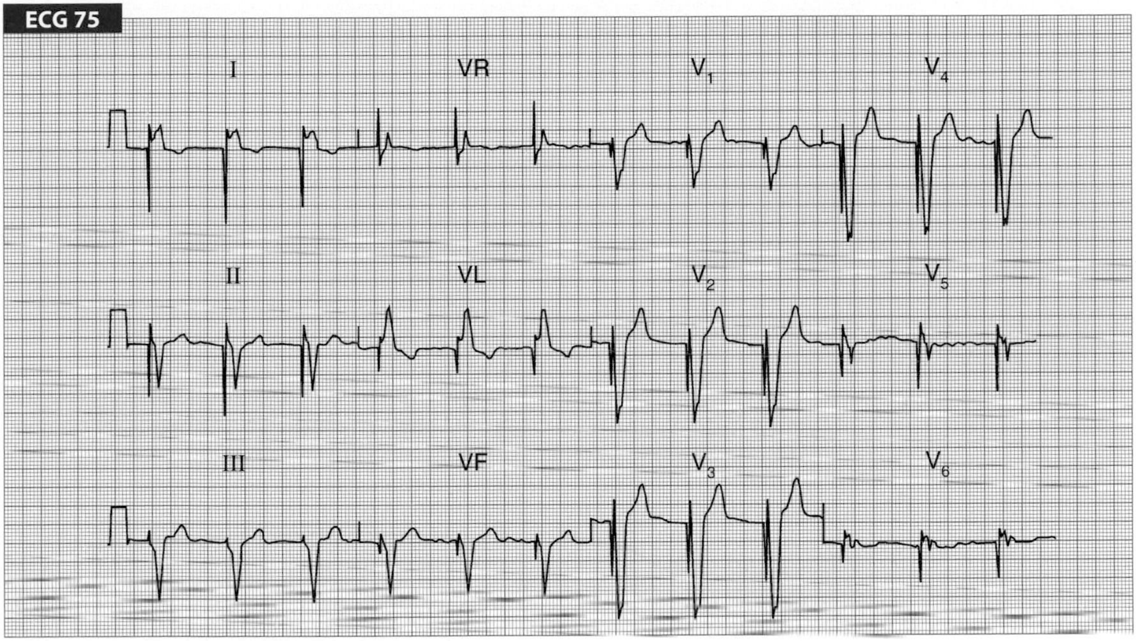

An elderly woman is admitted to hospital unconscious, evidently having had a stroke. No cardiac abnormalities are noted, but this is her ECG. What has been missed?

ANSWER 75

The ECG shows:

- No P waves; irregular baseline suggesting atrial fibrillation
- Regular QRS complexes; rate 73/min
- Left axis deviation
- Wide QRS complexes of an indeterminate pattern, with inverted T waves in some leads
- Each QRS complex is preceded by a deep and narrow spike

Clinical interpretation

The narrow spike is due to a pacemaker, and someone has not noticed the permanent pacing battery, which is probably below the left clavicle. The pacing wire will be stimulating the right ventricle, giving rise to broad QRS complexes resembling a bundle branch block pattern. The underlying rhythm here is atrial fibrillation: the patient may have had atrial fibrillation with complete block, or there may simply have been a slow ventricular response to the atrial fibrillation.

What to do

The stroke may have been due to an embolus arising in the left heart as a result of atrial fibrillation. There may have been temporary pacemaker failure, but probably the stroke was not related to the pacemaker.

Summary ★★

Ventricular-paced rhythm and atrial fibrillation.

ECG ME See p. 167, 8E

ECG IP See p. 187, 6E

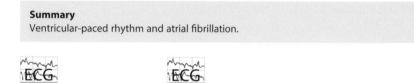

ECG 76

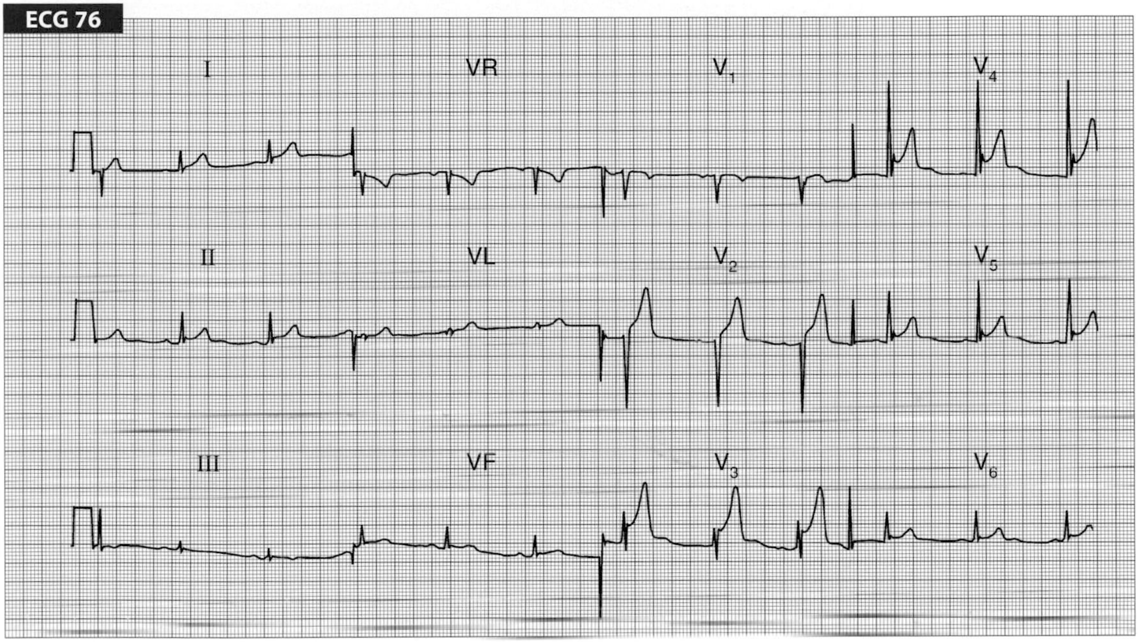

A 30-year-old man is seen in the A & E department with left-sided chest pain that appears to be pleuritic in nature. What does his ECG show?

ANSWER 76

The ECG shows:

- Sinus rhythm, rate 63/min
- Normal axis
- Normal QRS complexes
- Raised ST segments in leads II, V_3–V_6, in each case preceded by an S wave

Clinical interpretation

When a raised ST segment follows an S wave as shown here, it is called 'high take-off' of the ST segment. This is a normal variant, which must be distinguished from the changes associated with an acute infarction or pericarditis.

What to do

If the patient has chest pain that appears to be pleuritic, then pulmonary rather than cardiac causes of pain should be considered – infection, pulmonary embolus and pneumothorax. The ECG is completely unhelpful here.

Summary ★★

Normal ECG showing 'high take-off' ST segment.

ECG ME See p. 122, 8E

ECG IP See p. 31, 6E

ECG 77

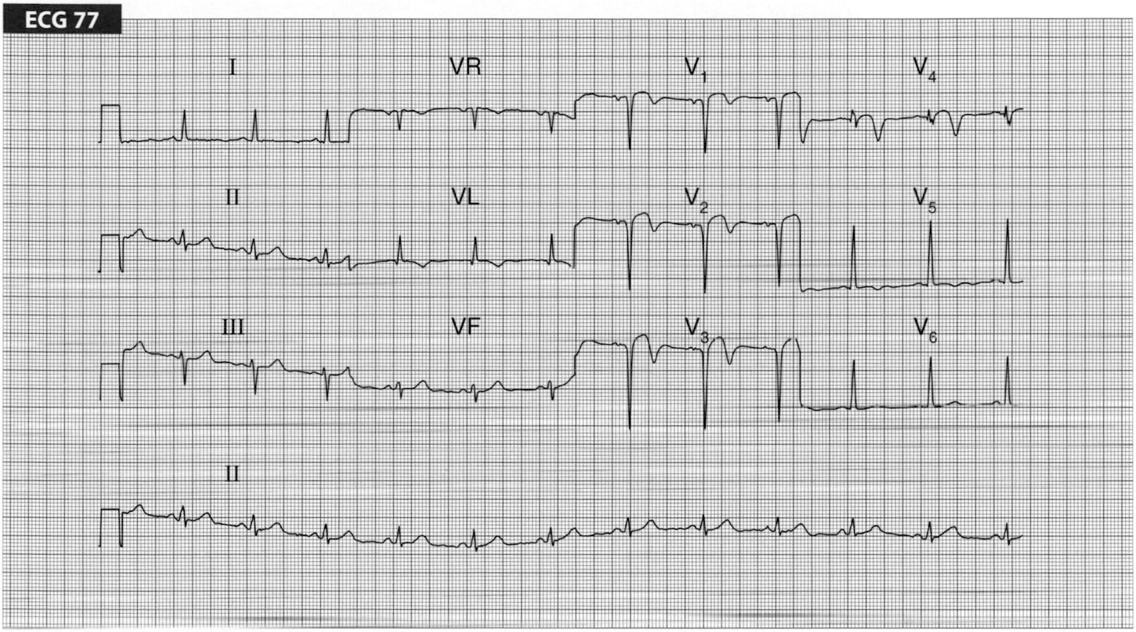

A 50-year-old man returned from holiday in Spain saying that while there he had had some bad indigestion, but was now perfectly well. This is his ECG: what does it show and what would you do?

ANSWER 77

The ECG shows:

- Sinus rhythm, rate 72/min
- Normal conduction
- Normal axis
- Q waves in leads V_2–V_3
- Elevated ST segments in leads V_2–V_4
- Inverted T waves in leads VL, V_1–V_5

Clinical interpretation

This ECG shows an old anterior myocardial infarction with lateral ischaemia. The elevation of ST segments might suggest an acute process if the pain were recent, but with this story the changes are almost certainly old. The persistence of ST segment elevation in the anterior leads may be due to a left ventricular aneurysm.

What to do

The assumption has to be that the 'indigestion' was actually a myocardial infarction. Since he is now well, the important thing is to ensure that he takes the appropriate steps to prevent a further attack – he must stop smoking and reduce weight if necessary, and he should be treated with aspirin, a beta-blocker, an angiotensin-converting enzyme inhibitor and a statin. In view of his age it might be worth doing an exercise test to ensure that there is no evidence of ischaemia at a low workload – if there were, an angiogram would be indicated.

Summary ★

Old anterior myocardial infarction.

ECG ME See p. 130, 8E

ECG IP See p. 225, 6E

ECG 78

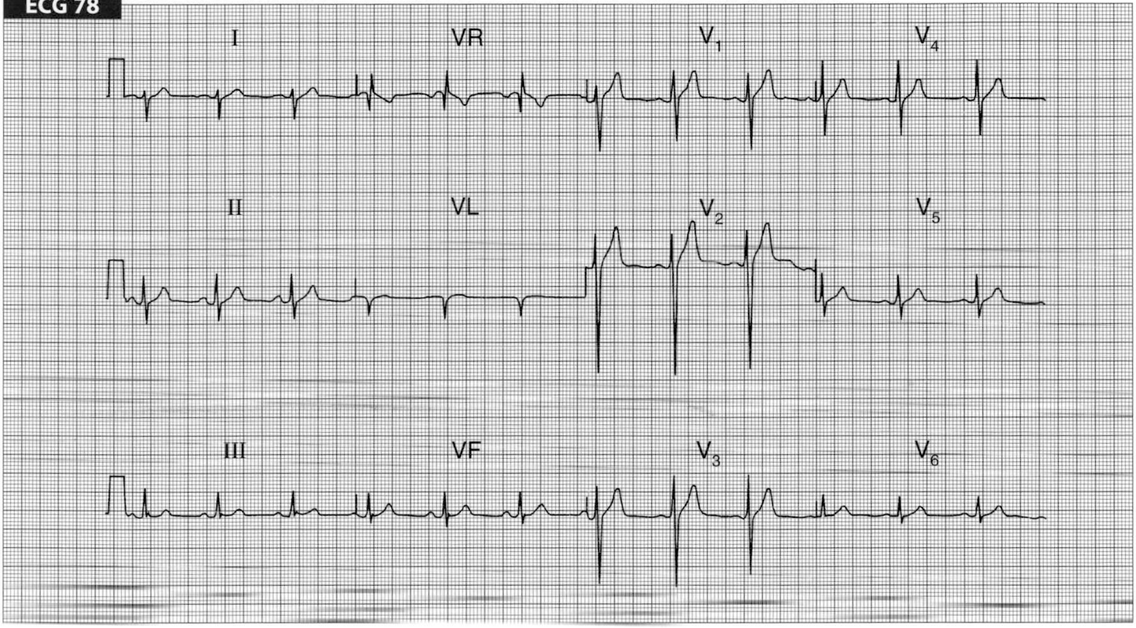

This ECG was recorded from an asymptomatic 30-year-old man at a routine examination. Is it normal?

ANSWER 78

The ECG shows:

- Sinus rhythm, rate 73/min
- Right axis deviation (S wave bigger than R wave in lead I, large R wave in lead VR, very small R wave and deep S wave in lead VL)
- Notched QRS complexes in lead III
- Otherwise entirely normal QRS complexes and T waves

Clinical interpretation

Right axis deviation can be a feature of right ventricular hypertrophy, but in tall, thin people it is a normal variant. The notched QRS complexes in lead III are normal, though if present in all leads they could be the 'J' waves of hypothermia.

What to do

Examine the patient and exclude right ventricular hypertrophy (you should have done this before recording the ECG!).

Summary ★

Normal ECG with right axis deviation.

ECG ME See p. 158, 8E

ECG IP See p. 15, 6E

ECG 79

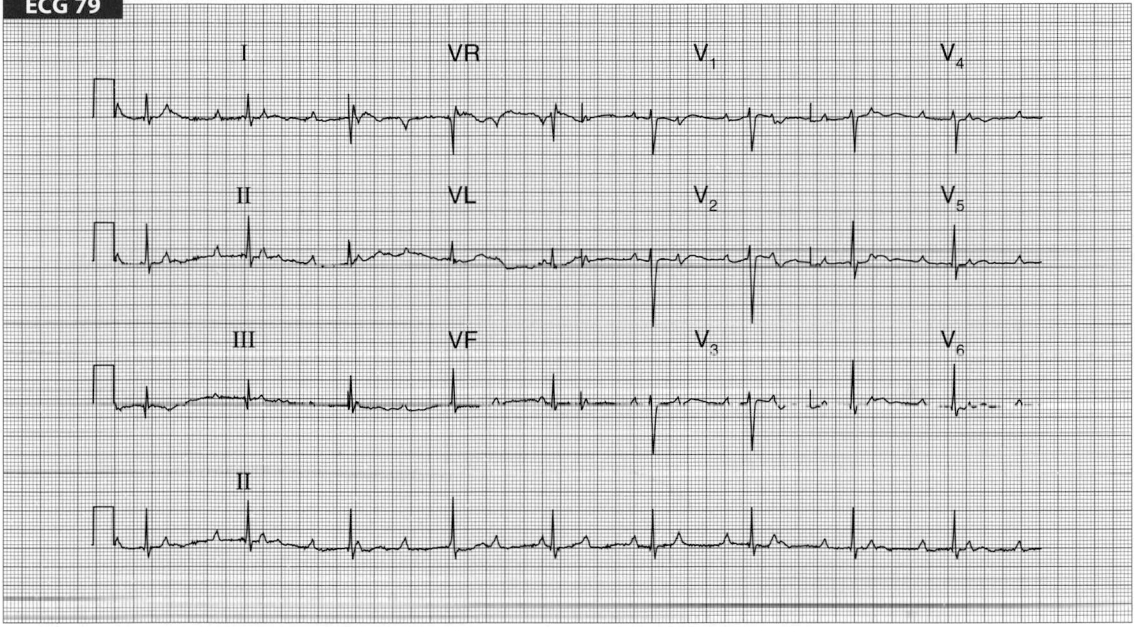

This ECG was recorded from a 70-year-old woman who had complained of attacks of dizziness for about a year. What is the problem, what might be its cause, and how should this woman be treated?

ANSWER 79

The ECG shows:

- Sinus rhythm with complete (third degree) block, rate 55/min
- Normal axis
- Normal QRS complexes and T waves

Clinical interpretation

This ECG shows complete heart block with a relatively low ventricular rate. The attacks of dizziness may be due to further slowing of the heart rate. Although at times there appears to be second degree (2 : 1) block, the lead II rhythm strip shows that what could be the PR interval is continually changing, and that there is actually no relationship between the P waves and QRS complexes. The QRS complex is narrow, and so must originate in the His bundle.

What to do

An ambulatory ECG, recorded over 24 h, may reveal the rhythm associated with the dizziness – but whatever the findings, the patient needs a permanent pacemaker. There are many causes of heart block, including ischaemia; association with aortic valve calcification; Lyme disease (*Borrelia burgdorferi*); His bundle interruption (due to surgery, trauma, parasites, tumours, abscesses, granulomata); and drugs (digoxin, beta-blockers, calcium-channel blockers). However, most cases of heart block are due to His bundle fibrosis, for which hypertension is a risk factor. An echocardiogram is necessary to study left ventricular function, and if this is impaired the patient needs an angiotensin-converting enzyme inhibitor.

Summary ★

Complete (third degree) block.

ECG ME See p. 41, 8E

ECG IP See p. 179, 6E

ECG 80

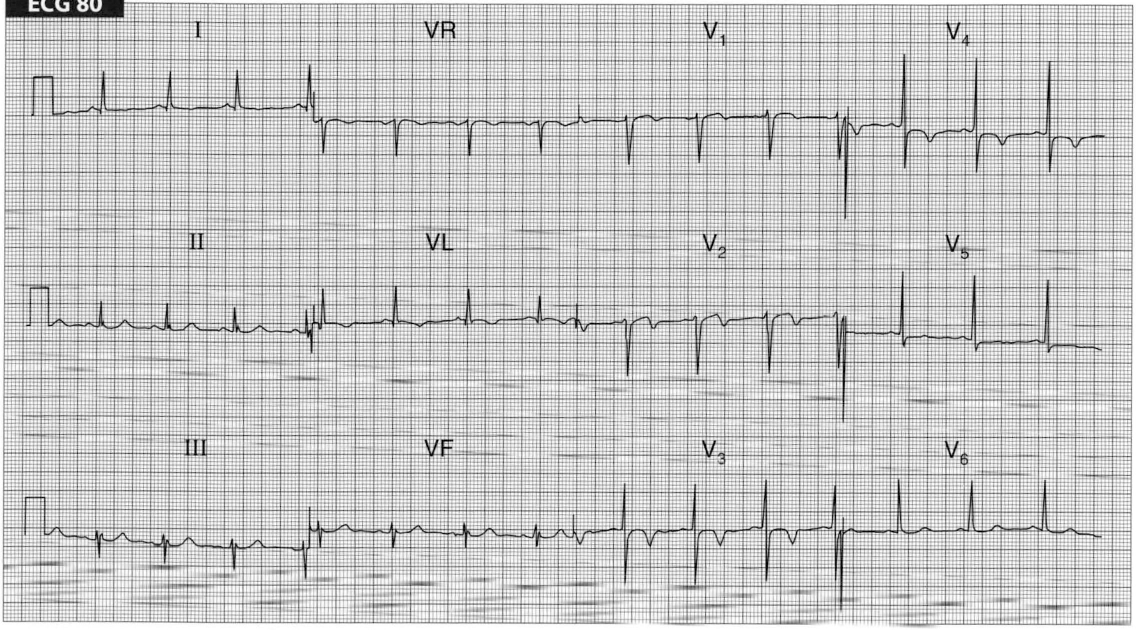

This ECG was recorded in the A & E department from a 60-year-old man who had had intermittent central chest pain for 24 h. What does it show and how should he be managed?

ANSWER 80

The ECG shows:

- Sinus rhythm, rate 81/min
- Normal conduction intervals
- Normal axis
- Normal QRS complexes
- Normal ST segments, with ST segment depression in lead V_4
- T wave inversion in leads VL, V_2–V_4

Clinical interpretation

This ECG shows an anterior non-ST segment elevation myocardial infarction (NSTEMI) of uncertain age.

What to do

This patient clearly has an acute coronary syndrome. He must be admitted to hospital and treated with low-molecular-weight heparin, a nitrate and a beta-blocker. If the pain does not settle quickly, the use of a glycoprotein IIb/IIIa inhibitor such as tirofiban or abciximab should be considered as a prelude to early percutaneous coronary intervention (PCI).

Summary ★
Anterior NSTEMI.

ECG ME See p. 142, 8E

ECG IP See p. 241, 6E

ECG 81

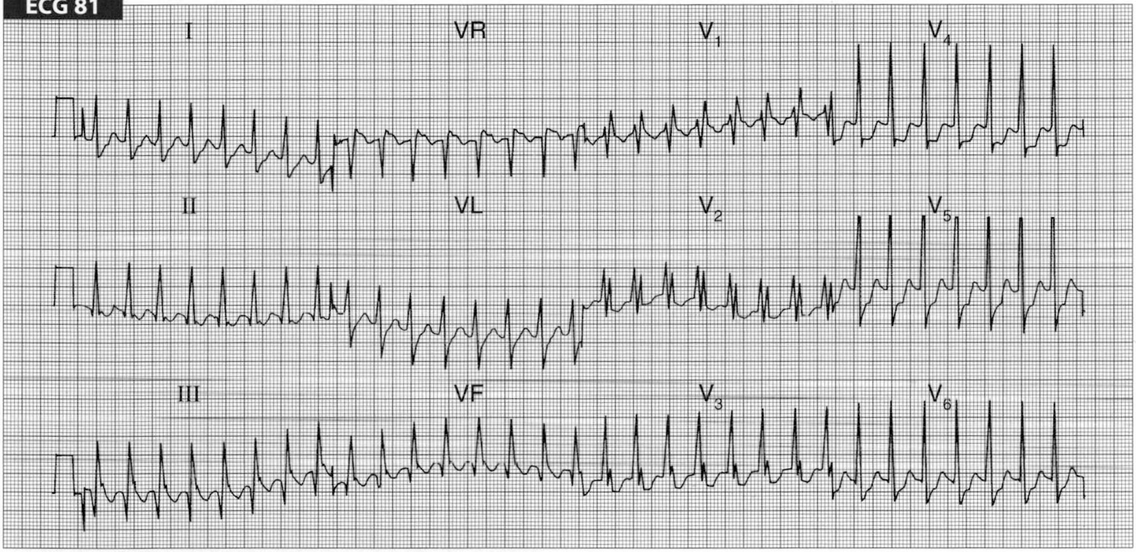

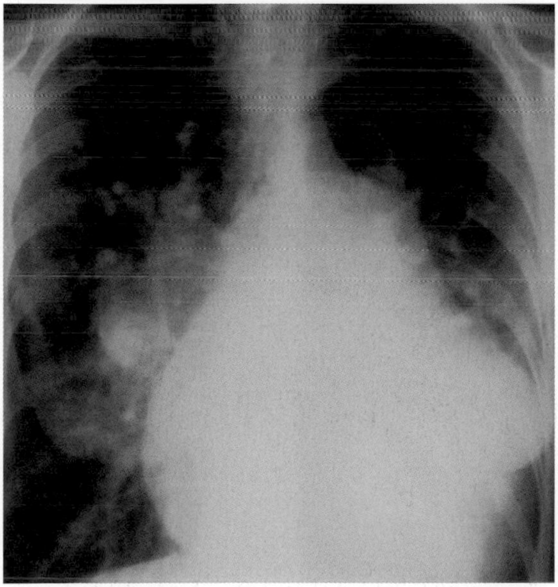

A 25-year-old man, known to have a heart problem for which he had refused surgery, was admitted to hospital as an emergency because of palpitations. His heart rate was 170/min, his blood pressure was 140/80 and there were no signs of heart failure. What is the cardiac rhythm and what would you do?

ANSWER 81

The ECG shows:

- Broad complex tachycardia, rate 170/min
- No clear P waves but possibly some P waves visible in lead VR
- Normal axis
- Right bundle branch block (RBBB) pattern
- Horizontal ST segment depression, best seen in lead V_4

The chest X-ray shows a very large heart with prominence of the right ventricle and pulmonary outflow, and large peripheral pulmonary arteries indicating a right-to-left shunt. These features are compatible with a large atrial septal defect.

Clinical interpretation

The QRS complex duration is 120 ms, the axis is normal, and the QRS complexes show the classic RBBB pattern. It is likely that this is a supraventricular tachycardia with RBBB, and this diagnosis would be certain if we were sure of the existence of P waves in lead VR. This is either an atrial or an atrioventricular nodal re-entry (junctional) tachycardia (AVNRT). The ST segment depression suggests ischaemia.

What to do

If the patient has an atrial septal defect, he is likely to have RBBB, and this could be confirmed from pre-existing hospital records. The initial treatment is carotid sinus massage, and if this proves ineffective, intravenous adenosine.

Summary ★★★

Supraventricular tachycardia (possibly atrial, possibly AVNRT) with RBBB; atrial septal defect.

ECG ME See p. 81, 8E

ECG IP See p. 145, 6E

ECG 82

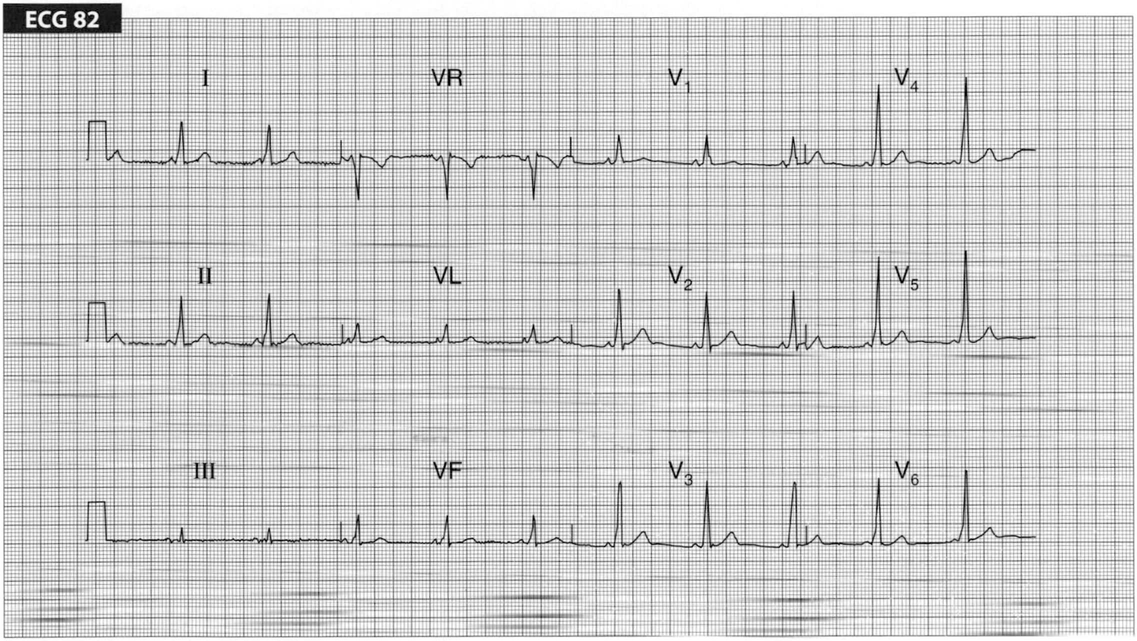

A 30-year-old woman, who had a baby 3 months previously, complains of breathlessness, and this is her ECG. What is the problem?

ANSWER 82

The ECG shows:

- Sinus rhythm, rate 64/min
- Short PR interval at 100 ms
- Normal axis
- Normal QRS complex duration
- Slurred upstroke to QRS complexes (delta wave)
- Dominant R wave in lead V_1
- Normal ST segments and T waves

Clinical interpretation

This ECG shows the Wolff–Parkinson–White (WPW) syndrome type A, which is characterized by a dominant R wave in lead V_1.

What to do

The catch here is that the dominant R wave in lead V_1 may be mistakenly thought to be due to right ventricular hypertrophy. In a young woman who complains of breathlessness after a pregnancy, pulmonary embolism is obviously a possibility, and this might well cause ECG evidence of right ventricular hypertrophy – but in the presence of the WPW syndrome this would be very difficult to diagnose from the ECG. The only thing that might help the diagnosis would be the appearance of right axis deviation, which is not part of the WPW syndrome, and is not present here. So, look for another cause of breathlessness, such as anaemia.

Summary ★★

The WPW syndrome type A.

ECG ME See p. 154, 8E

ECG IP See p. 69, 6E

ECG 83

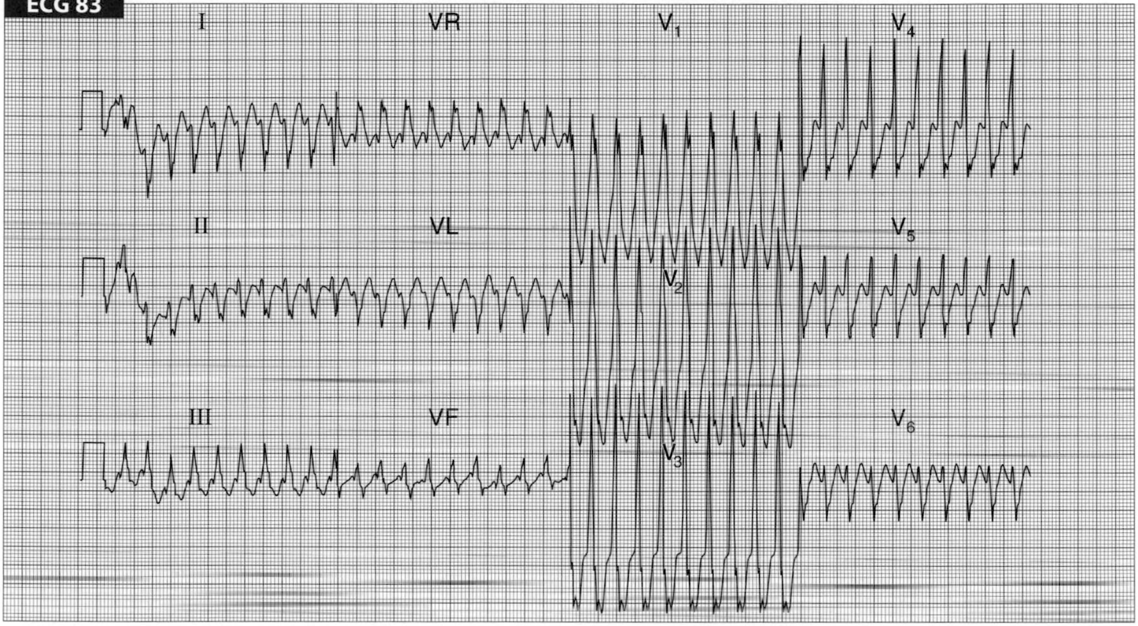

A 30-year-old man, who had had brief episodes of palpitations for at least 10 years, was seen during an attack in the A & E department and this is his ECG. What is the rhythm, and what would you do immediately, and in the long term?

ANSWER 83

The ECG shows:

- Broad complex tachycardia at about 230–240/min
- No P waves visible
- Right axis deviation
- QRS complex duration of about 180 ms
- QRS complexes point upwards in lead V_1 and downwards in lead V_6 – no concordance
- QRS complex configuration characteristic of right bundle branch block – but in lead V_1 the first R wave peak is higher than the second peak

Clinical interpretation

There are essentially three causes of a broad complex tachycardia: ventricular tachycardia, supraventricular tachycardia with bundle branch block, and the Wolff–Parkinson–White (WPW) syndrome. The key to the diagnosis lies in the ECG when the heart is in sinus rhythm, but this is not always available. Patients with a broad complex tachycardia in the context of an acute myocardial infarction must be assumed to have a ventricular tachycardia, but that does not apply here. In this record the QRS complexes are not very broad, the axis is to the right, and there is no concordance of the QRS complexes – all pointing to a supraventricular origin. In favour of a ventricular tachycardia is the fact that the height of the primary R wave in lead V_1 is greater than that of the secondary R wave. However, taking these features together with the clinical picture, the rhythm is probably supraventricular.

What to do

Carotid sinus pressure is the first move. If there is severe haemodynamic compromise the patient may need urgent electrical cardioversion, but intravenous flecainide would be a reasonable first choice. In fact, in this case the arrhythmia terminated spontaneously, revealing a short PR interval and a QRS complex with a delta wave. So this patient had the WPW syndrome, and needed an electrophysiological study with a view to ablation of the accessory tract.

See p. 75, 8E

See p. 145, 6E

Summary ★★★

Broad complex tachycardia (eventually shown to be due to the WPW syndrome).

ECG 84

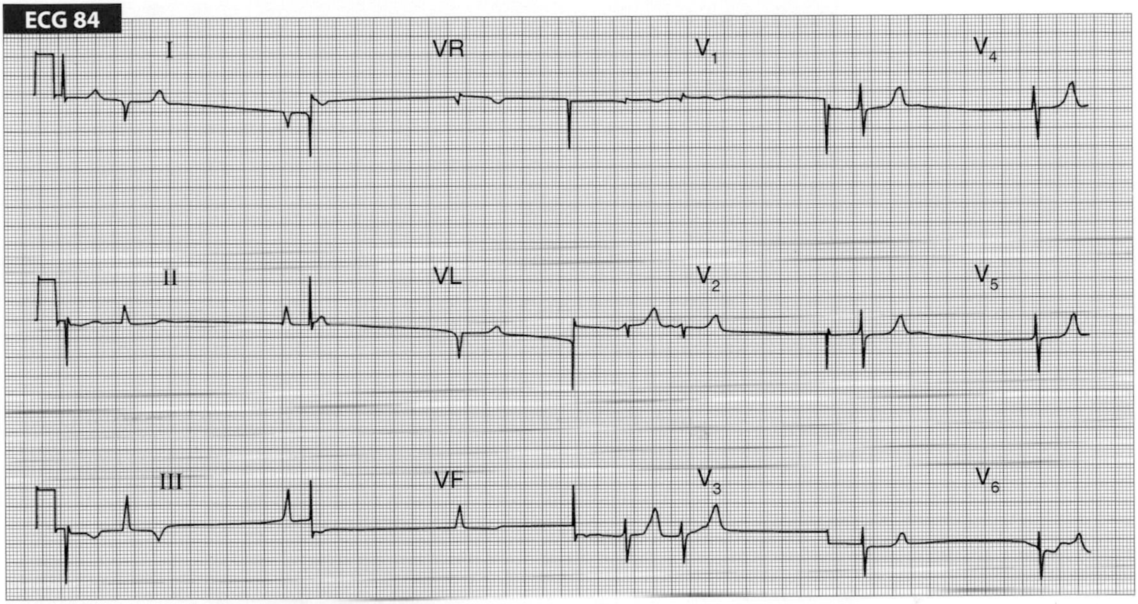

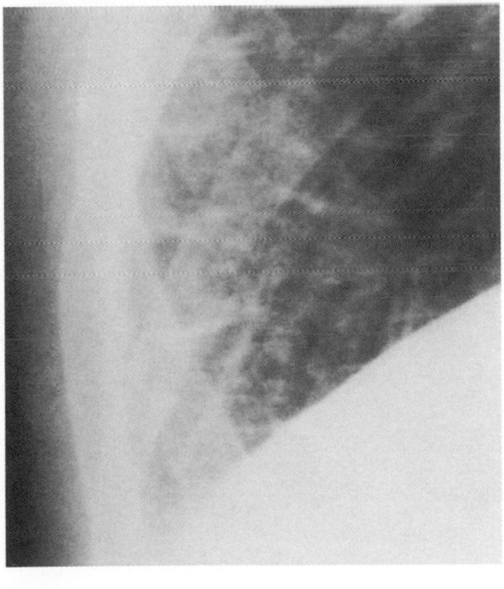

A 65-year-old woman with rheumatic heart disease, who had had severe heart failure for years, was admitted to hospital with increasing breathlessness and ankle swelling. Despite having been treated with angiotensin-converting enzyme inhibitors and diuretics, there was evidence of severe heart failure. Having seen the ECG and chest X-ray, what more do you want to know?

ANSWER 84

The ECG shows:

- Uncertain rhythm – no P waves; irregular QRS complexes; but no 'fibrillation' activity
- Right axis deviation
- Normal QRS complexes except for a small Q wave in lead V_1 and a deep S wave in lead V_6
- Symmetrically peaked T waves
- Inverted T waves in leads III, VF

The X-ray shows the right lung base. There is interstitial pulmonary oedema and 'Kerley B' lines (fluid in the lymphatics) can be seen, indicating left heart failure.

Clinical interpretation

The absence of atrial activity and the peaked T waves are consistent with hyperkalaemia. The right axis deviation and deep S waves in lead V_6 could indicate right ventricular hypertrophy and could result from chronic lung disease. The inverted T waves in leads III and VF suggest ischaemia.

What to do

Find out what the patient's medication has been and check her serum electrolyte levels. This woman had been treated with a combination of captopril 25 mg, three times daily (which tends to raise the serum potassium level) and three co-amilofruse tablets per 24 h (furosemide 40 mg plus amiloride 5 mg in each tablet). The combination of captopril and amiloride causes marked potassium retention, and in this case the serum potassium level was 7.4 mmol/l.

When the hyperkalaemia was corrected, sinus rhythm with clear P waves was restored and the peaked T waves became normal. The right axis deviation, clockwise rotation and inverted T waves in the inferior leads persisted.

Summary ★★★
Hyperkalaemia.

ECG ME See p. 101, 8E

ECG IP See p. 331, 6E

ECG 85

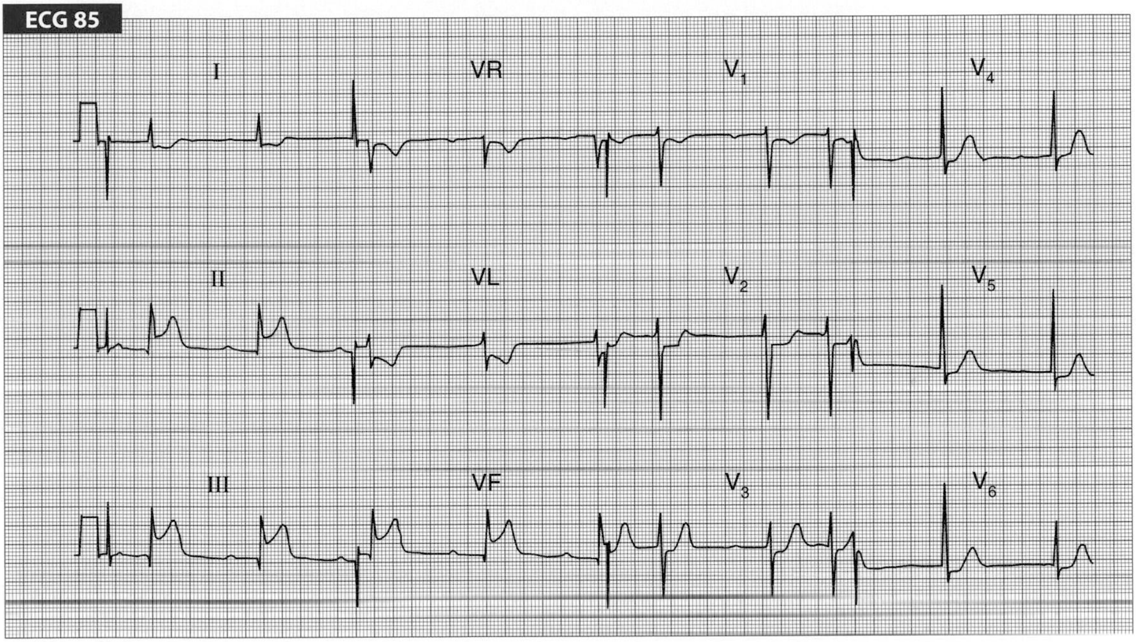

This ECG was recorded from a 55-year-old man who was admitted to hospital as an emergency with severe central chest pain that had been present for about an hour. He was pale, cold and clammy; his blood pressure was 100/80, but there were no signs of heart failure. What does this ECG show? Does anything about it surprise you?

ANSWER 85

The ECG shows:

- Sinus rhythm, rate 50/min
- First degree block (PR interval 350 ms)
- Normal axis
- Small Q waves in leads II, III, VF
- Raised ST segments in leads II, III, VF
- Depressed ST segments and inverted T waves in leads I, VL
- Slight ST segment depression in the chest leads

Clinical interpretation

Acute inferior ST segment elevation myocardial infarction (STEMI) with antero-lateral ischaemia, and first degree block. Patients who are in pain with an acute myocardial infarction usually have a sinus tachycardia, but here vagal overactivity is causing a bradycardia.

What to do

First degree block is not important in itself, but with evidence of vagal overactivity, atropine should be given. Otherwise this patient can be treated in the usual way with pain relief, aspirin, and percutaneous coronary intervention (PCI) or thrombolytics.

Summary ★

Acute inferior STEMI with first degree block.

ECG ME See p. 91, 8E

ECG IP See p. 215, 6E

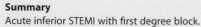

ECG 86

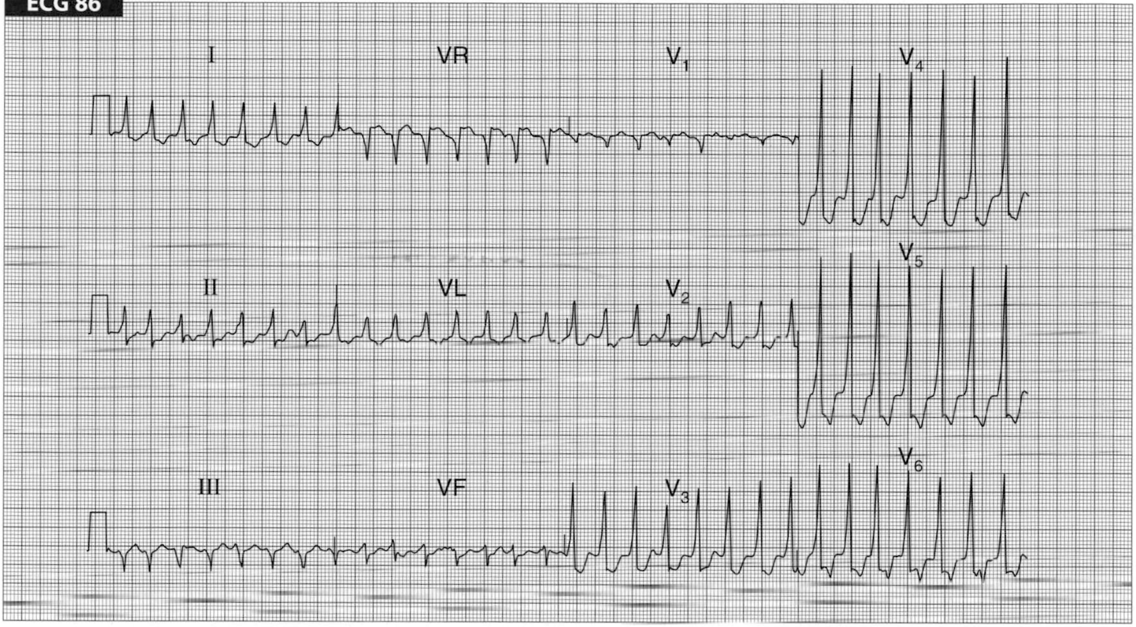

A 35-year-old woman, who had had attacks of what sounded like a paroxysmal tachycardia for many years, was seen in the A & E department, and this ECG was recorded. What is the diagnosis?

ANSWER 86

The ECG shows:

- Narrow complex tachycardia at about 170/min
- No P waves visible
- Normal axis
- QRS complex duration 112 ms
- Slurred upstroke to QRS complexes, best seen in leads V_3–V_6
- Depressed ST segments in leads V_3–V_6
- Inverted T waves in the lateral leads

Clinical interpretation

This is a narrow complex tachycardia, so it is supraventricular. The slurred upstroke to the QRS complex suggests the Wolff–Parkinson–White (WPW) syndrome, so this is a re-entry tachycardia, with depolarization spreading down the accessory pathway. The absence of a dominant R wave in lead V_1 indicates that this is WPW syndrome type B. This diagnosis is consistent with the patient's history.

What to do

Carotid sinus pressure is always the first thing to try in patients with a supraventricular tachycardia. In most such patients, adenosine is the first drug to use, but in cases of the WPW syndrome it must be used with caution. It can block the atrioventricular node and increase conduction through the accessory pathway, and if atrial fibrillation is present this can lead to ventricular fibrillation. Digoxin, verapamil and lidocaine can have the same effect. The safe drugs in this situation are the beta-blockers, flecainide and amiodarone.

Summary ★★

Supraventricular tachycardia and the WPW syndrome type B.

ECG ME See p. 155, 8E

ECG IP See p. 69, 6E

ECG 87

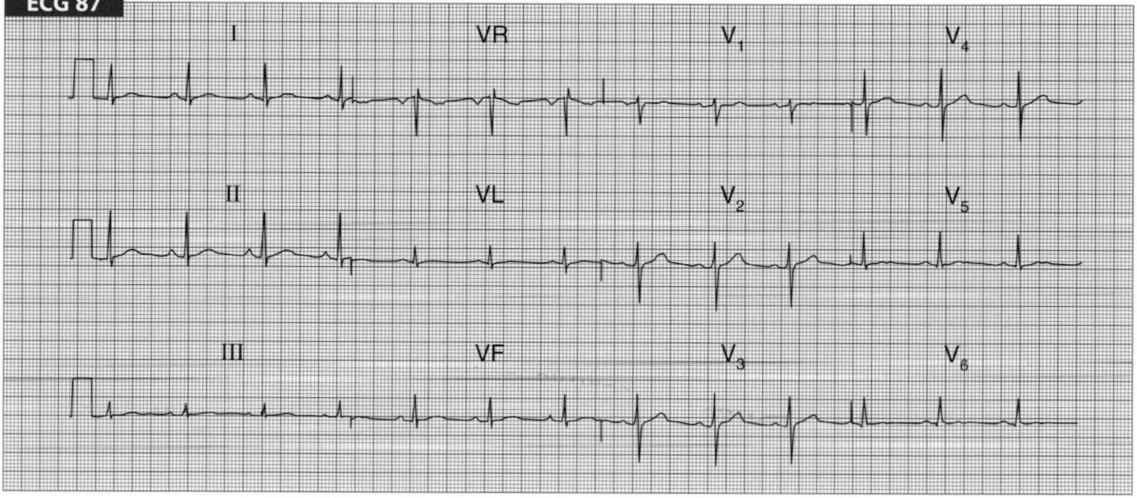

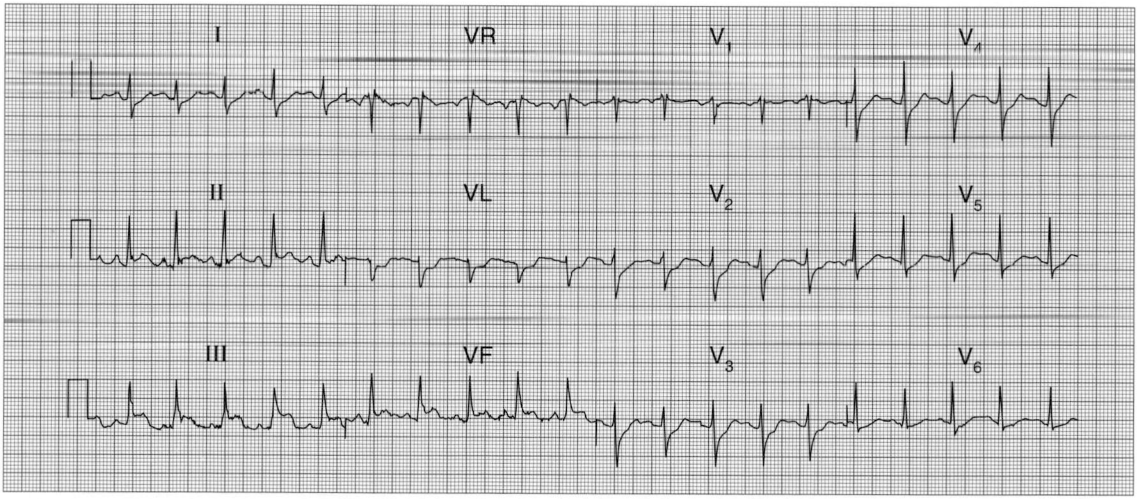

A 50-year-old man complains of pain in the front of his chest, which is predictably induced by walking uphill, especially in cold weather. The pain is sometimes caused by excitement. He has never had any pain without some precipitating cause. The upper ECG shows a recording made at rest, and the lower record comes from his exercise test, after 5 min of the Bruce protocol. What do the ECGs show?

ANSWER 87

Upper ECG

The upper ECG shows:

- Sinus rhythm with a rate of 75/min
- Normal axis
- Normal QRS complexes
- Normal ST segments
- Flat T wave in lead VL; flat and possibly biphasic T wave in lead V_6

Clinical interpretation

The T wave changes are very nonspecific, and the trace could well be normal. However, since the patient's story is highly suggestive of angina, an exercise test is necessary.

Exercise test

The lower ECG shows:

- Sinus rhythm with a rate of about 110/min
- ST segment depression in leads V_2–V_4, with a maximum in lead V_3
- ST segment elevation in leads II, III, VF

Clinical interpretation

The ST segment depression in leads V_2–V_4 is upward-sloping, so does not allow a confident diagnosis of ischaemia. The ST segment elevation in leads II, III and VF is suggestive of an acute inferior myocardial infarction. In this case, the ST segment elevation cleared immediately on resting – elevation like this is an occasional manifestation of ischaemia rather than infarction.

What to do

The patient's angina can be treated medically in the usual way. He needs long-term management with aspirin, and probably a statin and an angiotensin-converting enzyme inhibitor, and risk factors must be addressed. Since the exercise test was positive at a low exercise level, a coronary angiogram is indicated.

See p. 144, 8E ECG ME

See p. 275, 6E ECG IP

Summary ★★

Normal ECG at rest; ST segment elevation on exercise.

ECG 88

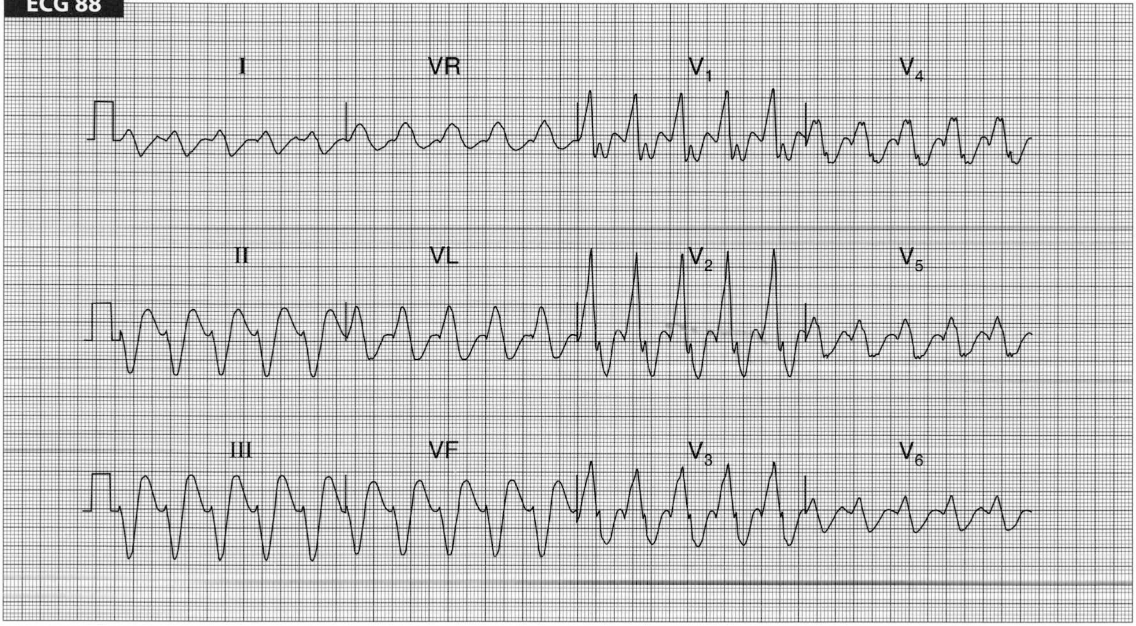

A 60-year-old man, who had been well apart from mild breathlessness on exertion, was admitted to hospital with the sudden onset of pulmonary oedema, and this is his ECG. He had no pain. What is the rhythm, and how would you treat him?

ANSWER 88

The ECG shows:

- Broad complex rhythm at 120/min
- No P waves
- Left axis deviation
- QRS complex duration 200 ms
- QRS complexes show a right bundle branch block (RBBB) configuration
- QRS complexes in the anterior leads are not concordant

Clinical interpretation

The very broad QRS complexes and left axis deviation suggest that this is a ventricular tachycardia. However, the lack of concordance (i.e. the QRS complexes in leads V_1–V_3 are upright, while those in leads V_5–V_6 are predominantly downward) and the RBBB pattern, with the secondary R wave peak taller than the primary peak, suggest that this could be a supraventricular rhythm with bundle branch block. Comparison with the patient's ECG when in sinus rhythm is the only way of being certain what the rhythm is.

What to do

If the patient has pulmonary oedema, preparations for DC cardioversion should be made immediately. While waiting for this he should be treated with diamorphine, intravenous diuretics and lidocaine or intravenous amiodarone. The ECG following cardioversion is shown in the next example (ECG 89).

Summary ★★★
Broad complex tachycardia of uncertain aetiology.

ECG ME See p. 75, 8E

ECG IP See p. 145, 6E

ECG 89

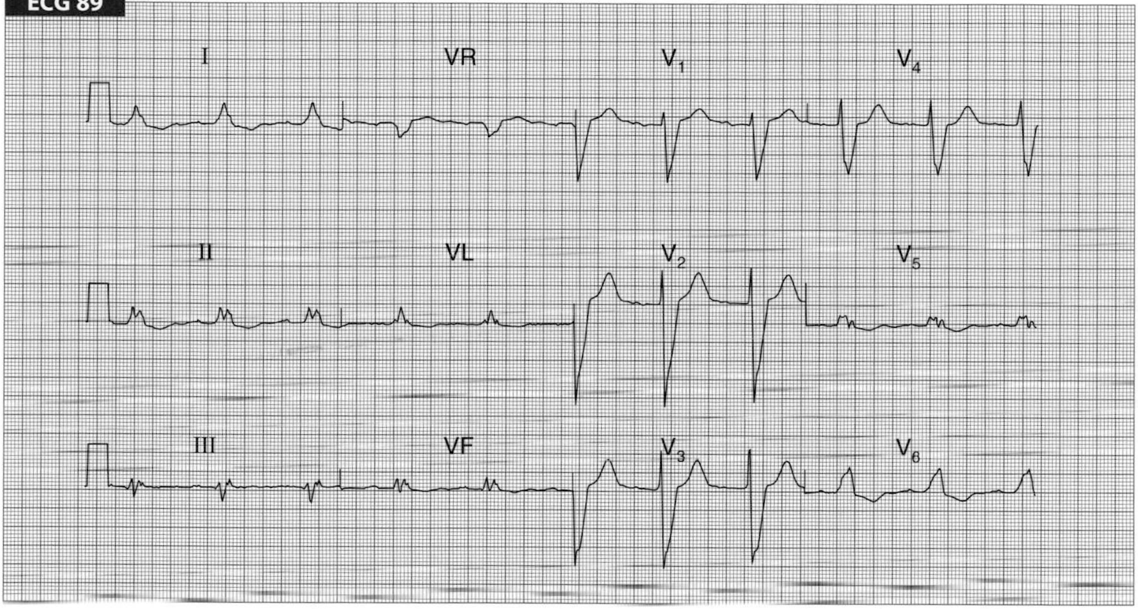

This is another ECG from the 60-year-old man who was admitted to hospital with a broad complex tachycardia (see the previous example – ECG 88). This ECG was recorded after cardioversion, when he was well. His serum troponin level remained normal following admission, so he had not had a myocardial infarction. How would you report on this ECG, and what do you think the underlying disease is?

ANSWER 89

The ECG shows:

- Sinus rhythm, rate 63/min
- First degree block (PR interval 220 ms)
- Normal axis
- Broad QRS complexes (200 ms)
- Left bundle branch block (LBBB)

Clinical interpretation

Comparison with this patient's previous ECG (see ECG 88) shows that when he had the tachycardia there was a change in axis and in QRS complex configuration. The broad complex tachycardia was therefore almost certainly ventricular in origin. He now has evidence of conduction tissue disease, with first degree block and LBBB. Since chest pain has not been a feature of his illness, it seems likely that he has a dilated cardiomyopathy.

What to do

If after treatment with an angiotensin-converting enzyme inhibitor and amiodarone the patient has another episode of ventricular tachycardia, an implanted defibrillator may be needed.

Summary ★★

First degree block and LBBB.

ECG ME See p. 43, 8E

ECG IP See p. 179, 6E

ECG 90

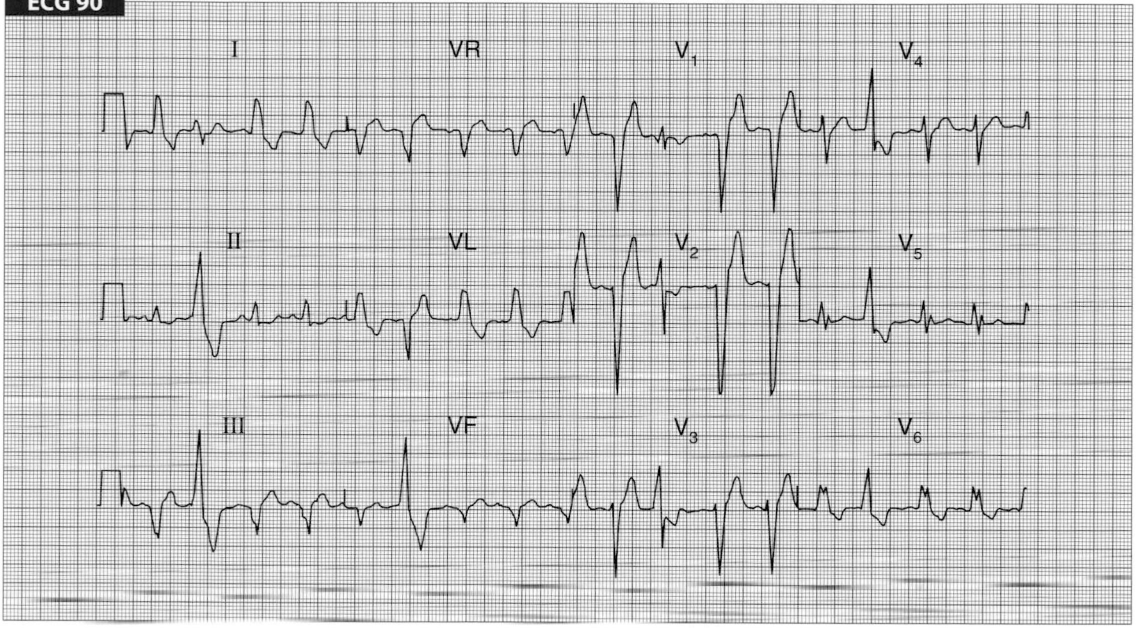

This ECG was recorded from a 50-year-old man admitted to hospital following 2 h of central chest pain that was characteristic of a myocardial infarction. His ECG had been normal 6 months ago. What does this record show and what would you do?

ANSWER 90

The ECG shows:

- Sinus rhythm, rate about 107/min
- Ventricular extrasystoles
- Normal axis
- Wide QRS complexes, with 'M' pattern in lead V_6, and inverted T waves in leads I, VL, V_5–V_6 – indicating left bundle branch block (LBBB) in the sinus beats

Clinical interpretation

The ventricular extrasystoles can be identified because they have a different morphology from the LBBB pattern, and because they have no preceding P waves. LBBB masks any changes there might be as the result of a myocardial infarction.

What to do

The LBBB has evidently developed in the last 6 months, and the history suggests a myocardial infarction. Provided there are no contraindications, percutaneous coronary intervention (PCI) or a thrombolytic agent is indicated. The ventricular extrasystoles should not be treated.

Summary ★★★

Sinus rhythm with LBBB and ventricular extrasystoles.

ECG ME See p. 43, 64, 8E

ECG IP See p. 235, 6E

ECG 91

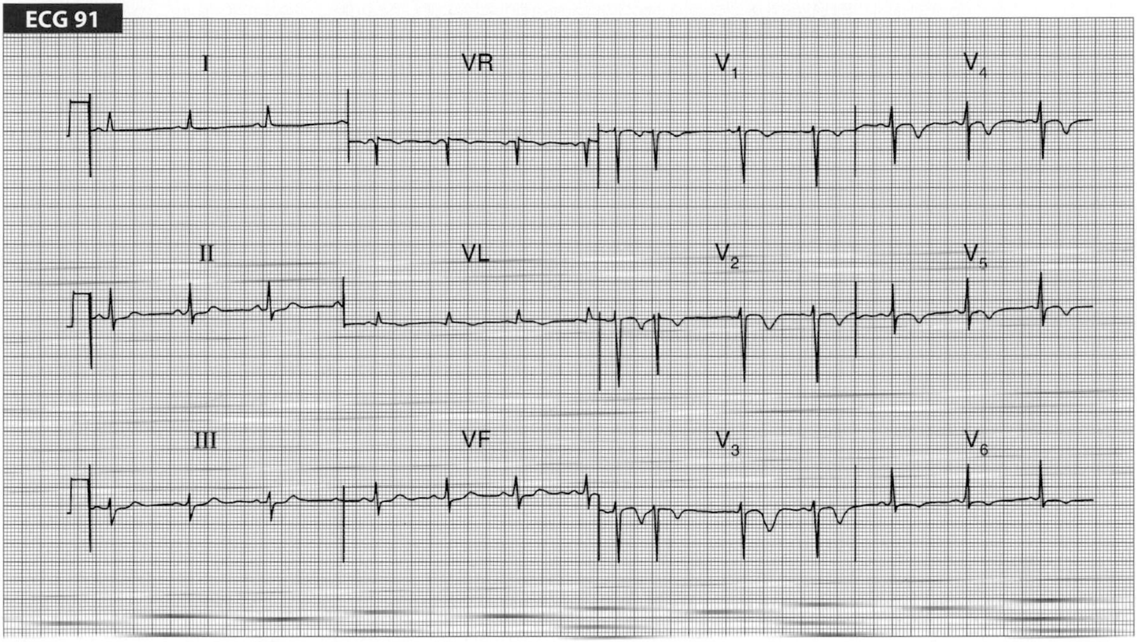

A 50-year-old man was admitted to hospital as an emergency, having had central chest pain for 1 h. By the time he was seen in the A & E department he was pain-free and there were no abnormalities on examination. This is his ECG. What does it show, and what would you do?

ANSWER 91

The ECG shows:

- Sinus rhythm, average rate 75/min, with one supraventricular extrasystole; there appears to be an abnormal P wave in lead V_1, so the extrasystole is atrial in origin
- Normal axis
- Normal QRS complexes
- Inverted T waves in leads VL, V_1–V_6

Clinical interpretation

There are many causes of inverted T waves, and ECGs should always be interpreted as part of the overall clinical picture. In this case the history suggests a myocardial infarction, and the ECG is characteristic of an acute anterior non-ST segment elevation myocardial infarction (NSTEMI).

What to do

The immediate risk is low and there is no evidence for the likelihood of benefit from thrombolysis. Although the patient is now asymptomatic he should remain in hospital for observation and the plasma troponin level should be checked 12 h after the onset of pain. The risk of reinfarction in the next 3 months is relatively high compared with the risk following an ST segment elevation myocardial infarction, and coronary angiography is needed.

Summary ★
Anterolateral NSTEMI.

ECG ME See p. 129, 8E

ECG IP See p. 241, 6E

ECG 92

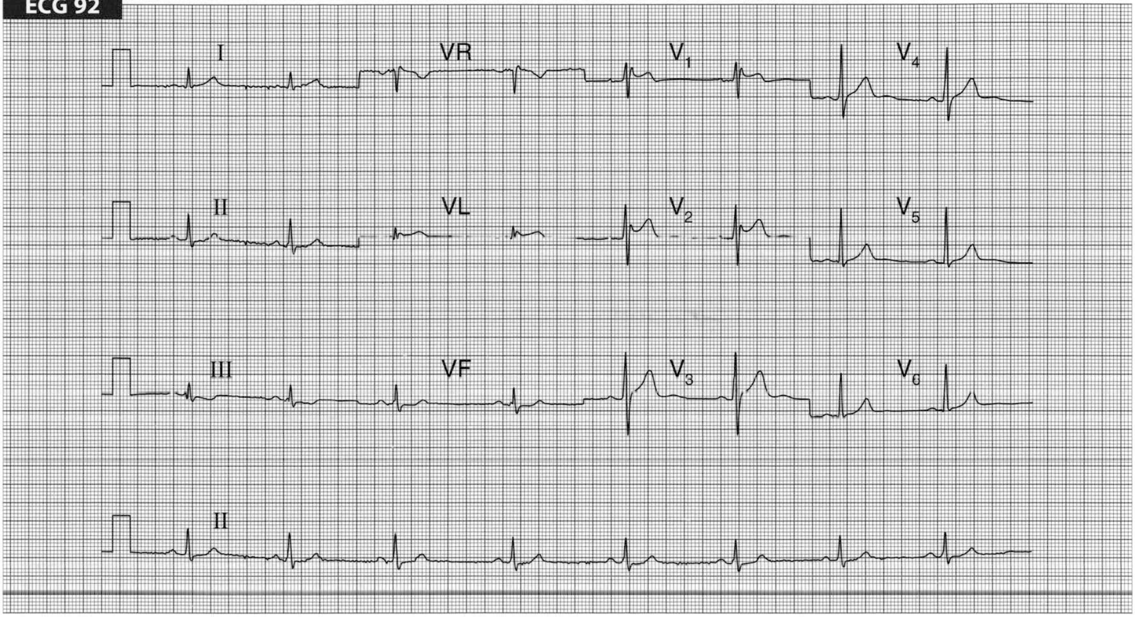

This ECG was recorded as part of the routine preoperative assessment of a 65-year-old man who had no cardiovascular symptoms, and whose heart was clinically normal. What does it show? Is any action necessary?

ANSWER 92

The ECG shows:

- Sinus rhythm, rate 50/min
- Normal axis
- QRS complex duration 110 ms, with an RSR^{1} pattern in leads V_1 and V_2 – partial right bundle branch block (RBBB)

Clinical interpretation

The QRS complex duration is at the upper limit of normal, so this is partial rather than complete RBBB. It is seldom of any clinical significance.

What to do

In the absence of symptoms or abnormal signs, no action is necessary.

Summary ★
Partial RBBB.

ECG ME See p. 44, 8E

ECG IP See p. 25, 6E

ECG 93

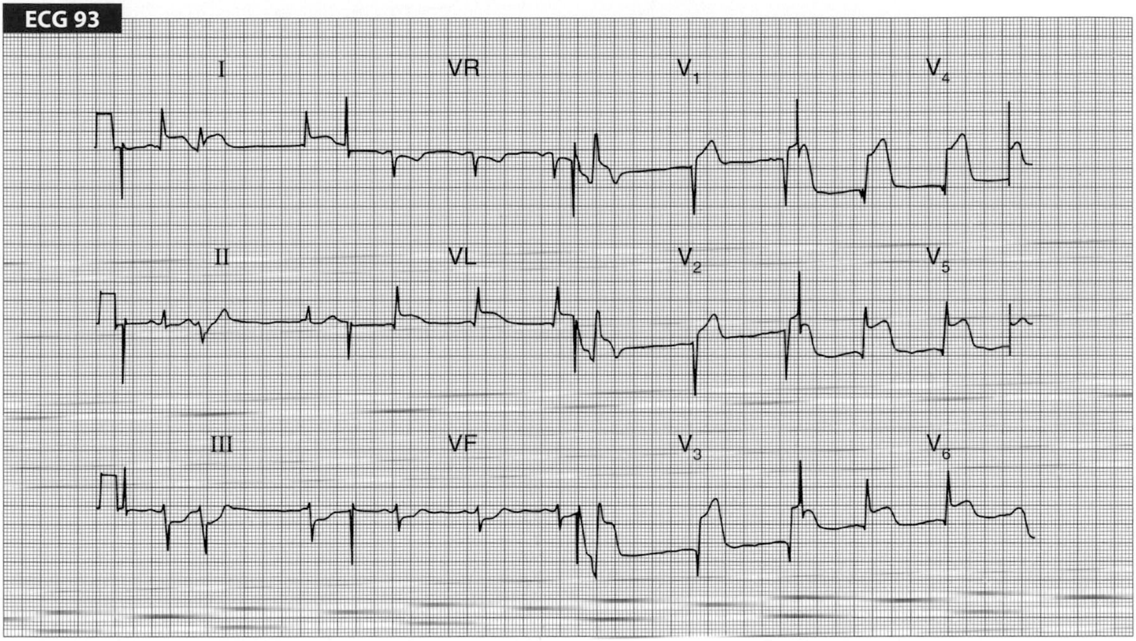

This ECG was recorded from a 50-year-old man who had had severe chest pain for 1 h. What does it show and what would you do?

ANSWER 93

The ECG shows:

- Sinus rhythm, rate 70/min, with ventricular extrasystoles
- Normal axis
- Q waves in leads V_3–V_5; small Q waves in leads VL and V_6
- Raised ST segments in leads I, VL, V_3–V_6
- Depressed ST segments in leads III, VF

Clinical interpretation

Ventricular extrasystoles associated with an acute anterolateral ST segment elevation myocardial infarction (STEMI).

What to do

The patient should be given diamorphine and aspirin immediately, and percutaneous coronary intervention (PCI) or thrombolysis as soon as possible. The extrasystoles should not be treated.

Summary ★

Acute anterolateral STEMI with ventricular extrasystoles.

ECG ME See p. 91, 8E

ECG IP See p. 217, 6E

ECG 94

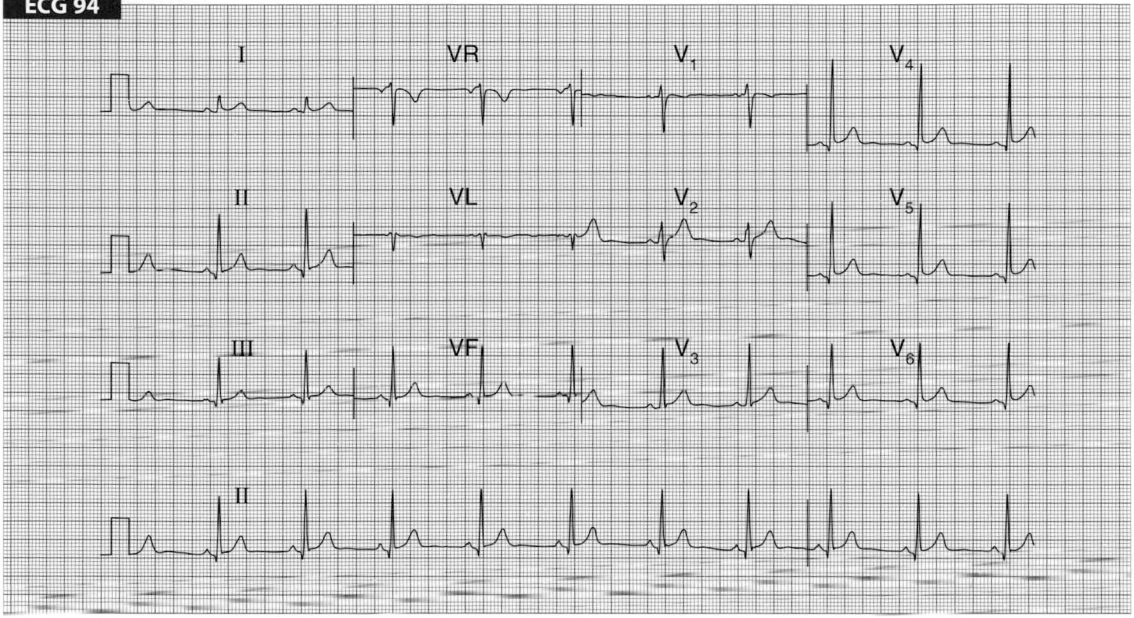

This ECG was recorded from a 30-year-old man who complained of chest pain: the pain did not appear to be cardiac in origin, and the physical examination was normal. Can this man be allowed to hold a commercial driving licence?

ANSWER 94

The ECG shows:

- Sinus rhythm, rate 62/min
- Normal axis
- Small Q waves, especially prominent in leads II, III, VF, V_4–V_6
- Otherwise normal QRS complexes, ST segments and T waves

Clinical interpretation

These Q waves are quite deep but only 40 ms in duration, and they are most prominent in the lateral leads. They represent septal depolarization, not an old lateral infarction.

What to do

The ECG is normal, and if the man has no other evidence of heart disease he can hold a commercial driving licence. If in doubt, an exercise test should be performed.

Summary ★
Normal ECG.

ECG ME See p. 17, 8E

ECG IP See p. 29, 6E

ECG 95

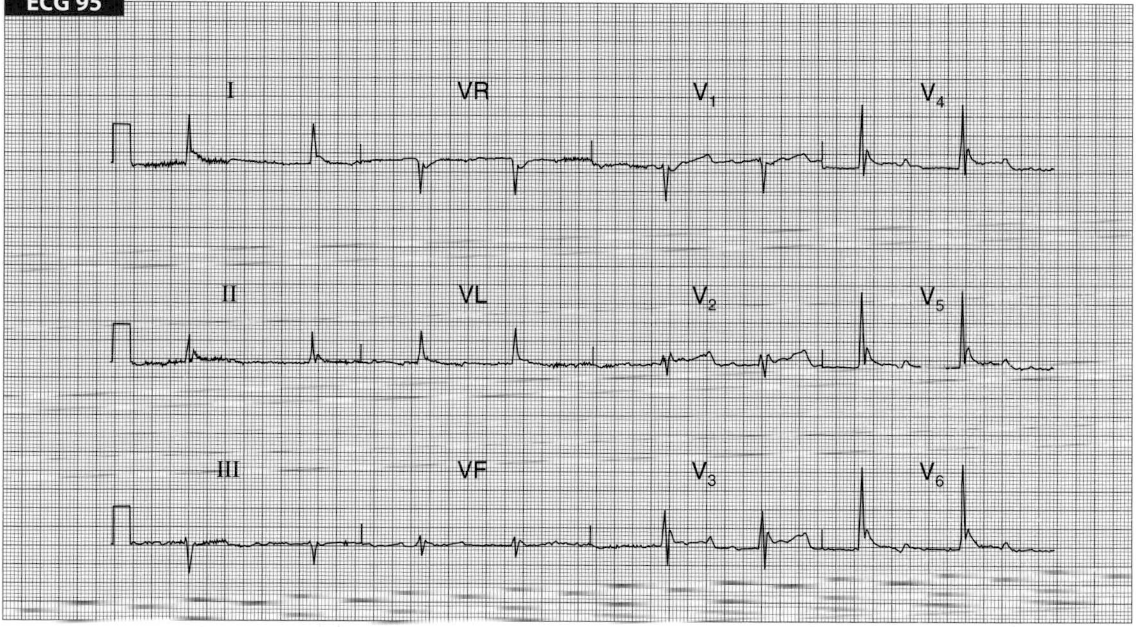

This ECG was recorded from an 80-year-old woman who had been found unconscious with physical signs suggesting a stroke. Any comments?

ANSWER 95

The ECG shows:

- Atrial fibrillation with a ventricular rate of about 55/min
- QRS complex duration prolonged at 200 ms
- Prominent 'J' waves, best seen in leads V_3–V_6
- Widespread but nonspecific ST segment/T wave changes

Clinical interpretation

The atrial fibrillation may or may not be related to her stroke – she may have had a cerebral embolus, or she may have both coronary and cerebrovascular disease. The slow ventricular rate and the 'J' waves indicate hypothermia, and her core temperature was 25°C. ECGs from hypothermic patients seldom show 'J' waves as clearly as this because there are too many artefacts due to shivering – but this patient was too cold to shiver. She did not survive.

Summary ★★★

Atrial fibrillation and hypothermia.

ECG IP See p.317, 6E

ECG 96

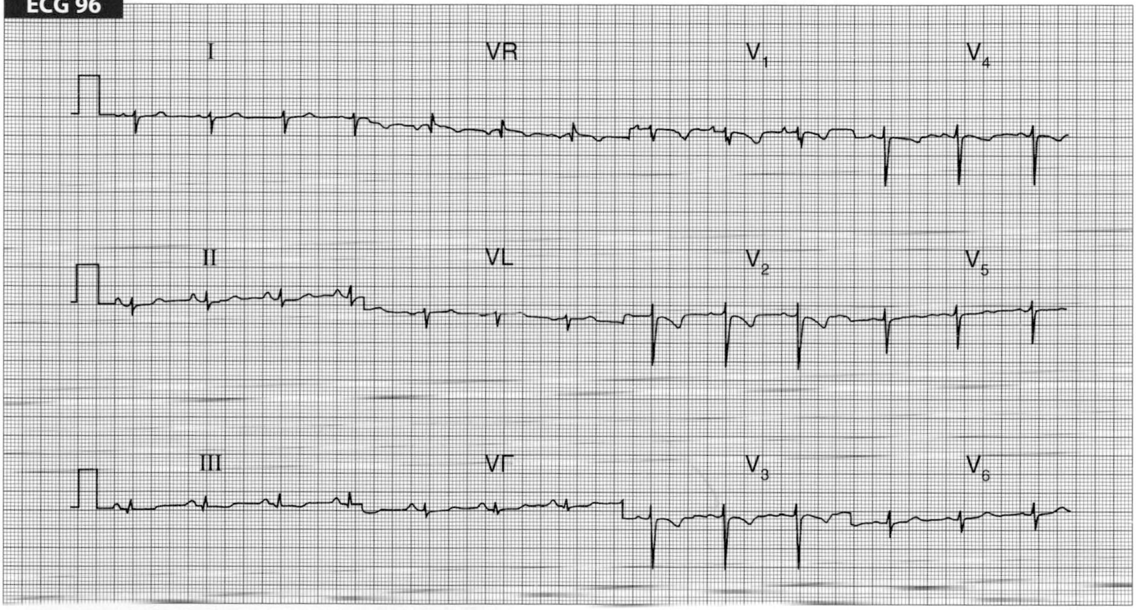

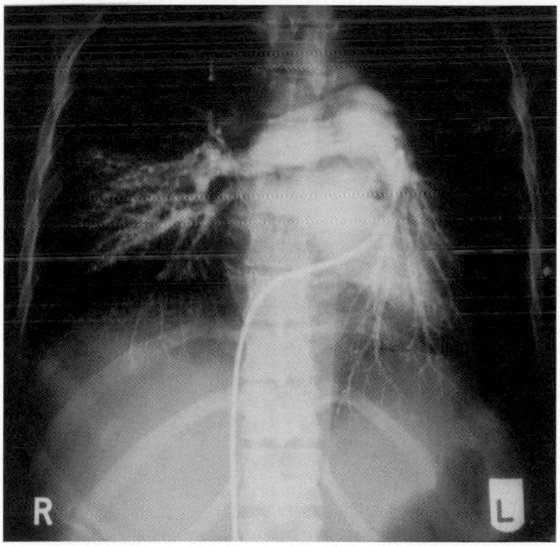

A 32-year-old woman, who had had a normal pregnancy and delivery 3 months previously, was seen in the outpatient department complaining of severe breathlessness and dizziness on exertion. She had some chest pain on both sides, which sounded pleuritic. Does her ECG help with her diagnosis and treatment?

A pulmonary angiogram was performed as part of a series of investigations.

ANSWER 96

The ECG shows:

- Sinus rhythm, rate 79/min
- Right axis deviation
- Normal QRS complexes, except for an RSR^1 pattern in lead V_1 and deep S waves in lead V_6
- Inverted T waves in leads V_1–V_4

The pulmonary angiogram shows clots within the main pulmonary arteries. The right mid-zone is perfused, but the rest of the lung fields have poor or no perfusion due to multiple pulmonary emboli.

Clinical interpretation

The right axis deviation, the deep S waves in lead V_6 ('clockwise rotation') and the inverted T waves in the chest leads are all characteristic of marked right ventricular hypertrophy: the only missing feature is the absence of dominant R waves in lead V_1. Note how the T wave inversion is at a maximum in lead V_1 and becomes progressively less marked from lead V_2 to V_4.

What to do

In the context of a delivery 3 months previously, this ECG pattern of right ventricular hypertrophy almost certainly indicates multiple pulmonary emboli causing pulmonary hypertension. The pulmonary angiogram confirms this diagnosis. Anticoagulants, and possibly thrombolysis, are needed urgently.

Summary ★★

Right ventricular hypertrophy due to pulmonary embolism.

ECG ME See p. 89, 8E

ECG IP See p. 305, 6E

ECG 97

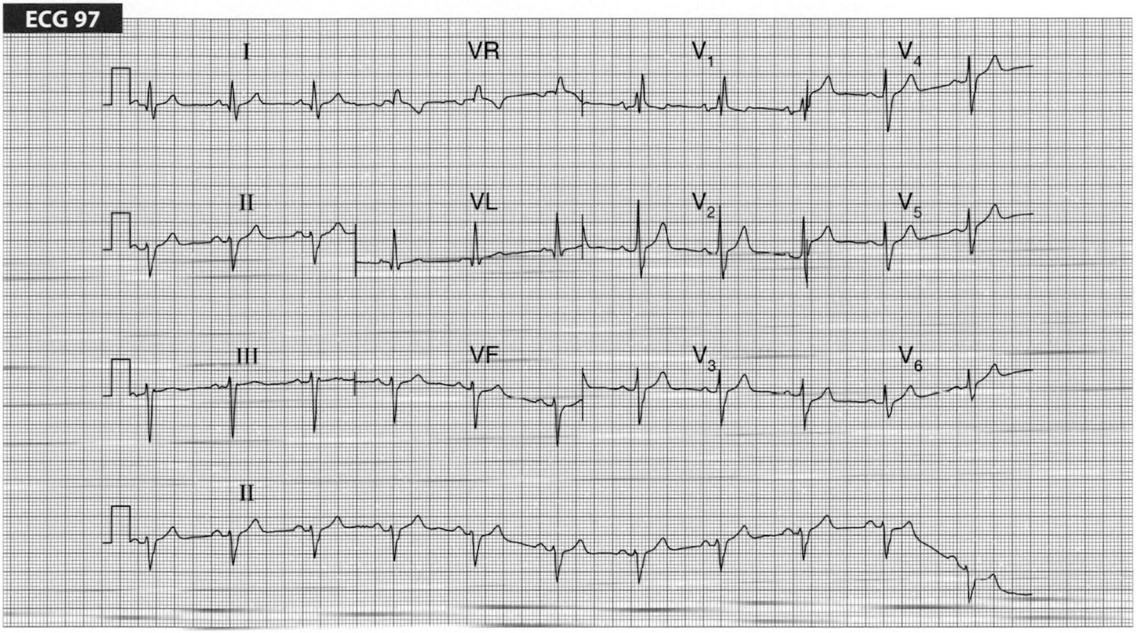

This ECG was recorded from a fit 60-year-old man at a routine medical examination. What does it show and what would you recommend?

ANSWER 97

The ECG shows:

- Sinus rhythm, rate 65/min
- Normal PR interval
- Left axis deviation – left anterior hemiblock
- QRS complex duration just over 120 ms, with an RSR^1 complex in lead V_1 – right bundle branch block (RBBB)

Clinical interpretation

The combination of left anterior hemiblock and RBBB is called bifascicular block. Atrioventricular conduction occurs via the posterior fascicle of the left bundle branch.

What to do

Progression to complete block can occur but is relatively rare. In the absence of symptoms, standard UK practice would be not to insert a permanent pacemaker; however, any symptoms suggestive of a bradycardia should be investigated immediately.

Summary ★★

Left axis deviation and RBBB – bifascicular block.

ECG ME See p. 51, 8E

ECG IP See p. 89, 6E

ECG 98

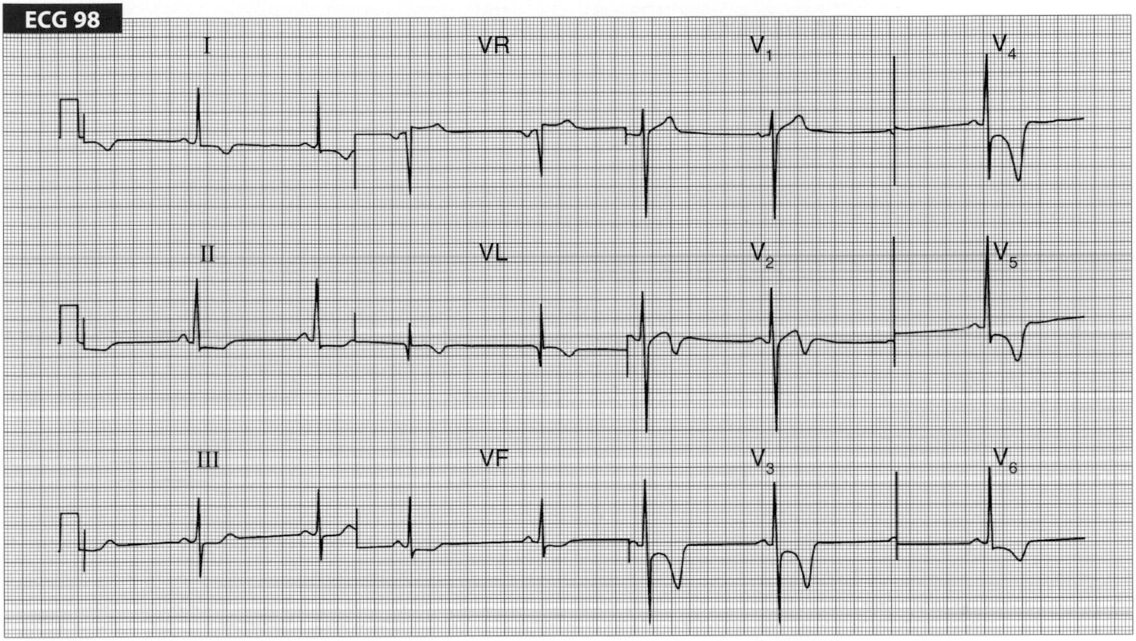

This ECG was recorded as part of a routine examination of a healthy 25-year-old professional athlete. There were no abnormal physical findings. What does it show and what would you do?

ANSWER 98

The ECG shows:

- Sinus rhythm, average rate 44/min
- Normal axis
- Normal QRS complexes, apart from narrow Q waves in lead VL
- Marked T wave inversion in leads I, VL, V_2–V_6

Clinical interpretation

If this ECG had been recorded from a middle-aged man presenting with acute chest pain, the diagnosis would be an anterior non-ST segment elevation myocardial infarction. The ECGs of athletes can show ST segment and T wave changes due to left ventricular hypertrophy, but anteroseptal T wave inversion of this degree in a healthy young man almost certainly represents hypertrophic cardiomyopathy.

What to do

Echocardiography will confirm the diagnosis. Ambulatory ECG recording will show whether the patient is having ventricular arrhythmias. He must not play competitive sports, and his close relatives should be screened.

Summary ★★★
Probable hypertrophic cardiomyopathy.

ECG ME See p. 152, 8E

ECG IP See p. 68, 6E

ECG 99

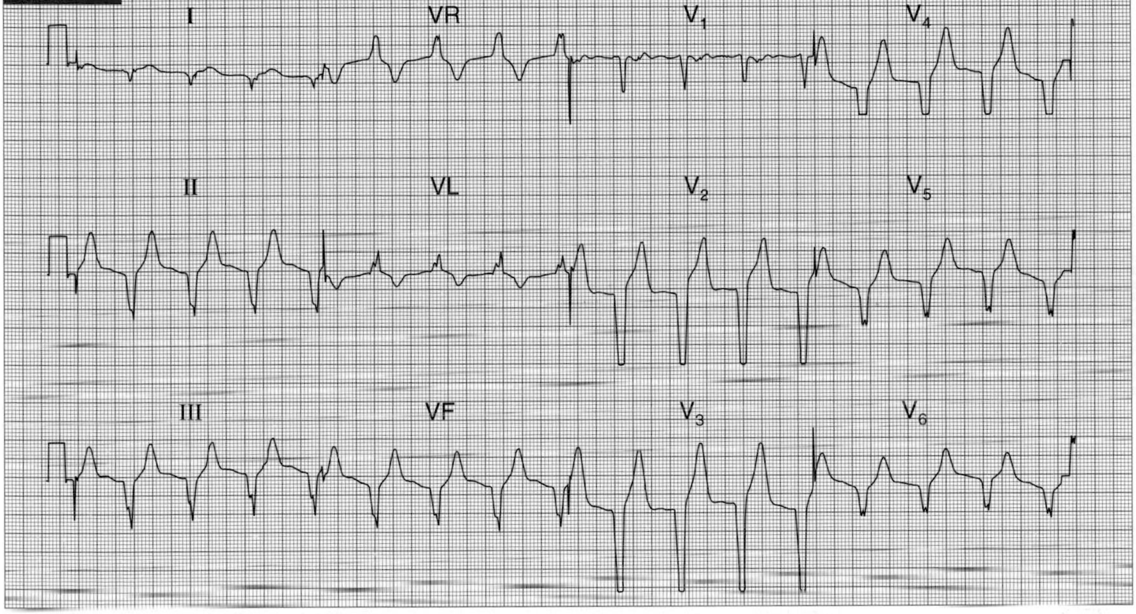

This ECG was recorded from a 45-year-old man, who had been admitted to a coronary care unit with a myocardial infarction and who was recovering well. What is the rhythm, and what would you do?

ANSWER 99

The ECG shows:

- Broad complex rhythm, rate 90/min
- No P waves
- Marked left axis deviation
- QRS complex duration 160 ms
- All chest leads show a downward QRS complex (concordance)

Clinical interpretation

If the heart rate were fast there would be little difficulty in recognizing this as ventricular tachycardia, and this rhythm used to be called 'slow VT'. It is, however, an accelerated idioventricular rhythm.

What to do

This rhythm is quite commonly seen in patients with an acute myocardial infarction, and indeed is not uncommon in ambulatory ECG records from normal people. It never causes problems, and it is important not to attempt to treat it: suppressing any 'escape' rhythm may lead to a dangerous bradycardia.

Summary ★★★

Accelerated idioventricular rhythm.

ECG ME See p. 60, 8E

ECG IP See p. 29, 6E

ECG 100

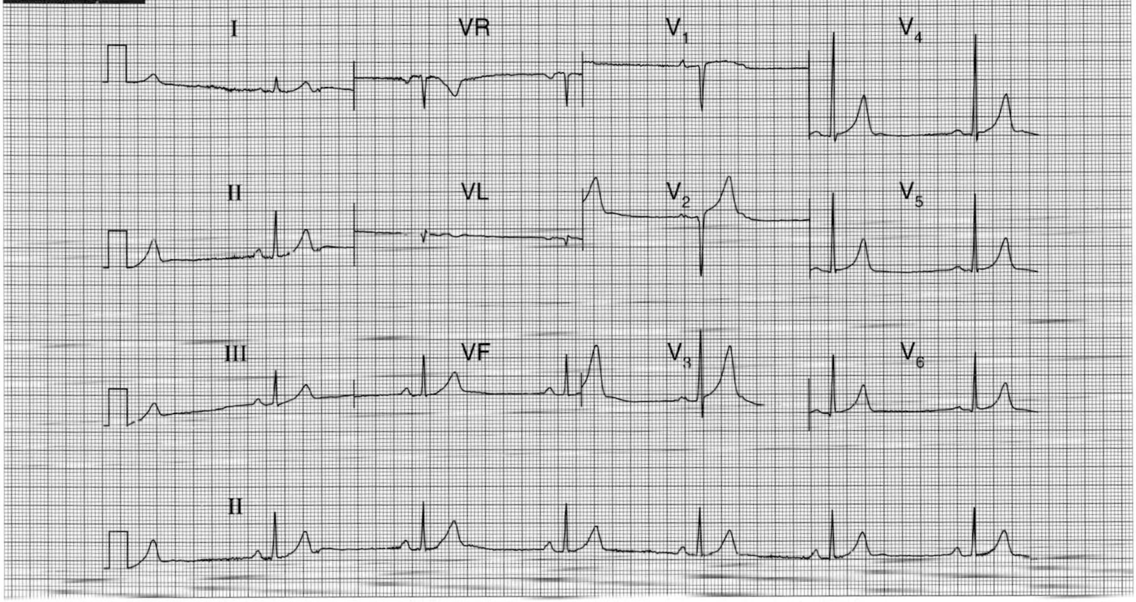

This ECG was recorded from a 40-year-old man who had hypertension but was otherwise well and ran marathons. Despite showing four possible 'abnormalities', is the trace actually normal?

ANSWER 100

The ECG shows:

- Sinus rhythm, average rate 39/min
- Bifid P waves, best seen in the anterior chest leads
- Normal axis
- QRS complexes show left ventricular hypertrophy on voltage criteria (R wave in lead V_4 = 2.5 mm)
- Peaked T waves

Clinical interpretation

Sinus bradycardia can be due to physical fitness, vagal overactivity or myxoedema. In a hypertensive patient, beta-blocker treatment is a possible explanation. The bifid P waves may indicate left atrial hypertrophy ('P mitrale'), but can be normal. Voltage criteria for left ventricular hypertrophy are extremely unreliable when there is no other evidence of this. The peaked T waves could be due to hyperkalaemia but are more often a normal variant.

What to do

All these possible abnormalities are seen in normal athletes, and the likelihood is that they are of no significance. In a patient with hypertension, beta-blocker treatment could be the cause of the bradycardia.

Summary ★★

Normal ECG for an athlete.

ECG ME See p. 125, 8E

ECG IP See p. 48, 6E

ECG 101

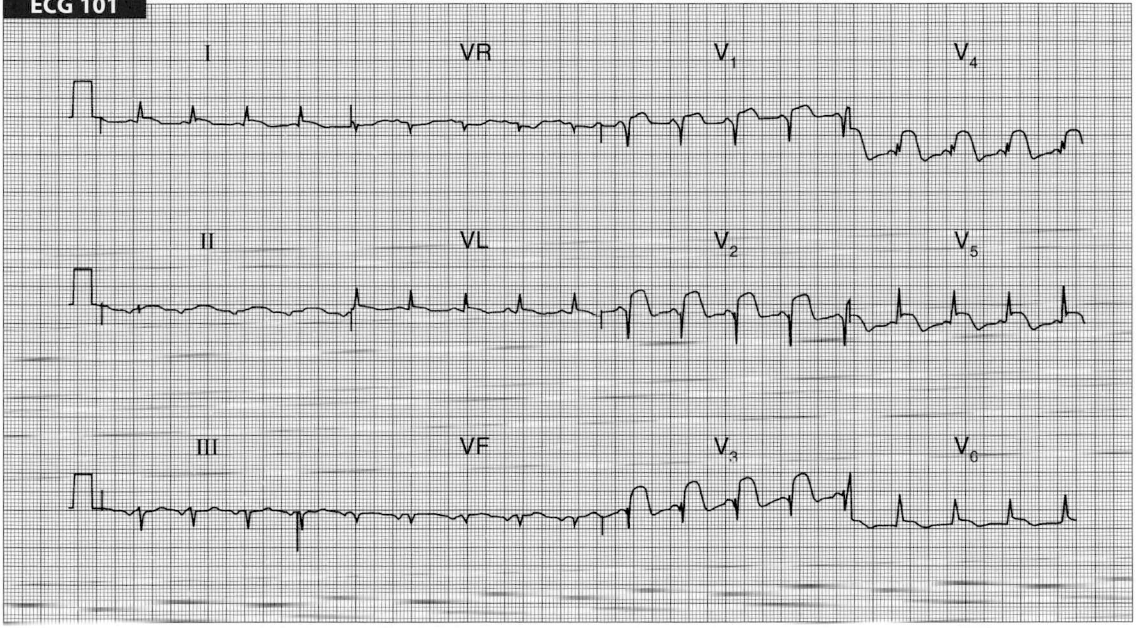

A 48-year-old man is seen in the A & E department with a history of severe chest pain which began 24 h previously, but has now cleared. He is now breathless. What does this ECG show and what treatment is needed?

ANSWER 101

The ECG shows:

- Sinus rhythm, rate 103/min
- Normal axis
- Normal QRS complexes
- Raised ST segments in leads I, VL, V_1–V_6

Clinical interpretation

The ECG has the classic appearance of an acute anterolateral ST segment elevation myocardial infarction (STEMI).

What to do

Since this patient's chest pain began more than 24 h ago, immediate percutaneous coronary intervention (PCI) or thrombolysis is not indicated. The breathlessness suggests that he may have developed left ventricular failure, and he must be admitted to hospital and treated with diuretics and if necessary intravenous nitrates to induce vasodilation. The patient will need long-term treatment with an angiotensin-converting enzyme inhibitor: the best time to begin treatment is a matter for debate but it should be within 2 or 3 days of the onset of the infarction. He will also need long-term treatment with aspirin, as a prophylactic against further infarction.

Summary ★
Acute anterolateral STEMI.

ECG ME See p. 91, 8E

ECG IP See p. 217, 6E

ECG 102

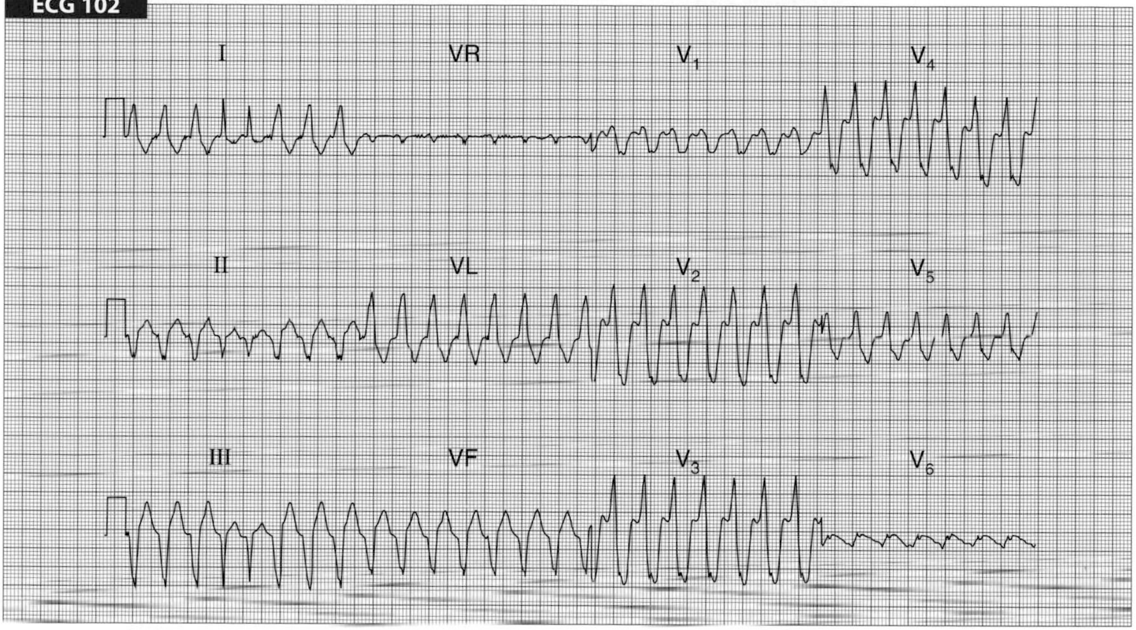

A 70-year-old woman, admitted to hospital because of increasing heart failure of uncertain cause, collapsed and was found to have a very rapid pulse and a low blood pressure. This is her ECG. She recovered spontaneously. What is this rhythm, and what would you do?

ANSWER 102

The ECG shows:

- Broad complex tachycardia at about 188/min
- No P waves visible
- Left axis deviation
- QRS complex duration about 140 ms
- Narrow fourth and fifth QRS complexes
- QRS complexes that are probably concordant (in the chest leads all point upwards) though it is difficult to be certain

Clinical interpretation

Broad complex tachycardias may be ventricular, supraventricular with bundle branch block, or due to the Wolff–Parkinson–White syndrome. We have no ECG from this patient recorded in sinus rhythm, which is always the most helpful thing in deciding between these possibilities. The complexes are not very wide, which would be consistent with a supraventricular origin with aberrant conduction, but the left axis deviation and (probable) concordance point to ventricular tachycardia. The key is the two narrow complexes near the beginning of the record: these are slightly early and are probably capture beats. They indicate that with an early supraventricular beat the conducting system can function normally; by implication, the broad complexes must be due to ventricular tachycardia.

What to do

An elderly patient with heart failure is more likely to have ischaemic disease than anything else, but all the possible causes of heart failure must be considered. The sudden onset of an arrhythmia could be due to a myocardial infarction. Pulmonary emboli can cause sudden arrhythmias, though these are more often supraventricular than ventricular. It is important to consider whether this rhythm change is related to treatment, in which case it could be due to an electrolyte imbalance or to the pro-arrhythmic effect of a drug the patient is taking.

Summary ★★★

Ventricular tachycardia.

ECG ME See p. 73, 8E

ECG IP See p. 142, 6E

ECG 103

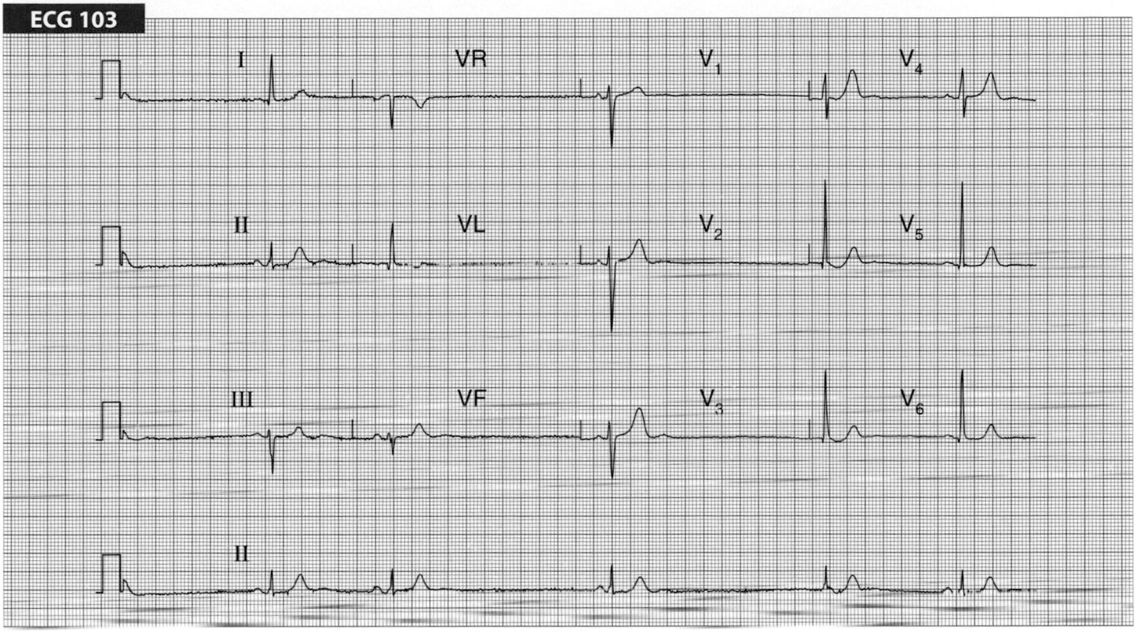

This is the ECG from a 25-year-old man who complained of episodes of fast, regular, palpitations associated with breathlessness and dizziness. There were no abnormalities on examination other than a slow and irregular pulse. What is the diagnosis and how can his problem be treated?

ANSWER 103

The ECG shows:

- Variable QRS complex rate, average 31/min
- Normal P waves in the first three beats; in the fourth beat the P wave immediately follows the QRS complex
- Normal QRS complexes and T waves

Clinical interpretation

This is the 'sick sinus syndrome' or 'sinoatrial disease'. The record shows sinus rhythm with a junctional escape beat, in which the atrium is activated retrogradely. The palpitations described by the patient are probably due to a paroxysmal supraventricular tachycardia, so he probably has the 'bradycardia–tachycardia' variant of sinoatrial disease.

What to do

Ambulatory ECG recording will confirm the cause of the patient's palpitations. Even though his bradycardia is asymptomatic, he will need a permanent pacemaker because antiarrhythmic agents given for the tachycardia may make his bradycardia worse.

Summary ★★★

Sinoatrial disease with sinus rhythm and a junctional escape beat.

ECG ME See p. 160, 8E

ECG IP See p. 171, 6E

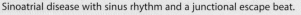

ECG 104

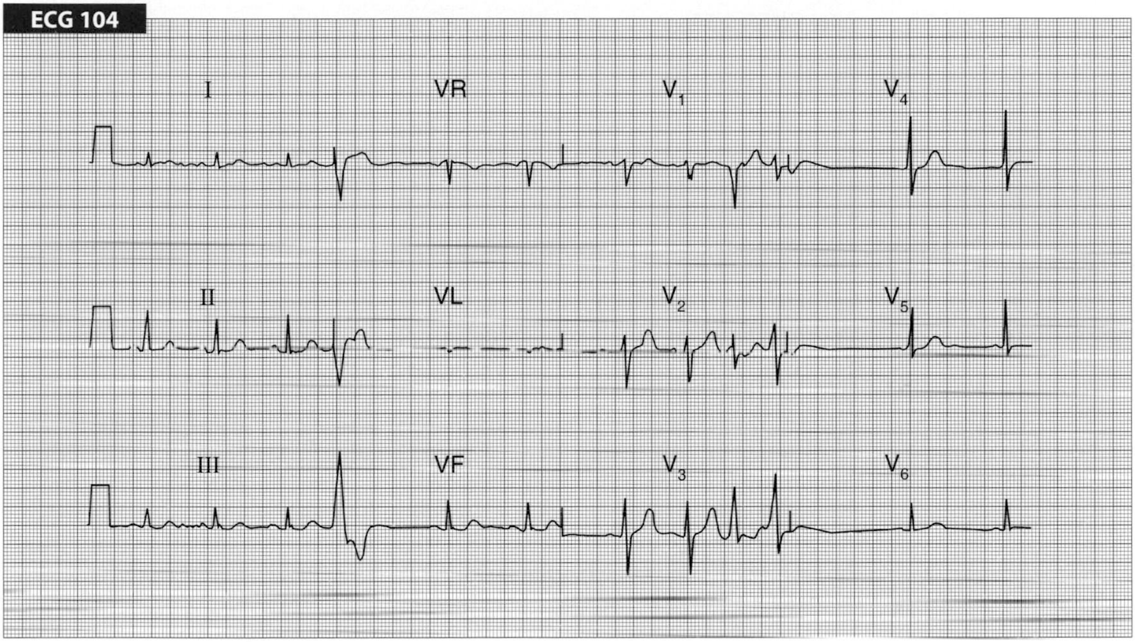

This ECG was recorded from an 80-year-old man during a routine preoperative assessment. What does it show? What are the implications for surgery?

ANSWER 104

The ECG shows:

- Sinus rhythm, rate about 77/min, with ventricular extrasystoles
- Ventricular extrasystoles are of two types, seen best in lead V_3
- Normal axis
- Normal QRS complexes in the sinus beats
- ST segments and T waves are normal in the sinus beats

Clinical interpretation

Sinus rhythm, with multifocal ventricular extrasystoles but otherwise normal.

What to do

In large groups of patients, ventricular extrasystoles are correlated with heart disease of all types. In individuals, however, extrasystoles may well occur in a perfectly normal heart – indeed, virtually everyone has extrasystoles at times. Ventricular extrasystoles become more common with increasing age, and this patient is 80 years old. In the absence of symptoms or clinical signs suggesting cardiovascular disease, the extrasystoles do not have any great significance and should not materially affect the patient's fitness for surgery. They should not be treated.

Summary ★
Sinus rhythm with multifocal ventricular extrasystoles.

ECG ME See p. 64, 8E

ECG IP See p. 56, 6E

ECG 105

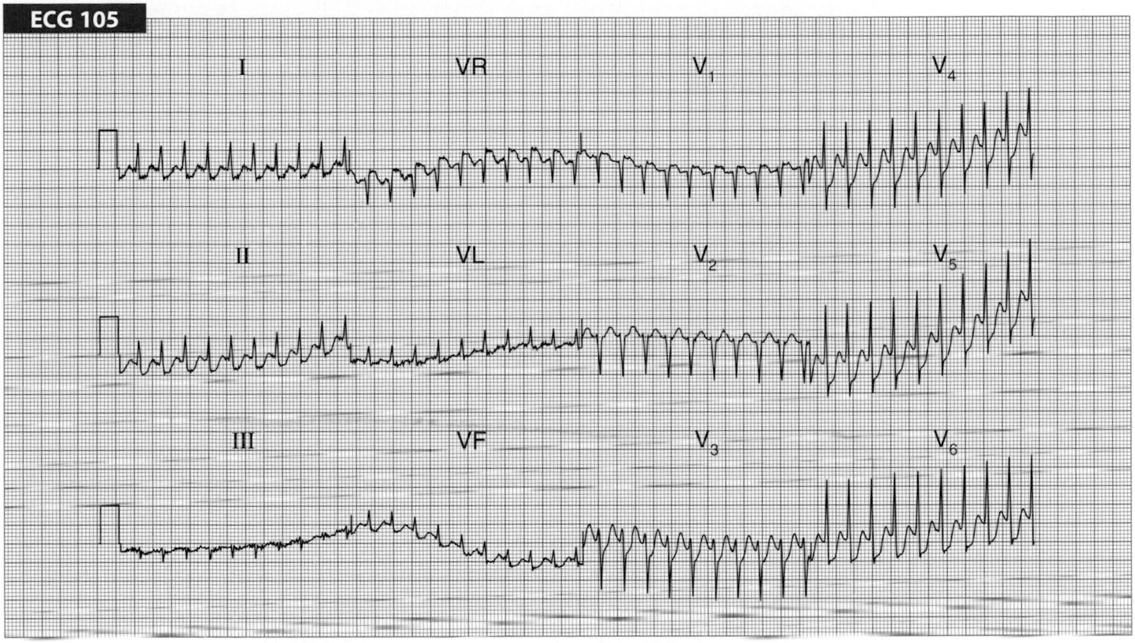

A 50-year-old man was admitted to hospital as an emergency with chest pain; he was not aware of a rapid heart rate. He had had several episodes of pain that appeared to be due to ischaemia, but they had no clear relationship with exertion. Shortly after this ECG was recorded, his heart rate suddenly slowed and his ECG was then normal. What does this record show, and what would you do?

ANSWER 105

The ECG shows:

- Narrow complex tachycardia, rate about 230/min
- No P waves
- Normal axis
- Normal QRS complexes
- Horizontal ST segment depression, most marked in leads V_4–V_6

Clinical interpretation

Narrow complex tachycardia without P waves – atrioventricular nodal re-entry (junctional) tachycardia (AVNRT). Ischaemic ST segment depression, accounting for his pain.

What to do

Not all patients with a paroxysmal tachycardia complain of palpitations; this patient's recurrent chest pain may well have been due to this arrhythmia. He should be taught the methods of inducing vagal activity, but prophylactic drug therapy will be needed: a beta-blocker or verapamil should be tried first. Electrophysiological investigation, with a view to ablating an abnormal pathway, may be needed.

Summary ★
Atrioventricular nodal re-entry (junctional) tachycardia (AVNRT) with ischaemia.

ECG ME See p. 81, 8E

ECG IP See p. 106, 6E

ECG 106

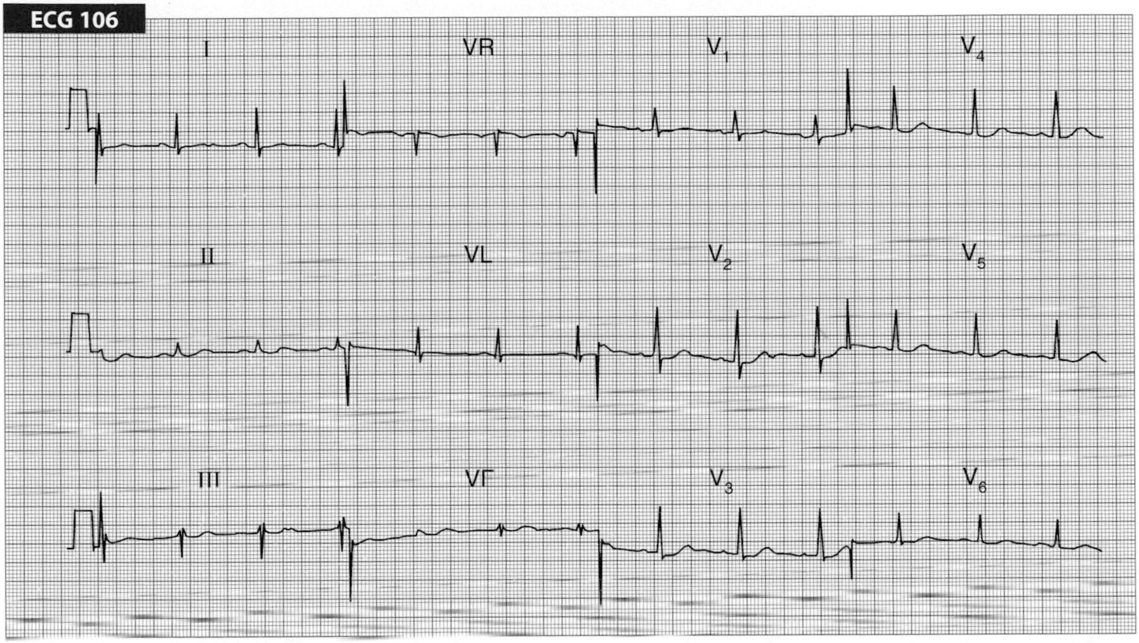

A 40-year-old man is seen in the outpatient department with a history that suggests a myocardial infarction 3 weeks previously. There are no abnormalities on examination, and this is his ECG. There are two possible explanations for the abnormality it shows, though only one of these would explain his history. What is the likely diagnosis?

ANSWER 106

The ECG shows:

- Sinus rhythm, rate 71/min
- Normal axis
- Dominant R waves in lead V_1
- ST segment depression in leads V_2–V_3
- Nonspecific T wave flattening in leads I, VL

Clinical interpretation

The dominant R waves in lead V_1 might indicate right ventricular hypertrophy, but there are none of the other features that would be associated with this – right axis deviation, and T wave inversion in leads V_1, V_2 and possibly V_3. The changes are therefore probably due to a posterior myocardial infarction, which would fit the history of chest pain 3 weeks previously.

What to do

It is important not to miss a diagnosis of pulmonary embolism. The patient should be re-examined to ensure that there is no clinical evidence of right ventricular hypertrophy. A chest X-ray examination should be carried out, and an echocardiogram may be helpful.

Summary ★★

Probable posterior myocardial infarction.

ECG ME See p. 91, 140, 8E

ECG IP See p. 226, 6E

ECG 107

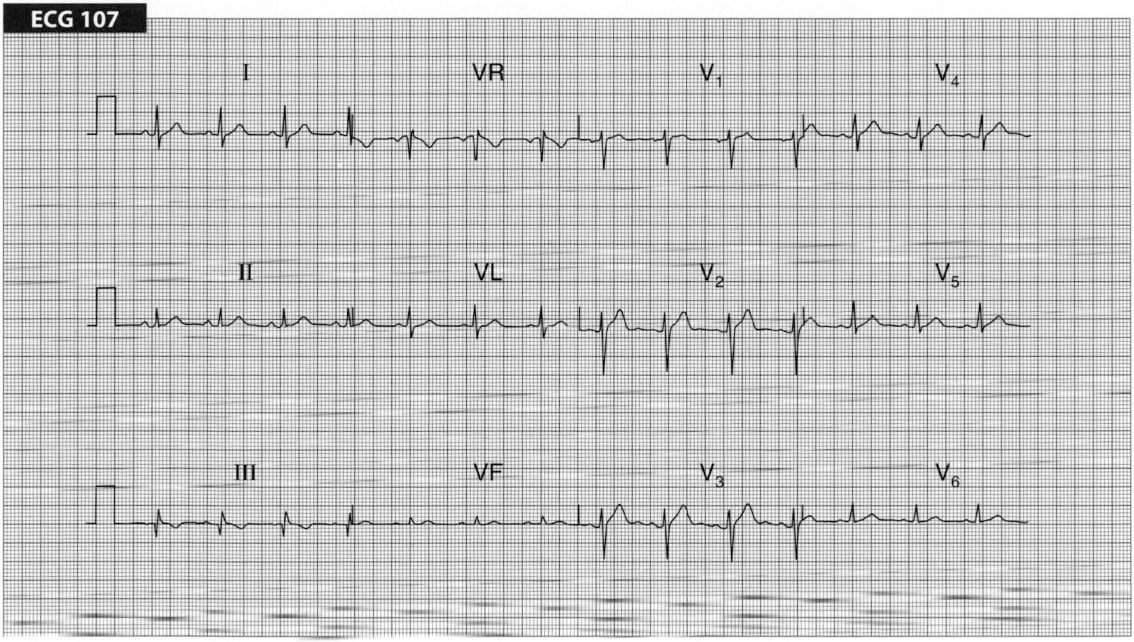

This ECG was recorded from a 60-year-old man with no symptoms, who wanted a private pilot's licence. Is the ECG normal? What would you tell the licensing authority?

ANSWER 107

The ECG shows:

- Sinus rhythm, rate 88/min
- Normal conduction
- Normal axis
- Q wave in lead III but not in lead VF
- Inverted T wave in lead III but not in lead VF
- U waves in leads V_2–V_3 (normal)

Clinical interpretation

A Q wave and/or an inverted T wave in lead III, but not in lead VF, is a normal variant. If lead III is recorded with the patient taking a deep breath in, the changes will often normalize as shown below.

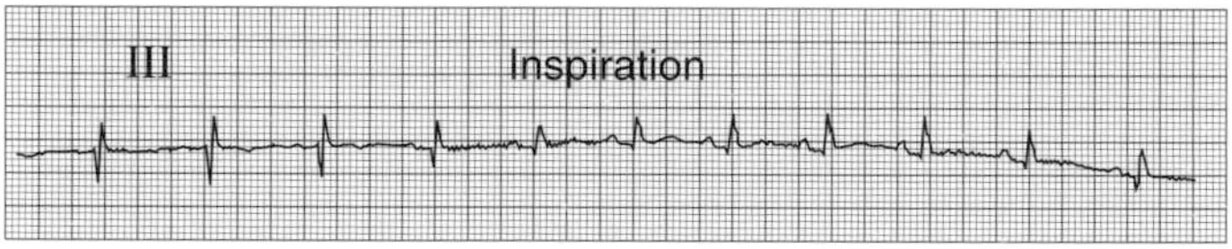

Summary ★★

Normal record with Q waves and inverted T waves in lead III.

ECG ME See p. 120, 8E

ECG IP See p. 39, 6E

ECG 108

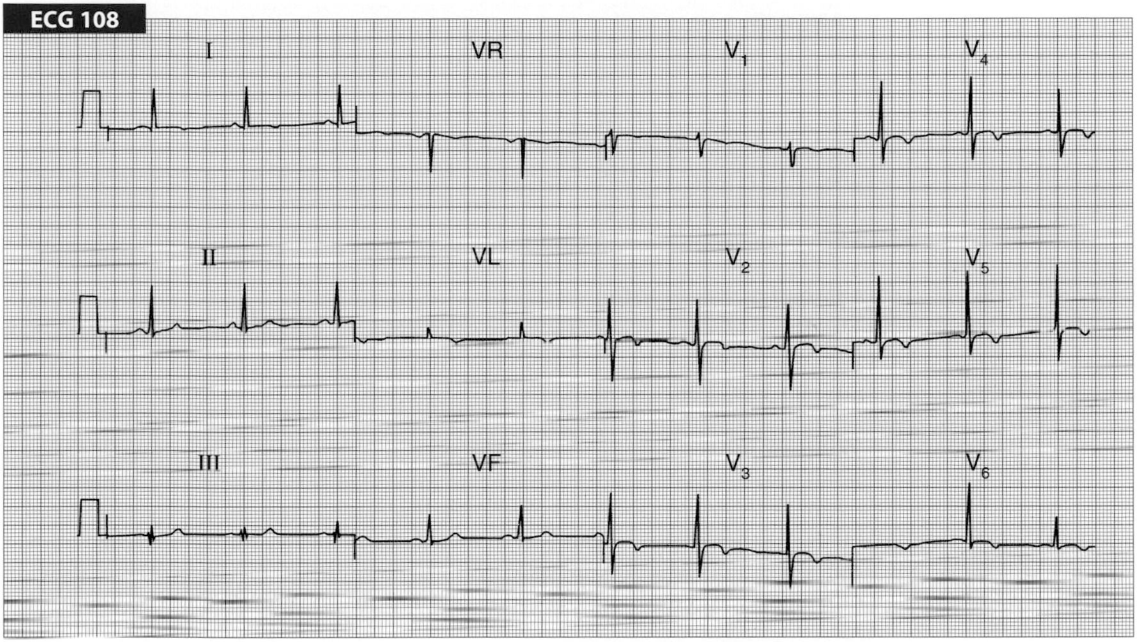

This ECG was recorded from a 55-year-old black woman who had been complaining for several years of chest pain, and was admitted to hospital with persistent pain that was not characteristic of ischaemia. How would you have managed her?

ANSWER 108

The ECG shows:

- Sinus rhythm, rate 60/min
- Normal axis
- Normal QRS complexes; variation in the complexes in lead V_6 is probably due to an artefact
- T wave inversion in leads I, VL, V_2–V_6

Clinical interpretation

With this history, an anterolateral non-ST segment elevation myocardial infarction has to be the first diagnosis, but T wave 'abnormalities' are common in black people, and this ECG could be normal.

What to do

In this patient the diagnosis of an acute infarction was excluded when the plasma troponin levels were found to be normal. An exercise test was performed, but was limited by breathlessness without further ECG change. A coronary angiogram was completely normal. The chest pain was therefore thought to be musculoskeletal in origin, and the T wave changes were presumably due to her ethnicity.

Summary ★★

Widespread T wave 'abnormalities', normal in a black woman.

ECG ME See p. 124, 8E

ECG IP See p. 39, 6E

ECG 109

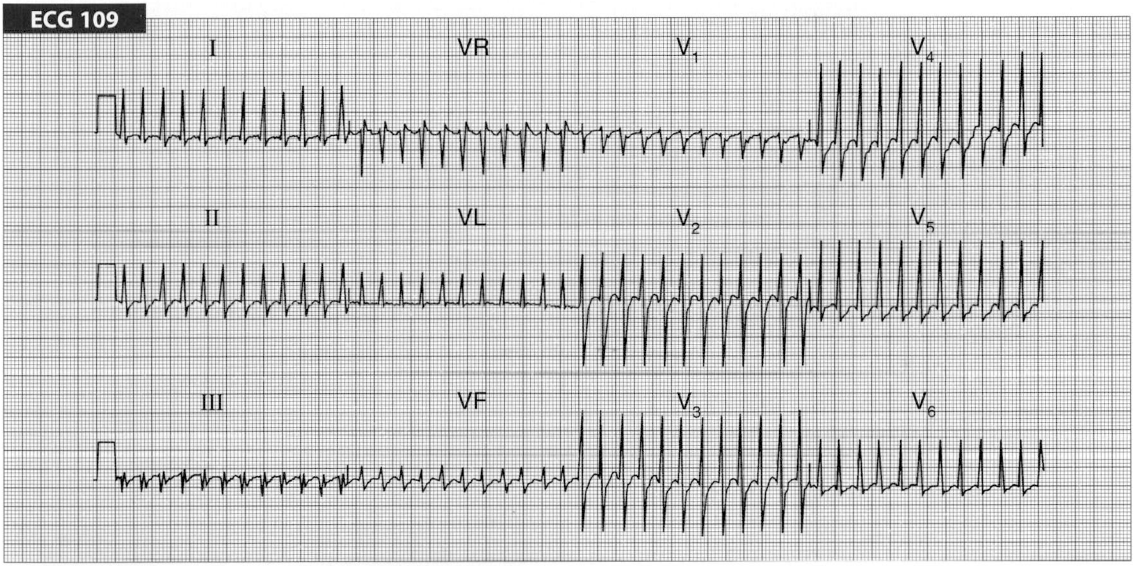

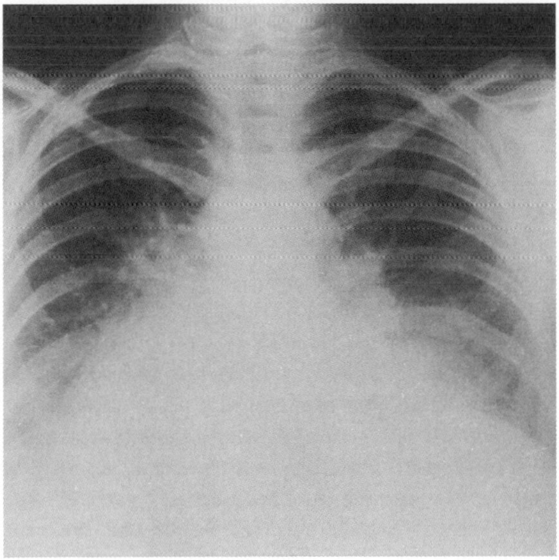

A 50-year-old man, who had complained of attacks of dizziness and palpitations for several years, collapsed at work and was brought to the A & E department. He was cold and clammy. His heart rate was rapid and his blood pressure was unrecordable. There were signs of left ventricular failure. These are his ECG and chest X-ray. What do they show and what would you do?

ANSWER 109

The ECG shows:

- Narrow complex tachycardia, rate just under 300/min
- No definite P waves
- Normal QRS complexes
- ST segment depression in leads V_4–V_6

The chest X-ray shows pulmonary oedema.

Clinical interpretation

A regular narrow complex tachycardia at 300/min probably represents atrial flutter with 1 : 1 conduction (i.e. each atrial activation causes ventricular activation).

What to do

The cardiovascular collapse results from the rapid heart rate, with a loss of diastolic filling. Carotid sinus pressure may temporarily increase the degree of block and establish the diagnosis, but it is unlikely to convert atrial flutter to sinus rhythm. Intravenous adenosine is likely to have the same effect as carotid sinus pressure. A patient who is haemodynamically compromised by a tachycardia should be treated with immediate DC cardioversion.

Summary ★★
Probable atrial flutter with 1 : 1 conduction.

ECG ME See p. 67, 8E

ECG IP See p. 117, 6E

ECG 110

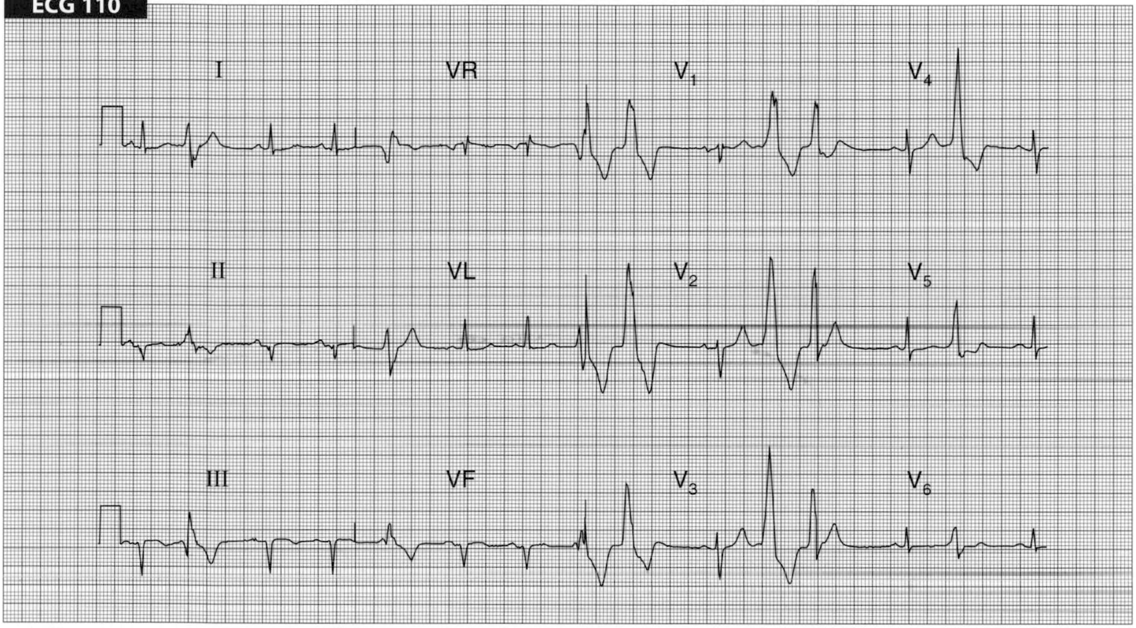

A 70-year-old man, who had had angina for several years, began to complain of attacks of dizziness. This is his ECG. What does it show and what would you do?

ANSWER 110

The ECG shows:

- Sinus rhythm, rate 88/min, with frequent multifocal ventricular extrasystoles
- Normal PR interval
- Normal axis
- Q waves in leads II, III, VF
- T waves flattened or inverted in the sinus beats in leads II, III, V_5–V_6

Clinical interpretation

The ECG shows a probable old inferior myocardial infarction, which accounts for his angina. Ventricular extrasystoles are in themselves usually not important, but in a patient complaining of attacks of dizziness, ventricular extrasystoles that are frequent and multifocal may be causing haemodynamic impairment.

What to do

It would be worth recording an ambulatory ECG to see if the patient is having runs of ventricular tachycardia, but the extrasystoles probably do need suppressing. A beta-blocker would be the first drug to try, and then amiodarone.

Summary ★★

Old inferior myocardial infarction and frequent multifocal ventricular extrasystoles.

ECG ME See p. 139, 8E

ECG IP See p. 152, 6E

ECG 111

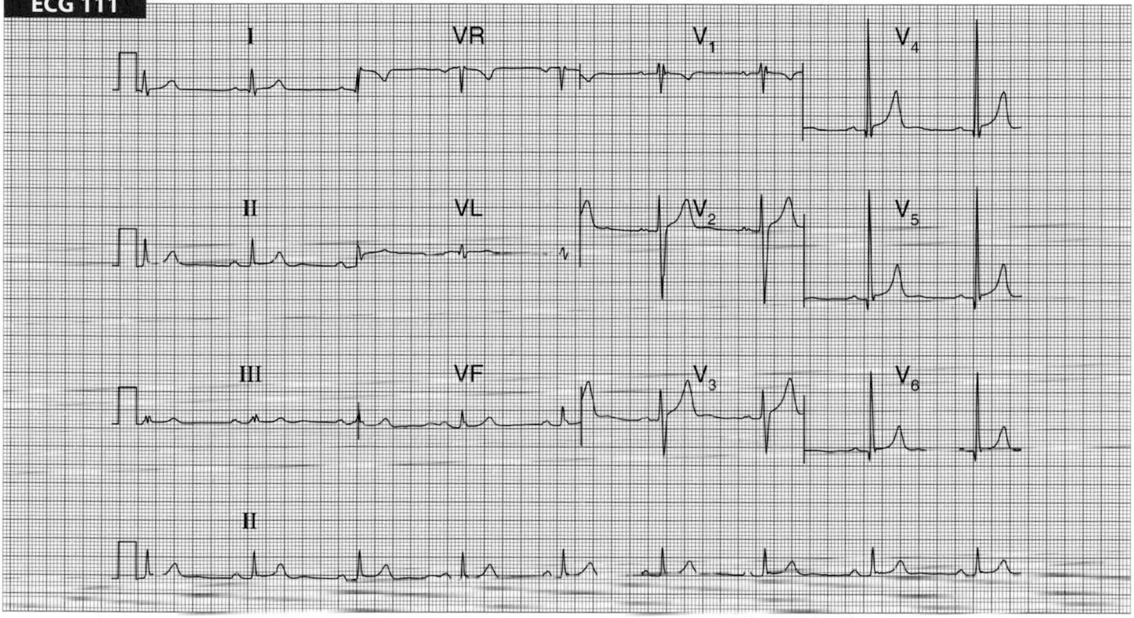

This ECG was recorded from a 50-year-old woman who complained of breathlessness and palpitations. What physical signs would you look for, and what is the next stage in her management?

ANSWER 111

The ECG shows:

- Sinus rhythm, rate 52/min
- Broad notched P waves, best seen in leads V_2 and V_3
- Normal axis
- QRS complexes exhibiting left ventricular hypertrophy on voltage criteria – the S wave in lead V_2 is 20 mm deep and the R wave in lead V_5 is 30 mm tall; septal Q waves in leads V_4–V_6
- Partial RBBB pattern (RSR in V_1)
- Normal ST segments and T waves, apart from high take-off ST segments in leads V_4–V_5

Clinical interpretation

The broad P waves suggest left atrial hypertrophy. There is nothing other than the voltage criteria (which are unreliable) to suggest left ventricular hypertrophy, so mitral stenosis must be considered – although significant mitral stenosis usually causes right ventricular hypertrophy. The palpitations could be due to atrial fibrillation if the patient has mitral stenosis.

What to do

Look for the tapping apex beat, the loud first sound, the opening snap and the mid-diastolic murmur that are characteristic of mitral stenosis. Echocardiography will be helpful in distinguishing between valve disease and left ventricular hypertrophy as a cause of left atrial hypertrophy. Ambulatory ECG recording may be necessary to identify the cause of the palpitations. Treatments to be considered if she has mitral valve disease and atrial fibrillation are digoxin or a beta-blocker, anticoagulants, and mitral valve surgery. If the breathlessness turns out to be due to poor left ventricular function, an angiotensin-converting enzyme inhibitor is needed.

Summary ★★

Sinus rhythm with left atrial hypertrophy.

ECG ME See p. 86, 8E

ECG IP See p. 293, 6E

ECG 112

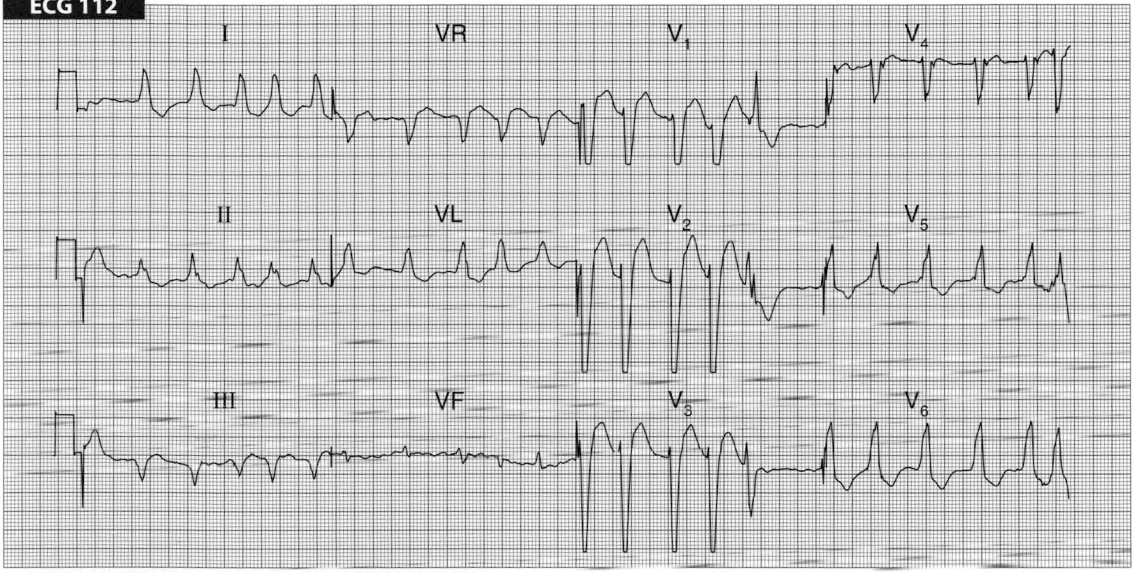

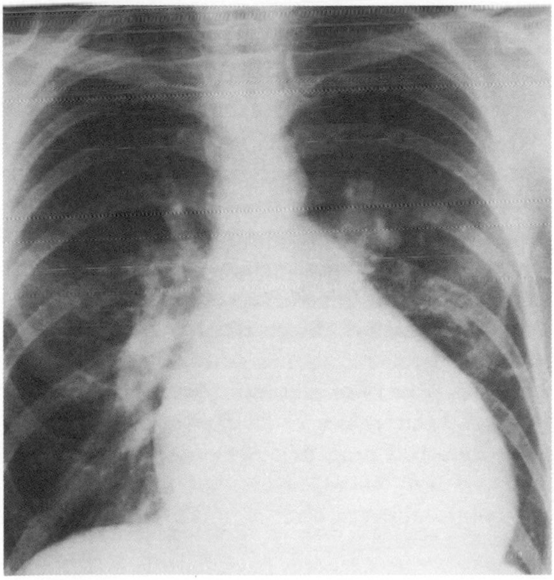

A 60-year-old man who complains of ankle swelling is found to have an irregular pulse, a blood pressure of 115/70, an enlarged heart, and signs of congestive cardiac failure. These are his ECG and chest X-ray. What do they show? He is untreated – how would you manage him?

ANSWER 112

The ECG shows:

- Atrial fibrillation, ventricular rate about 100/min, with one ventricular extrasystole
- Normal axis
- Broad QRS complexes, with 'M' pattern in the lateral leads indicating left bundle branch block (LBBB); bottom of S waves flattened in leads V_1–V_3 due to artefacts
- T waves inverted in lateral leads, as expected in LBBB

The chest X-ray shows a very large heart, all chambers being affected, and there is upper-zone blood diversion, indicating early heart failure.

Clinical interpretation

Atrial fibrillation and LBBB in a patient with an enlarged heart.

What to do

This patient has had no chest pain, but has developed a very large heart with atrial fibrillation; the ECG shows LBBB, which prevents any further interpretation. Ischaemia seems unlikely, and the diagnosis is almost certainly dilated cardiomyopathy of unknown cause. An echocardiogram may show some mitral regurgitation due to left ventricular dilatation, but the valves will probably be structurally normal. There will probably be globally reduced left ventricular function with a low ejection fraction. It is unlikely that a primary cause will be found, though alcoholism is the important one to exclude. A coronary angiogram should probably be performed to exclude 'silent' coronary disease, and an endomyocardial biopsy could be considered, to exclude the remote chance of a primary cardiomyopathy. Treatment would be the usual combination of diuretics, an angiotensin-converting enzyme inhibitor, digoxin, anticoagulants and ultimately cardiac transplantation.

Summary ★★

Atrial fibrillation and LBBB in a patient with dilated cardiomyopathy.

ECG ME See p. 43, 8E

ECG IP See p. 127, 6E

ECG 113

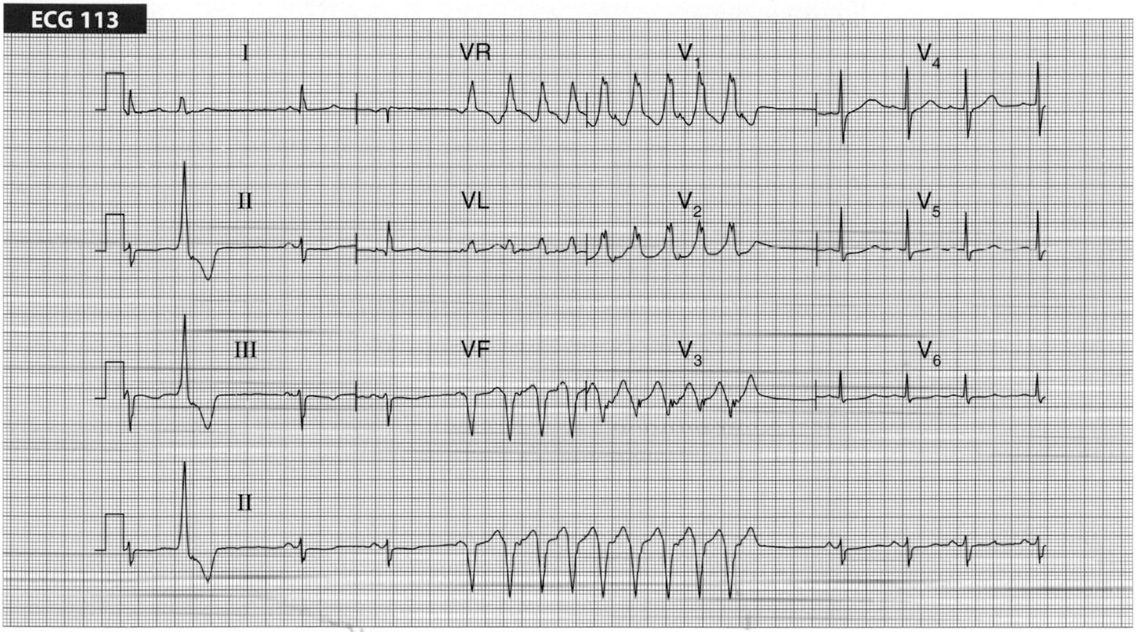

A 70-year-old man is sent to the outpatient department because of attacks of dizziness. What abnormalities does his ECG show, and what treatment is needed?

ANSWER 113

This ECG looks difficult to interpret because there is a nine-beat run of a broad complex tachycardia which occupies the whole of leads V_1–V_3. The key is to identify the rhythm first, from the lead II rhythm strip at the bottom. The ECG shows:

- The rhythm is basically sinus, with a rate varying between 65/min and 100/min
- One ventricular extrasystole, at the beginning of the record
- Broad complex tachycardia with an obviously different morphology from the sinus beats. The QRS complex duration is 160 ms, and in lead V_1 the R peak is higher that the R^1 peak. These features make it likely that the tachycardia is ventricular in origin
- Left axis deviation in the sinus beats (left anterior hemiblock)
- QRS complexes in the sinus beats otherwise appear normal
- Slight ST segment depression in leads II, III, V_5–V_6
- T wave inversion in leads II, III

Clinical interpretation

This ECG shows paroxysmal ventricular tachycardia, and probably underlying ischaemic disease.

What to do

This patient's attacks of dizziness may be due to the paroxysmal arrhythmia, which is life-threatening. The results of an ambulatory ECG recording and an exercise test would be interesting, but the patient needs immediate treatment, and amiodarone would probably be the drug of choice. A coronary angiogram should be considered because there may be one or more critical stenoses amenable to percutaneous coronary intervention (PCI), and this might abolish the ventricular tachycardia.

Summary ★★★

Sinus rhythm with paroxysmal ventricular tachycardia, and probable ischaemia.

ECG ME See p. 73, 8E

ECG IP See p. 155, 6E

ECG 114

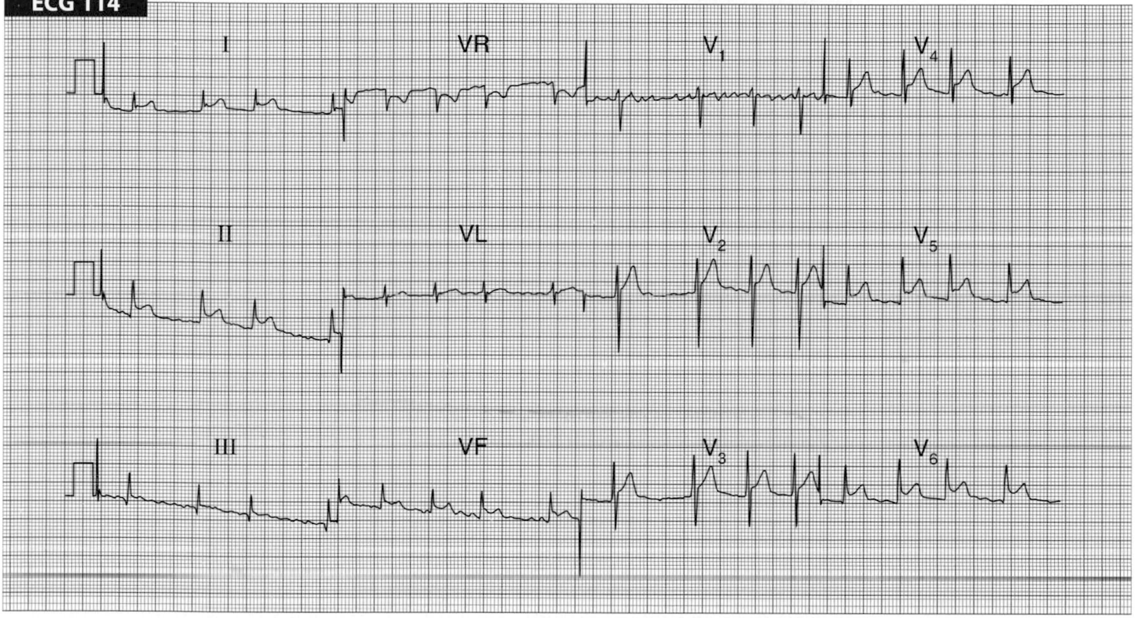

This ECG was recorded from a 30-year-old woman with severe rheumatoid arthritis, who was admitted to hospital with central chest pain. She was a non-smoker and had no risk factors for coronary artery disease. What do you think is going on?

ANSWER 114

The ECG shows:

- Atrial fibrillation, average rate about 100/min
- Normal axis
- Normal QRS complexes
- Raised ST segments in leads I, II, III, VF, V_2–V_6
- In leads V_3 and V_4 the raised ST segments seem to be due to 'high take-off'

Clinical interpretation

In a young woman with chest pain but no risk factors for a myocardial infarction, an ST segment elevation infarction is obviously possible, but other causes of raised ST segments must be considered. The 'high take-off' ST segments in leads V_3–V_4 (raised ST segment following an S wave) are a normal variant. The other raised ST segments, which are widespread, could well be due to pericarditis.

What to do

The patient should be examined lying flat, because this gives the best chance of hearing a pericardial friction rub – and this is what was found here. The pericarditis could, of course, be due to an infarction, but repeated ECGs showed no development of an infarction pattern, and the raised ST segments persisted for several days. An echocardiogram showed a pericardial effusion. The pericarditis, and presumably the associated atrial fibrillation, were due to the rheumatoid arthritis.

Summary ★★

Atrial fibrillation; ST segment elevation, partly 'high take-off' but mainly due to pericarditis.

ECG ME See p. 96, 8E

ECG IP See p. 251, 6E

ECG 115

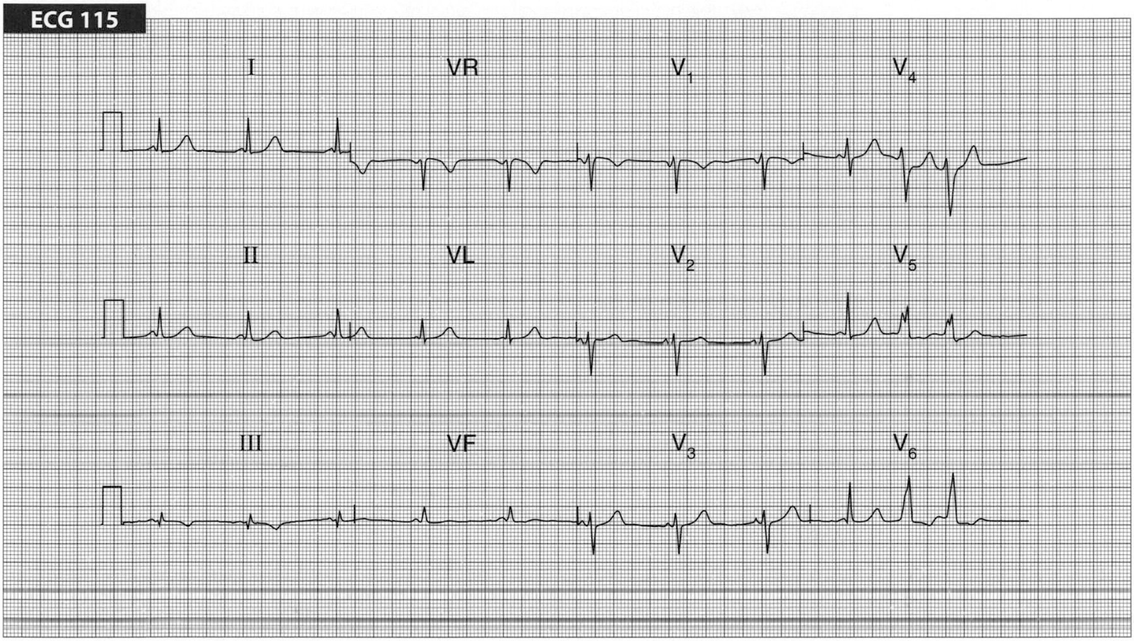

An 18-year-old student complains of occasional attacks of palpitations. These start suddenly without provocation; the heartbeat seems regular and is 'too fast to count'. During attacks she does not feel dizzy or breathless, and the palpitations stop suddenly after a few seconds. Physical examination is normal, and this is her ECG. What is the diagnosis and what advice would you give?

ANSWER 115

The ECG shows:

- Sinus rhythm, rate 64/min, with ventricular extrasystoles
- Very short PR interval
- Normal axis
- Normal QRS complexes and T waves, apart from a small Q wave and an inverted T wave in lead III

Clinical interpretation

This is the Lown–Ganong–Levine (LGL) syndrome. Unlike the Wolff–Parkinson–White (WPW) syndrome, in which there is an accessory pathway separate from the atrioventricular node and His bundle, in the LGL syndrome there is a bypass close to the atrioventricular node, connecting the left atrium and the His bundle. In the WPW syndrome the QRS complex shows an early delta wave, but in the LGL syndrome the QRS complex is normal.

What to do

Ambulatory ECG recording may confirm the diagnosis if attacks are frequent enough. Infrequent and short-lived attacks such as this patient describes are not dangerous, but she should be taught vagal-stimulating procedures such as Valsalva's manoeuvre and carotid sinus pressure. An electrophysiological study and ablation of the abnormal tract may be necessary. The ventricular extrasystoles are not important, but she should be advised not to smoke, and to avoid alcohol and caffeine.

Summary ★★★

The LGL syndrome.

ECG ME See p. 152, 8E

ECG IP See p. 72, 6E

ECG 116

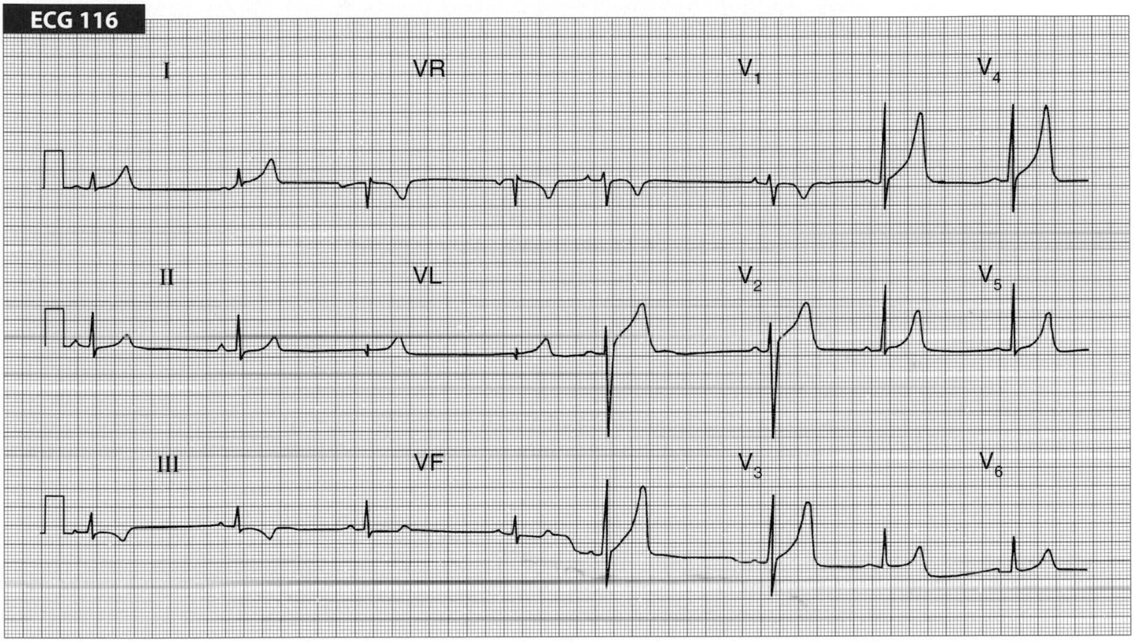

This ECG was recorded from a 37-year-old man admitted to hospital for a routine orthopaedic operation. The anaesthetist asks for comments.

ANSWER 116

The ECG shows:

- Sinus rhythm, average 45/min
- Normal axis
- Normal QRS complexes
- ST segment depression in lead VF
- Inverted T waves in leads III, VR, V_1
- Peaked T waves in the anterior leads

Clinical interpretation

Provided the patient is not taking a beta-blocker, the slow heart rate is probably a reflection of physical fitness. Inverted T waves in leads III, VR and V_1, and the depressed ST segments in lead VF, are probably normal. Peaked T waves are characteristic of hyperkalaemia, and are sometimes described as 'hyperacute' in ischaemia. However, when as large as this – and particularly when the patient is asymptomatic – peaked T waves are nearly always perfectly normal.

What to do

Ensure that the patient has no cardiac symptoms, and check his electrolyte levels preoperatively.

Summary ★★★
Normal ECG.

ECG ME See p. 57, 8E

ECG IP See p. 45, 6E

ECG 117

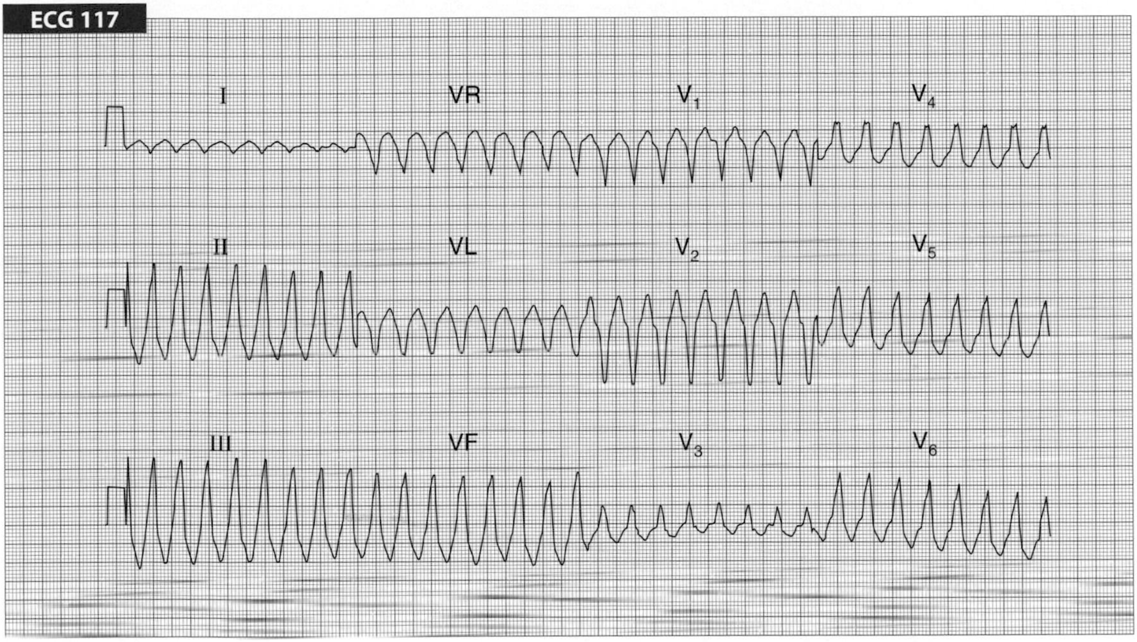

A 30-year-old man, who had had attacks of palpitations for several years, was seen during an attack, and this ECG was recorded. He was breathless and his blood pressure was unrecordable. What does the ECG show and how should he be treated?

ANSWER 117

The ECG shows:

- Broad complex tachycardia at 200/min
- No P waves visible
- Right axis deviation
- QRS complex duration 200 ms
- QRS complexes show no concordance
- Left bundle branch block (LBBB) pattern – QRS complexes show 'M' pattern, best seen in lead V_4

Clinical interpretation

A broad complex tachycardia like this is probably of ventricular origin. In this case, features against the rhythm being ventricular tachycardia are the right axis deviation and the lack of concordance in the QRS complexes (i.e. the complexes point downwards in leads V_1–V_2 and upwards in the other chest leads). The combination of right axis deviation and an LBBB pattern in a broad complex tachycardia suggests that the origin is in the right ventricular outflow tract.

What to do

Any patient with an arrhythmia and evidence of haemodynamic compromise (in this case, breathlessness and a very low blood pressure) needs immediate cardioversion. While preparations are being made, it would be reasonable to try intravenous lidocaine or amiodarone. Once the arrhythmia has been corrected, an electrophysiological study is needed, because right ventricular outflow tract tachycardia is the one variety of ventricular tachycardia that should be amenable to ablation therapy.

Summary ★★★

Ventricular tachycardia, probably originating in the right ventricular outflow tract.

ECG ME See p. 166, 8E

ECG IP See p. 144, 6E

ECG 118

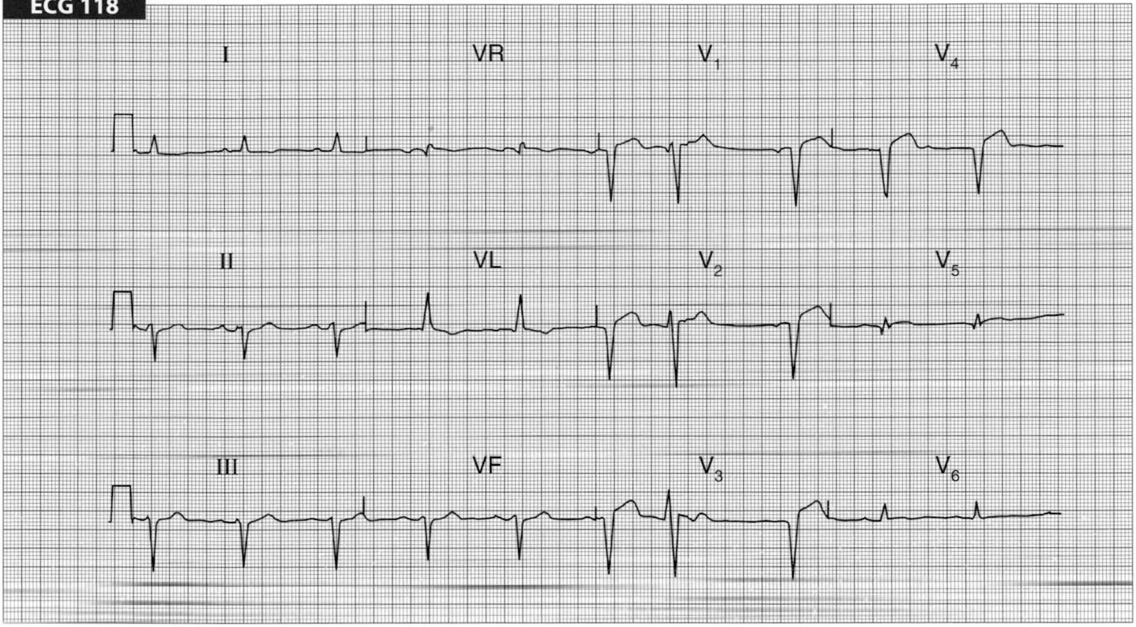

This ECG was recorded from a 75-year-old man with heart failure. He did not complain of chest pain. There are three main abnormalities. How should he be treated?

ANSWER 118

The ECG shows:

- Sinus rhythm, rate 60/min, with one ventricular extrasystole
- Left axis deviation
- Q waves in leads V_1–V_5 in the sinus beats
- Raised ST segments in the anterior leads
- Inverted T wave in lead VL; flattened T waves in leads I, V_6

Clinical interpretation

A 'silent' anterior infarction of uncertain age has caused left anterior hemiblock, which explains the left axis deviation. The lateral T wave changes are presumably due to ischaemia.

What to do

Ventricular extrasystoles should not be treated, and left anterior hemiblock is not an indication for pacing. In the absence of pain, the anterior infarction cannot be assumed to be new, so percutaneous coronary intervention (PCI) or thrombolysis should not be given. He needs an angiotensin-converting enzyme inhibitor and a diuretic.

Summary ★★

Left anterior hemiblock and anterior infarction of uncertain age; one ventricular extrasystole.

ECG ME See p. 49, 8E

ECG IP See p. 85, 6E

ECG 119

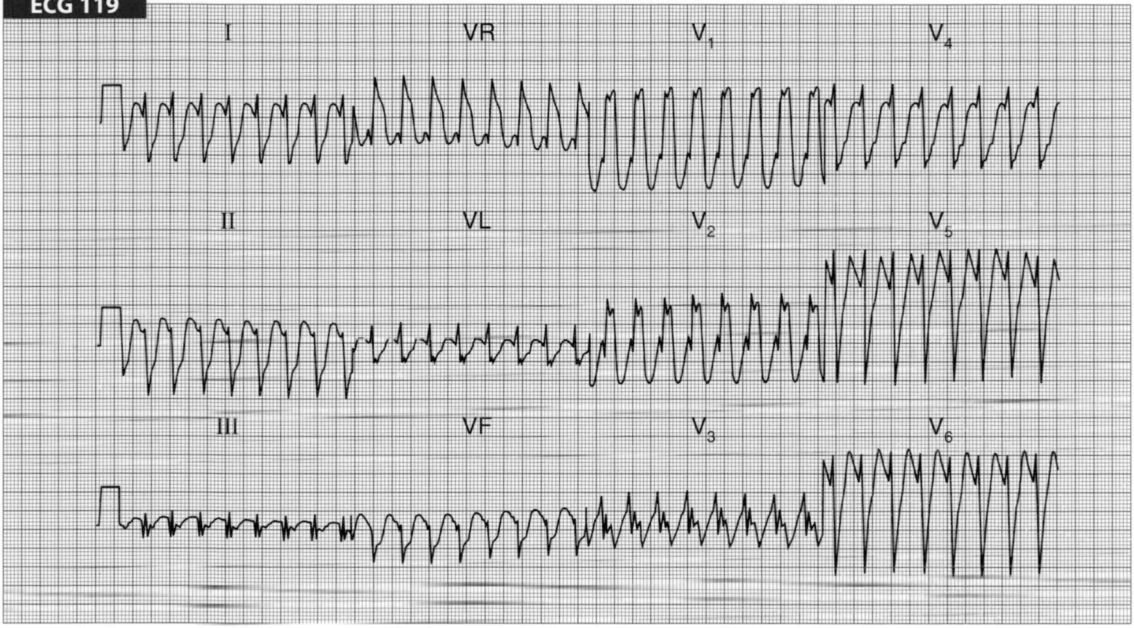

A 35-year-old woman, who had had palpitations for many years without any diagnosis being made, was eventually seen in the A & E department during an attack. She looked well and was not in heart failure, and her blood pressure was 120/70. This is her ECG. What is the rhythm, and what would you do?

ANSWER 119

The ECG shows:

- Broad complex tachycardia (QRS complex duration 200 ms), rate nearly 200/min
- No P waves visible
- Right axis deviation
- In lead V_1, the R^1 peak is higher than the R peak
- Right bundle branch block (RBBB) pattern
- No concordance of QRS complexes in the V leads

Clinical interpretation

The problem here is to distinguish between a supraventricular tachycardia with bundle branch block and a ventricular tachycardia. The clinical history is not helpful, nor is the fact that the patient is haemodynamically stable. The combination of right axis deviation, RBBB and the R^1 peak being higher than the R peak in lead V_1 make it likely that this is a supraventricular tachycardia with RBBB rather than ventricular tachycardia. However, the very broad QRS complex (>140 ms) would favour a ventricular origin for the arrhythmia.

What to do

Carotid sinus massage. If this has no effect, try intravenous adenosine, and if this is ineffective, try intravenous lidocaine.

Summary ★★★

Broad complex tachycardia with RBBB pattern, probably supraventricular in origin.

ECG ME See p. 166, 8E

ECG IP See p. 126, 6E

ECG 120

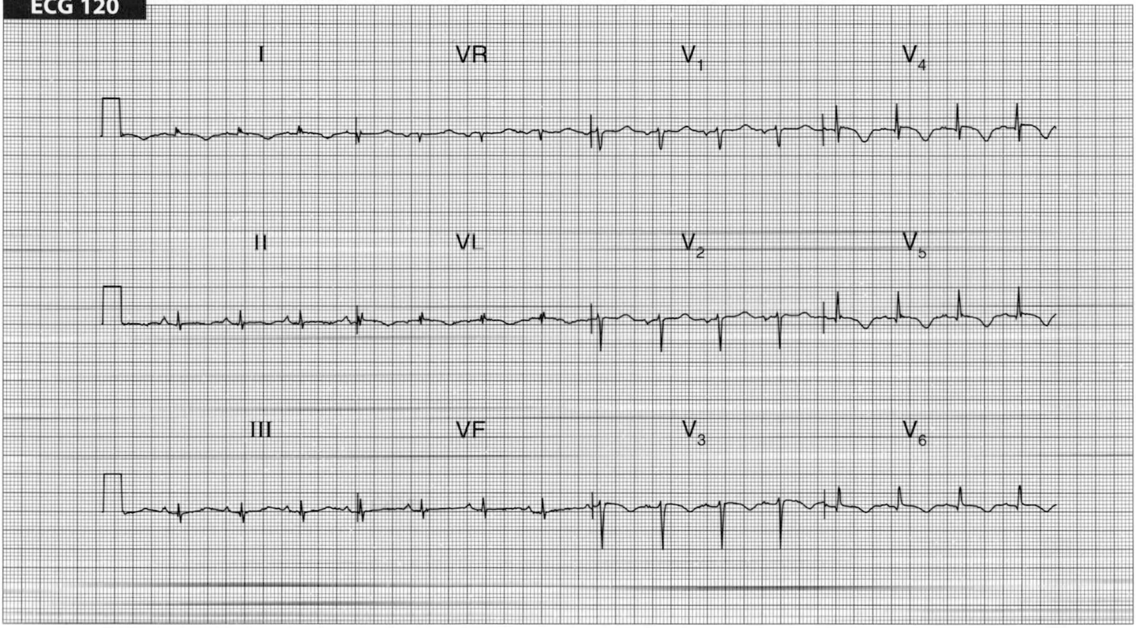

This ECG was recorded as part of the routine investigation of a 40-year-old man who was admitted to hospital following a first seizure. He was unconscious and had a stiff neck and bilateral extensor plantar responses. His heart was clinically normal. What do you think has happened?

ANSWER 120

This ECG shows:

- Sinus rhythm, rate 90/min
- Normal PR interval and QRS complex duration
- Normal axis
- Small Q waves in the lateral leads, probably septal
- Normal QRS complexes
- T wave inversion in leads I, VL, V_4–V_6
- Prolonged QT interval (QT_c 529 ms)

Clinical interpretation

The appearances here are suggestive of an anterolateral non-ST segment elevation myocardial infarction, but this does not correspond with the clinical picture and would not explain the long QT interval.

What to do

It is possible that this patient had a myocardial infarction which caused a cerebrovascular accident because of an arrhythmia or a cerebral embolus, and that the cerebrovascular accident caused the seizure. The unconsciousness and the bilateral extensor plantar responses could simply be post-ictal. However, such a sequence would not explain the stiff neck, which would seem to point to either a subarachnoid haemorrhage or meningitis. Changes like those in this ECG are common in subarachnoid haemorrhage, probably because of intense coronary vasospasm resulting from catecholamine release. Measurements of the blood troponin level are unlikely to help to differentiate between a primarily cardiac and a primarily neurological event. This patient did indeed have a subarachnoid haemorrhage, and the ECG eventually returned to normal.

Summary ★★★

Anterolateral T wave inversion due to subarachnoid haemorrhage.

ECG IP

See p. 345, 6E

ECG 121

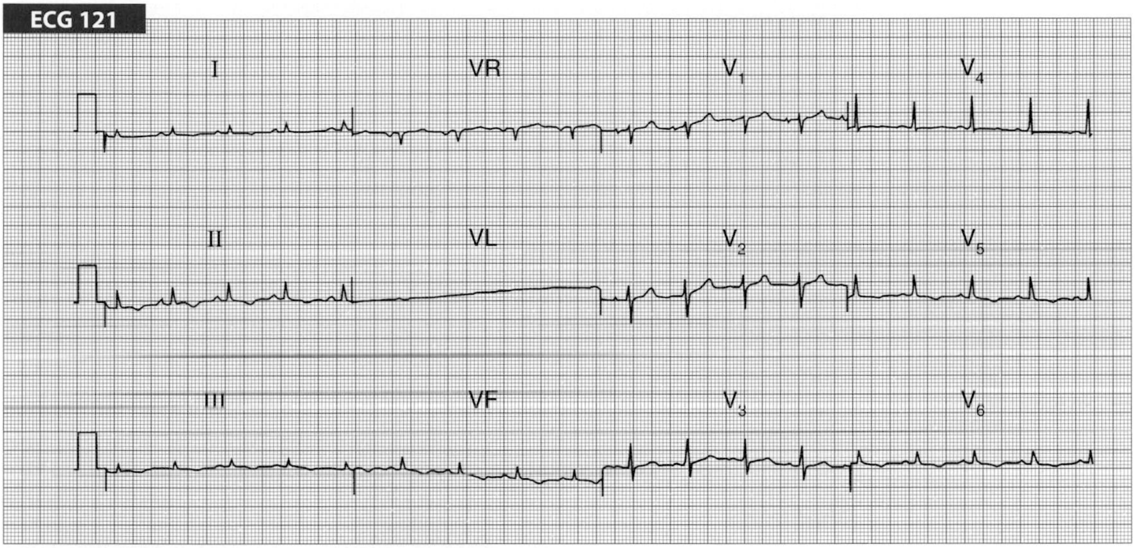

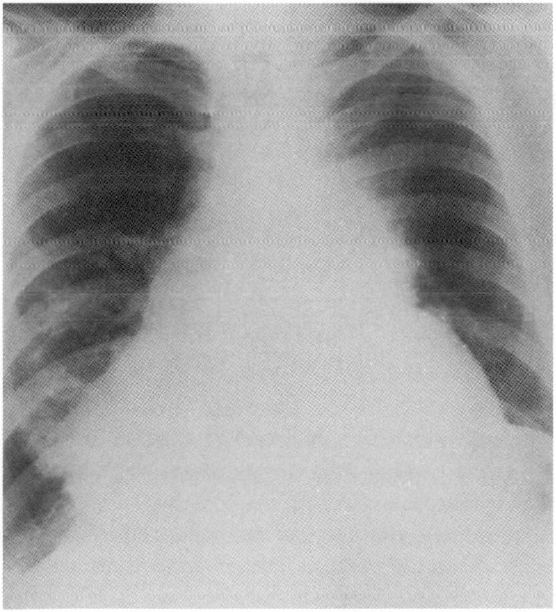

A 70-year-old man with lung cancer is admitted to hospital with abdominal pain and ankle swelling. He has a raised jugular venous pressure, a tender and distended liver, and marked peripheral oedema. Does this ECG help with the diagnosis and what might you need to do? What does the chest X-ray show?

ANSWER 121

The ECG shows:

- Sinus rhythm, rate 97/min
- Normal axis
- QRS complexes of normal width, but generally small
- T wave inversion in leads I, II, III, VF, V_5–V_6
- Loss of signal in lead VL – artefact

The chest X-ray shows an enlarged cardiac shadow with a triangular shape, suggesting a pericardial effusion.

Clinical interpretation

Small QRS complexes are seen with a pericardial effusion, and sometimes in patients with chronic lung disease. The widespread T wave changes would be consistent with pericardial disease. There is nothing in this record to suggest pulmonary disease.

What to do

The physical findings, the ECG and the chest X-ray would fit with a pericardial effusion associated with malignancy. You should look carefully at the jugular venous pressure to see if it rises with inspiration, indicating pericardial tamponade. Echocardiography is essential, and if there is evidence of right ventricular collapse in diastole, a pericardial drain should be inserted. The patient had a malignant pericardial effusion.

Summary ★★★

Small QRS complexes and widespread T wave changes consistent with a pericardial effusion.

ECG ME See p. 119, 8E

ECG IP See p. 329, 6E

ECG 122

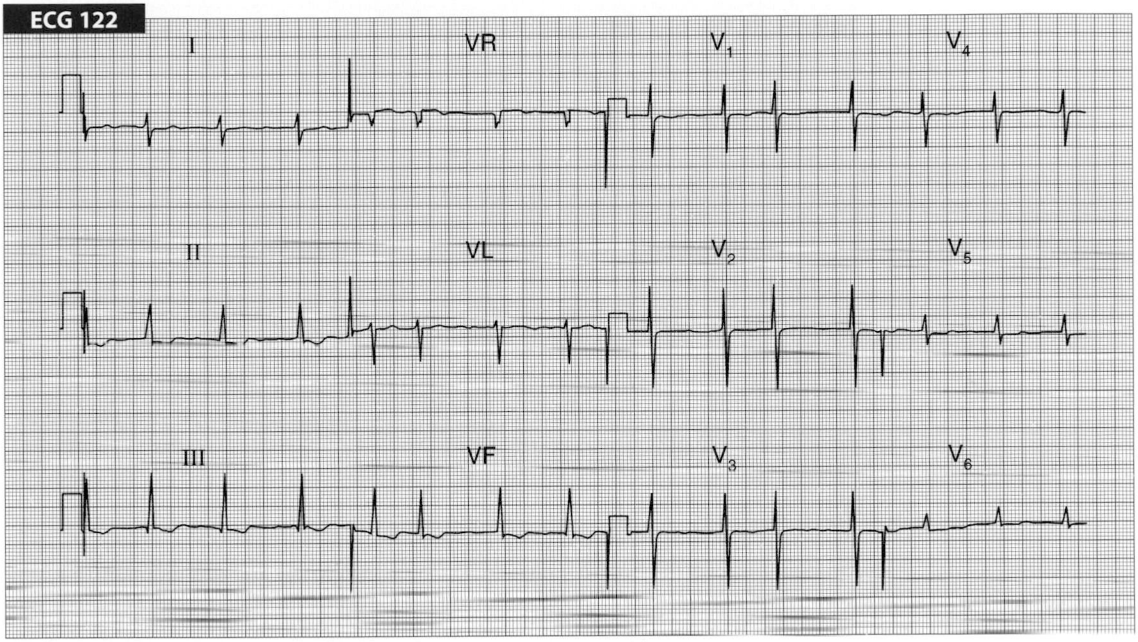

This ECG was recorded from a 65-year-old woman who had had a mitral valve replacement to treat rheumatic valve disease, and who was admitted to hospital with generalized lethargy, nausea and vomiting. What does the ECG show and what would you do? Unfortunately the chemical pathology laboratory burned down last night.

ANSWER 122

The ECG (*note*: chest leads at half sensitivity) shows:

- Atrial fibrillation
- Right axis deviation
- Normal QRS complexes, except for a tall R wave in lead V_1
- Downward-sloping ST segments, best seen in leads II, III, VF
- Generally flattened T waves
- U waves, best seen in leads V_4–V_5

Clinical interpretation

The atrial fibrillation, and the right axis deviation and tall R waves in lead V_1 (indicating right ventricular hypertrophy) probably pre-date the valve replacement. The flat T waves with obvious U waves suggest hypokalaemia. The downward-sloping ST segments suggest digoxin effect.

What to do

The clinical picture fits hypokalaemia and digoxin toxicity. Since the electrolyte and digoxin levels cannot be measured, stop the digoxin and any potassium-losing diuretics. Give the patient potassium orally. Monitoring the T and U waves is a crude but effective way of judging the serum potassium level.

Summary ★★★
Atrial fibrillation, hypokalaemia and digoxin effect.

ECG ME See p. 101, 8E

ECG IP See p. 331, 6E

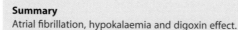

ECG 123

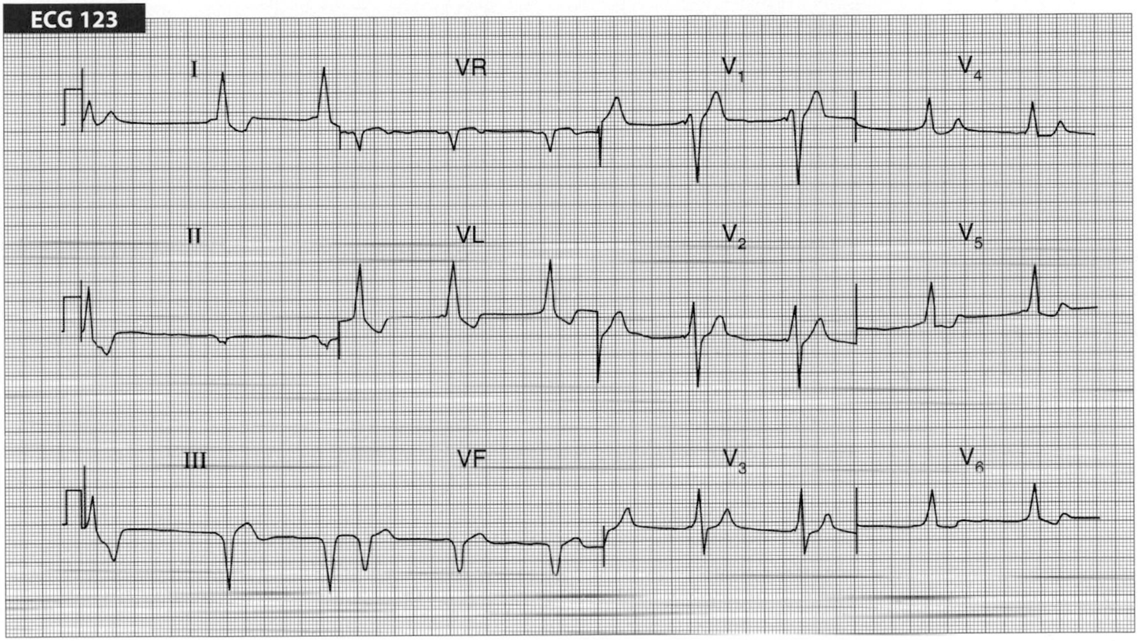

A 20-year-old man is seen in the A & E department with a head injury; there is a vague story of a collapse. What does the ECG show?

ANSWER 123

The ECG shows:

- Sinus rhythm, rate 55/min – P waves best seen in lead V_1
- The first complex is probably a ventricular systole
- Short PR interval
- Left axis deviation
- Broad QRS complexes (160 ms) with a slurred upstroke (delta wave), best seen in leads V_2–V_4
- Inverted T waves in leads I, II, VL; biphasic T waves in leads V_5–V_6
- The small second and third complexes in lead II appear to be due to a technical error

Clinical interpretation

The short PR intervals and the delta waves are characteristic of the Wolff–Parkinson–White (WPW) syndrome. Superficially, leads I, VL and V_5–V_6 might mistakenly be interpreted as suggesting left bundle branch block, but it is important to look at all the leads because the diagnosis here is best seen in lead V_2. In this case there is no dominant R wave in lead V_1, so the accessory conducting bundle is on the right side, and this is the WPW syndrome type B.

What to do

The WPW syndrome is associated with paroxysmal tachyarrhythmia, which may cause collapse. Asymptomatic WPW syndrome should be left untreated, but it is important in this case to establish – perhaps by ambulatory ECG recording and exercise testing – whether the patient was having paroxysmal tachycardia or not.

If there is reason to suppose that an arrhythmia caused his collapse and head injury he needs electrophysiological ablation of the abnormal conducting pathway.

Summary ★★★

The WPW syndrome type B.

ECG ME See p. 154, 8E

ECG IP See p. 69, 6E

ECG 124

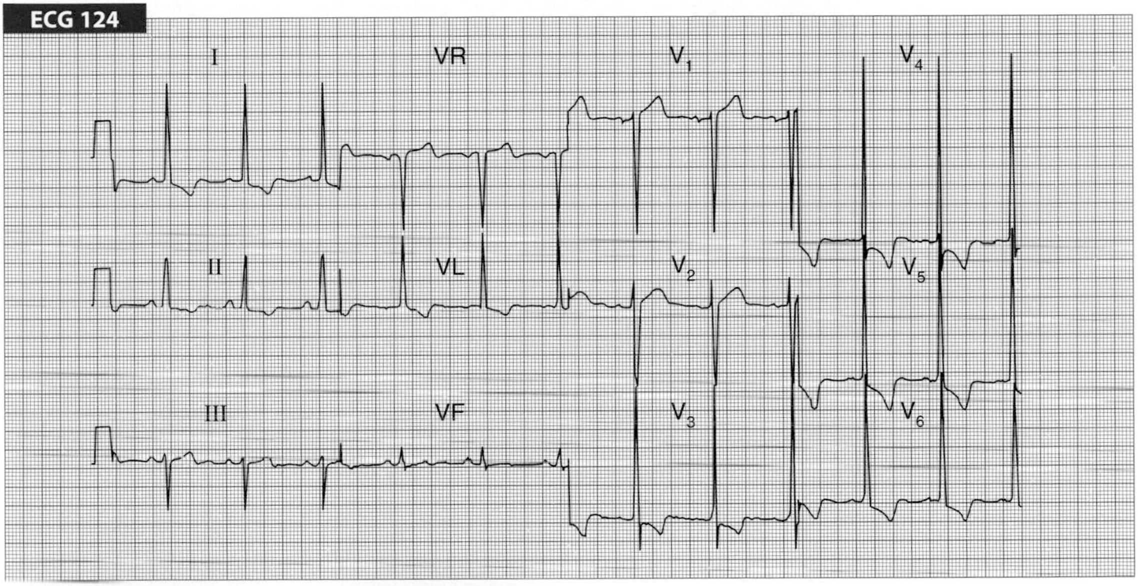

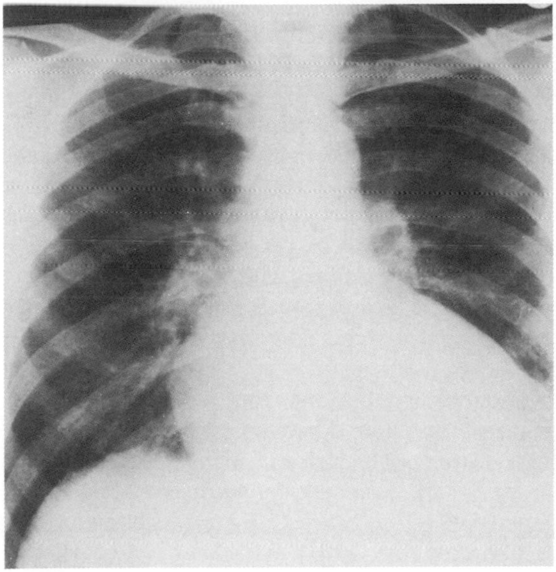

An 85 year-old man, who has had high blood pressure for many years, is seen in the outpatient department complaining of typical angina and of occasional dizziness when walking up hills. These are his ECG and chest X-ray. What is the diagnosis, and what would you do?

ANSWER 124

The ECG shows:

- Sinus rhythm, rate 71/min
- Normal axis
- Tall R waves and deep S waves in the chest leads
- ST segment depression in leads V_4–V_6
- Inverted T waves in leads I, II, VL, V_3–V_6

The chest X-ray shows a large heart, due to left ventricular hypertrophy.

Clinical interpretation

This is marked left ventricular hypertrophy. It can be difficult to distinguish between T wave inversion due to ischaemia and the T wave inversion of left ventricular hypertrophy, and when the T wave is inverted in the septal leads (V_3–V_4), ischaemia has to be considered. However, here the change is most marked in the lateral leads, and is associated with the 'voltage criteria' for left ventricular hypertrophy. Angina, dizziness and left ventricular hypertrophy in an 85-year-old may be due to tight aortic stenosis, though hypertension is a possibility.

What to do

Look for the signs of aortic stenosis ('plateau' pulse, narrow pulse pressure, displaced apex beat, aortic ejection systolic murmur) and confirm the valve gradient with echocardiography. In this patient the aortic valve gradient was 20 mmHg, indicating trivial stenosis of the valve, so the left ventricular hypertrophy must be due to the long-standing hypertension. The angina may well improve with adequate blood pressure control and the usual anti-anginal medication, but if it does not, then 85 years is not too old for coronary angiography with a view to percutaneous coronary intervention (PCI) or bypass surgery.

Summary ★
Left ventricular hypertrophy.

ECG ME See p. 118, 8E

ECG IP See p. 251, 6E

ECG 125

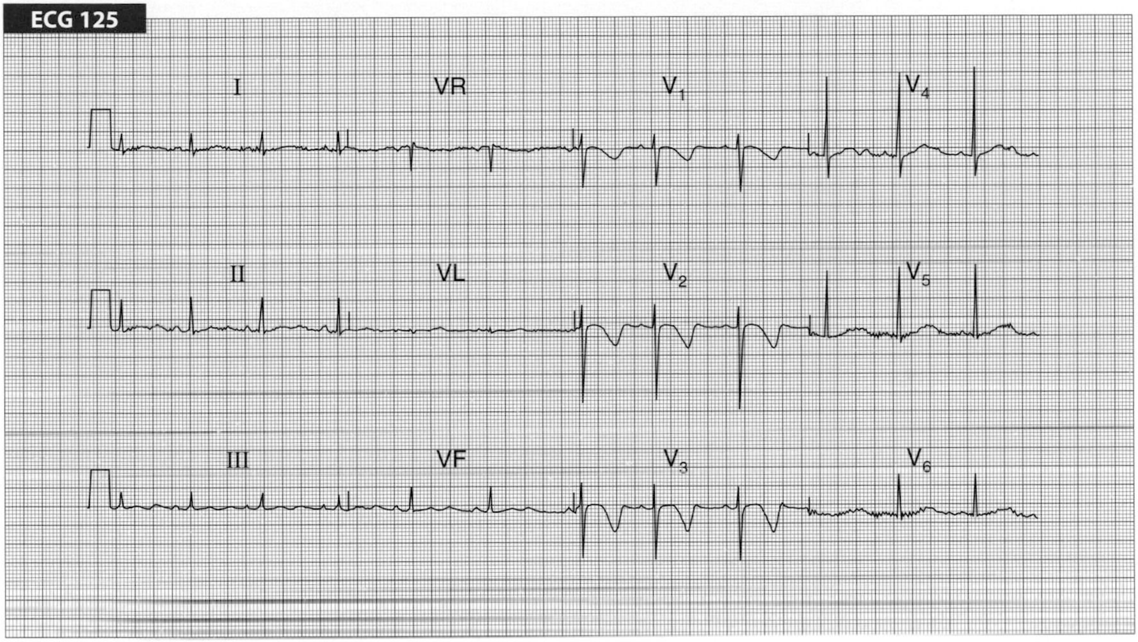

This ECG was recorded from a 15-year-old boy who collapsed while playing football, but was well by the time he was seen. What are the possible diagnoses?

ANSWER 125

The ECG shows:

- Sinus rhythm, rate 75/min
- Normal PR interval and QRS complex duration
- Normal axis
- Normal QRS complexes
- Inverted T waves in leads V_1–V_3
- Long QT interval (520 ms)

Clinical interpretation

A collapse during exercise raises the possibility of aortic stenosis, hypertrophic cardiomyopathy, or an exercise-induced arrhythmia. This ECG does not show the pattern of left ventricular hypertrophy, so aortic stenosis is unlikely. Anterior T wave inversion is characteristic of hypertrophic cardiomyopathy, but this does not normally cause a prolonged QT interval. Exercise-induced arrhythmias are typical of the familial long QT syndrome, and this boy's sister had died suddenly.

What to do

Initial treatment is with a beta-blocker, but an ICD (implantable cardioverter defibrillator) must be considered.

Summary ★★

The congenital long QT syndrome.

ECG ME See p. 157, 8E

ECG IP See p. 76, 6E

ECG 126

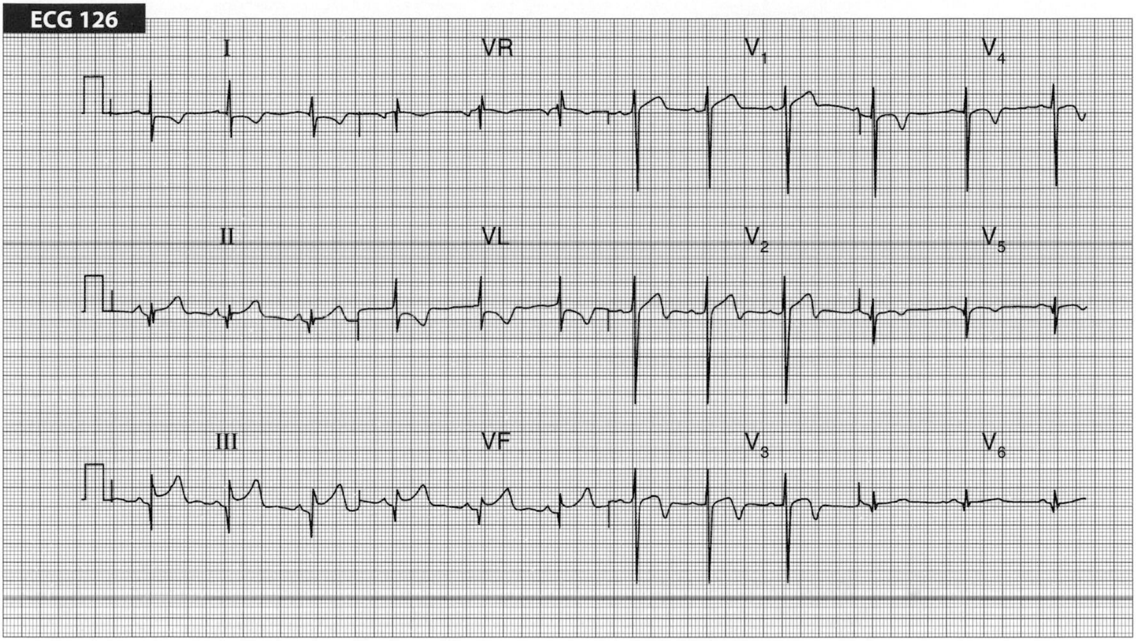

A 70-year-old man, who has had angina for 10 years, is admitted to hospital with severe central chest pain that has been present for 4 h. This is his ECG. What does it show and what would you do?

ANSWER 126

The ECG shows:

- Sinus rhythm, average rate 70/min
- Normal axis
- Q waves in leads III, VF
- Normal QRS complexes elsewhere
- Raised ST segments in leads II (following small S waves), III, VF
- Biphasic T waves in leads V_2–V_3
- Inverted T waves in leads V_4–V_5

Clinical interpretation

The inferior Q waves suggest an old infarction. The raised ST segments in leads III and VF would be compatible with an acute infarction, though the raised ST segment in lead II is a 'high take-off' segment because it follows an S wave, and this raises the possibility that the changes in leads III and VF may not be significant. The anterior changes suggest a non-ST segment elevation myocardial infarction (NSTEMI).

What to do

There is enough evidence here from leads III and VF to justify percutaneous coronary intervention (PCI) or thrombolysis – which should, of course, be combined with pain relief and aspirin.

Summary ★

Possible old and/or possible new inferior myocardial infarction; anterior NSTEMI.

ECG ME See p. 91, 98, 8E

ECG IP See p. 231, 6E

ECG 127

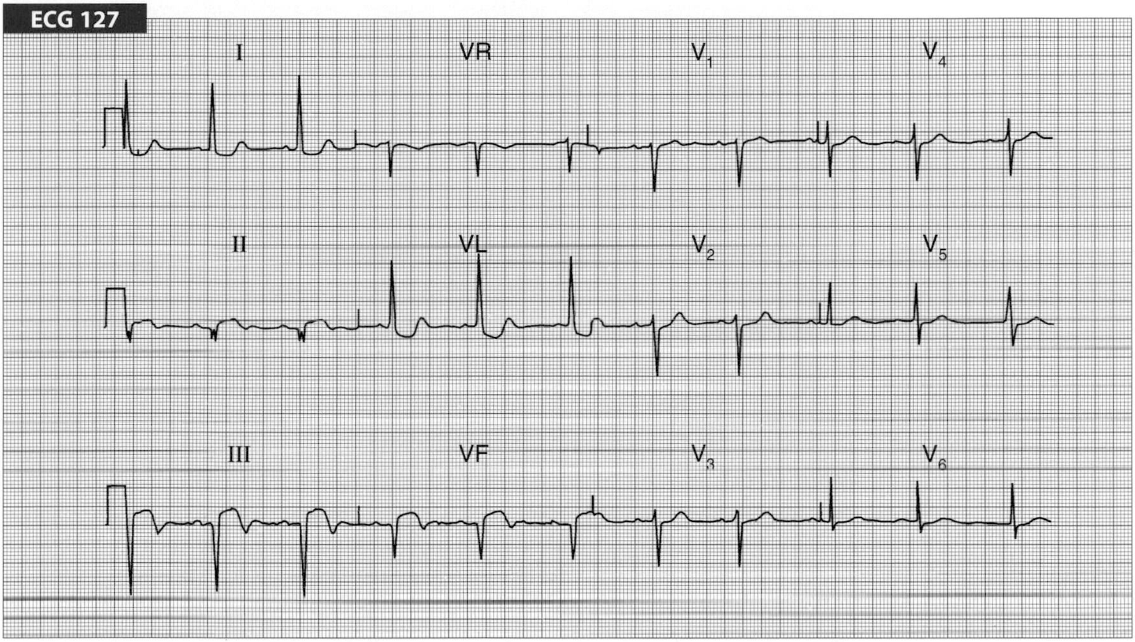

A 50-year-old man is admitted to hospital as an emergency, having had chest pain for 4 h. The pain is characteristic of a myocardial infarction. Apart from signs due to pain, the examination is normal. What does this ECG show and what would you do?

ANSWER 127

The ECG shows:

- Sinus rhythm
- Normal axis
- Q waves in leads II, III, VF
- Elevated ST segments in leads II, III, VF, with biphasic T waves
- Downward-sloping ST segments in lead VL
- Normal QRS complexes, ST segments and T waves in the chest leads

Clinical interpretation

This is an acute ST segment elevation inferior myocardial infarction. The rapidity of Q wave development is extremely variable, but the trace is certainly consistent with a 4 h history.

What to do

Pain relief is the most important part of the treatment. In the absence of contra-indications, the patient should be given aspirin immediately, and then thrombolysis or percutaneous coronary intervention (angioplasty) as soon as possible.

Summary ★
Acute inferior myocardial infarction.

ECG ME See p. 104, 8E

ECG IP See p. 215, 6E

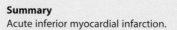

ECG 128

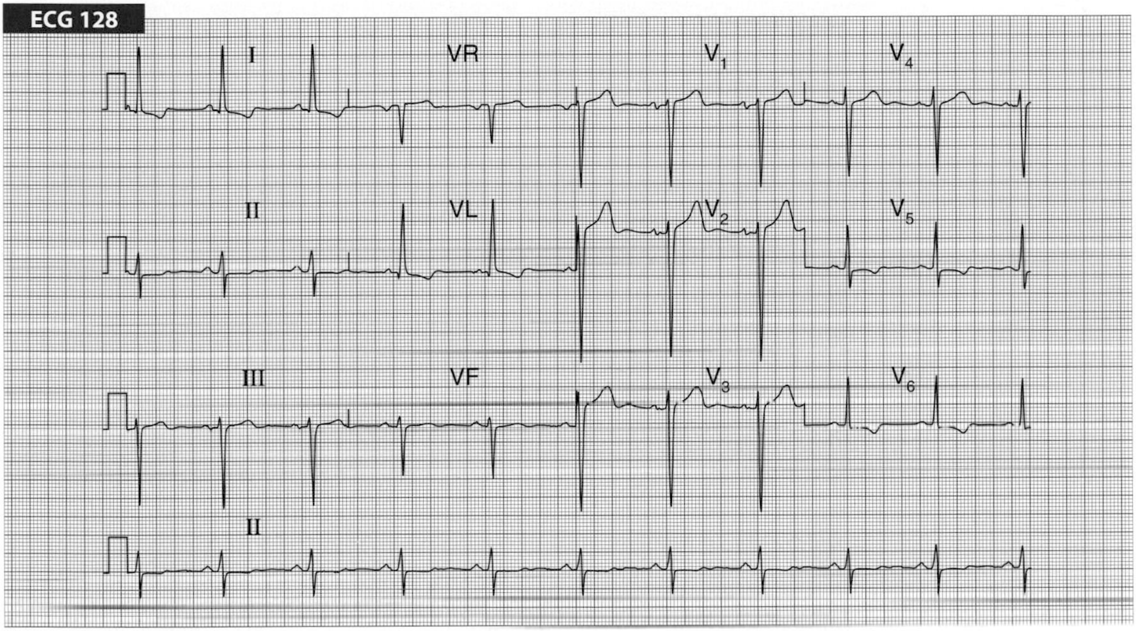

This ECG was recorded from a 60-year-old man admitted to hospital with severe heart failure and a heart murmur. What does it show and what would you do?

ANSWER 128

The ECG shows:

- Sinus rhythm, rate 60/min
- Bifid P wave (best seen in lead V_3) suggesting left atrial hypertrophy
- Left ventricular hypertrophy by 'voltage criteria' (height of R wave in lead V_6 plus depth of S wave in lead V_2 = 50 mm)
- Lateral T wave inversion

Clinical interpretation

These are the classic changes of left atrial and left ventricular hypertrophy. In a patient with heart failure and a heart murmur the likely diagnosis is severe aortic valve disease.

What to do

The heart failure must be treated with diuretics, but it is essential to establish the cause of the left ventricular hypertrophy before selecting long-term treatment. It could be due to aortic stenosis or regurgitation, to mitral regurgitation or to hypertension. While an angiotensin-converting enzyme inhibitor would be appropriate treatment for a patient with hypertension or mitral regurgitation, it would be potentially dangerous in a patient with aortic stenosis. An echocardiogram is the essential next step. This patient had severe aortic stenosis, and needed an aortic valve replacement.

Summary ★
Left atrial and left ventricular hypertrophy.

ECG ME See p. 86, 118, 8E

ECG IP See p. 293, 6E

ECG 129

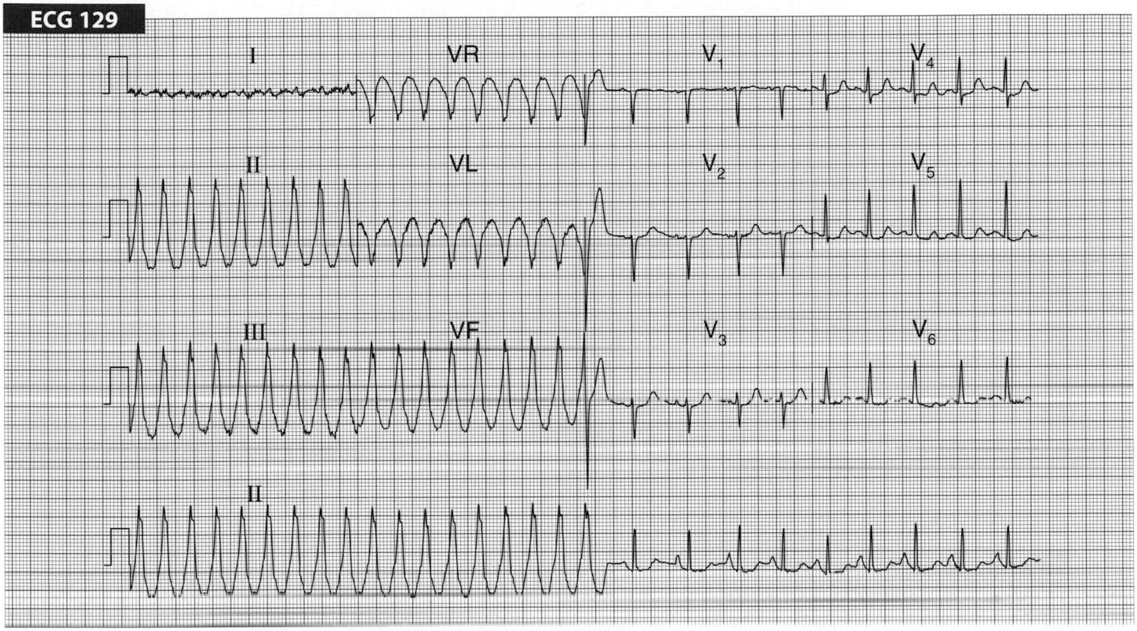

A 60-year-old man had complained of occasional episodes of palpitations for several years. Between attacks he was well, there were no physical abnormalities, and his ECG was normal. Eventually this ECG was recorded during one of his attacks. What is the arrhythmia and what would you do?

ANSWER 129

The lead II rhythm strip at the bottom of the record shows that the rhythm changes half way through the recording, and this makes interpretation difficult. However, the ECG shows:

- Regular broad complex tachycardia, rate 160/min, followed by sinus rhythm, rate 120/min
- Normal axis during the tachycardia
- Broad QRS complexes, duration 160 ms
- QRS complexes normal during sinus rhythm
- During sinus rhythm there is ST segment depression in leads V_4–V_5

Clinical interpretation

Without a full 12-lead record of the tachycardia it is difficult to be certain, but the complexes are very broad and have a totally different appearance from those in sinus rhythm, so this is almost certainly ventricular tachycardia. The ST segment depression in sinus rhythm is mild and not sufficient to make a confident diagnosis of ischaemia, but because the depression is horizontal, ischaemia seems likely.

What to do

Patients who have only occasional episodes of an arrhythmia, and who are otherwise well, are always difficult to manage. This patient should certainly have an echocardiogram to exclude a cardiomyopathy, and an exercise test to investigate the possibility of ischaemia and exercise-induced arrhythmias. At the age of 60 years, coronary angiography is probably indicated. Electrophysiological studies can be carried out to determine which antiarrhythmic agent to use in individual cases; however, in practice, amiodarone is just as effective as the agent selected by means of these studies. If the episodes were causing syncope, an implanted defibrillator could be considered.

Summary ★★
Paroxysmal ventricular tachycardia.

ECG ME See p. 164, 8E

ECG IP See p. 131, 6E

ECG 130

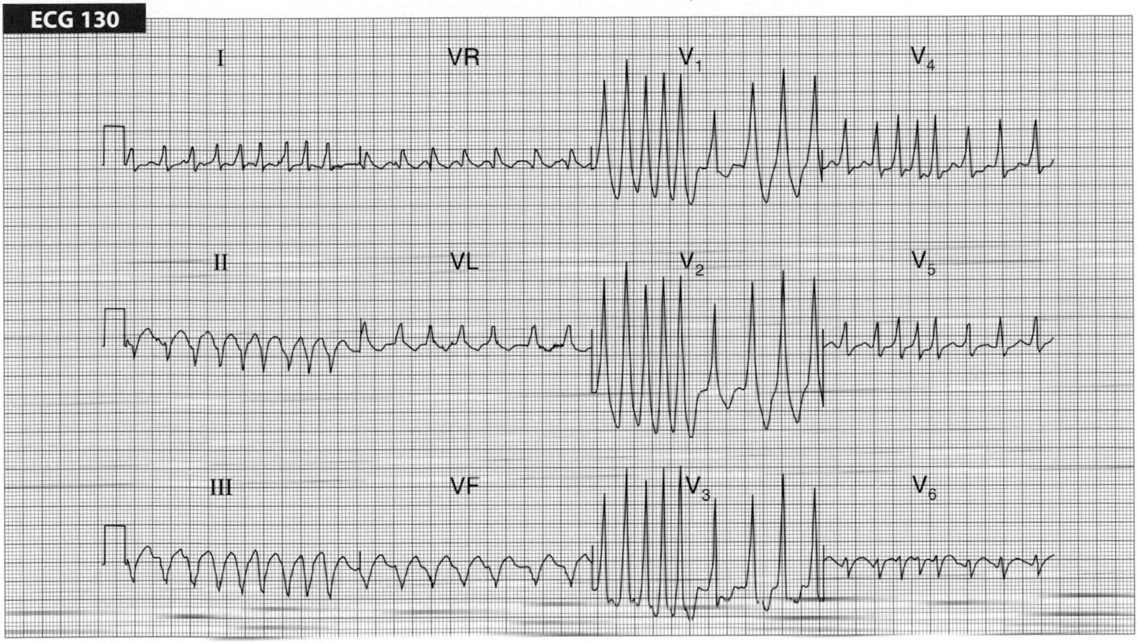

A 25-year-old woman, who had had episodes of what sound like a paroxysmal tachycardia for 10 years, produced this ECG when seen during an attack. What is the rhythm, and what is the underlying problem?

ANSWER 130

The ECG shows:

- Irregular tachycardia at about 200/min
- No consistent P waves visible
- Left axis deviation
- QRS complex duration varies between about 120 and 160 ms
- QRS complexes show a dominant R wave in lead V_1 and a prominent S wave in lead V_6
- After the longer pauses, the upstroke of the QRS complexes appears slurred

Clinical interpretation

The marked irregularity of this rhythm must be explained by atrial fibrillation. The broad QRS complexes might be due to right bundle branch block, but the dominant R wave in lead V_1, together with the slurred upstroke of the QRS complex in at least some leads, indicate the Wolff–Parkinson–White (WPW) syndrome type A.

What to do

A combination of the WPW syndrome and atrial fibrillation is very dangerous, because it can degenerate into ventricular fibrillation. The arrhythmia needs treating as an emergency, whatever the clinical state of the patient. It is important not to use drugs that may block the atrioventricular node and increase conduction through the accessory pathway, because this will increase the risk of ventricular fibrillation. Therefore, adenosine, digoxin, verapamil and lidocaine are contraindicated. The drugs that slow conduction in the accessory pathway, and are therefore safe, are the beta-blockers, flecainide and amiodarone. Thereafter, an electrophysiological study to identify and ablate the accessory pathway is essential.

Summary ★★★

Atrial fibrillation and the WPW syndrome type A.

ECG ME See p. 79, 154, 8E

ECG IP See p. 147, 6E

ECG 131

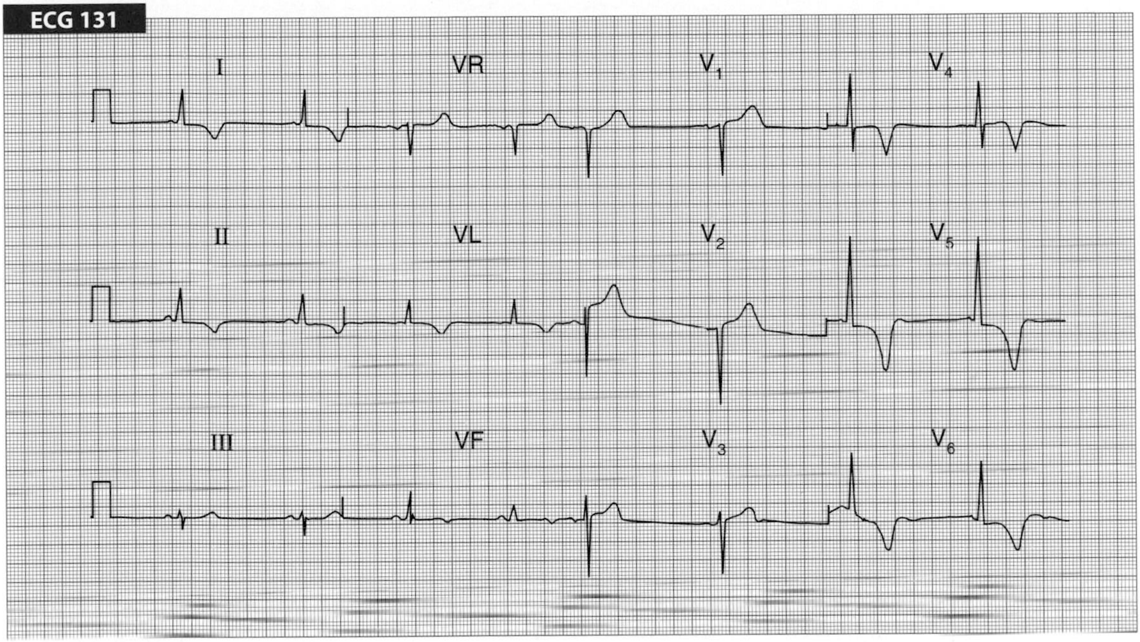

A 35-year-old white man is seen in the outpatient department complaining of chest pain on exertion, sometimes with exertion-induced dizziness, and this is his ECG. What is the likely diagnosis? What physical signs would you look for?

ANSWER 131

The ECG shows:

- Sinus rhythm
- Normal axis
- Normal QRS complexes
- Marked T wave inversion in leads I, II, VL, V_4–V_6

Clinical interpretation

Anterolateral T wave inversion as gross as this may be due to a non-ST segment elevation myocardial infarction, or even to left ventricular hypertrophy. However, there are no other features of left ventricular hypertrophy on this trace, which is fairly characteristic of hypertrophic cardiomyopathy. Myocardial infarction is uncommon in people of this age.

What to do

Physical signs of hypertrophic cardiomyopathy include a 'jerky pulse'; an aortic flow murmur which is characteristically louder after the pause that follows an extrasystole; and mitral regurgitation. Hypertrophic cardiomyopathy is best diagnosed by echocardiography, which will show asymmetric septal hypertrophy, systolic anterior movement of the mitral valve apparatus, and sometimes early closure of the aortic valve. This patient's echocardiogram showed all these features, confirming the diagnosis of hypertrophic cardiomyopathy.

Summary ★★★

Gross T wave inversion in the anterolateral leads, suggesting hypertrophic cardiomyopathy.

ECG ME See p. 153, 8E

ECG IP See p. 229, 6E

ECG 132

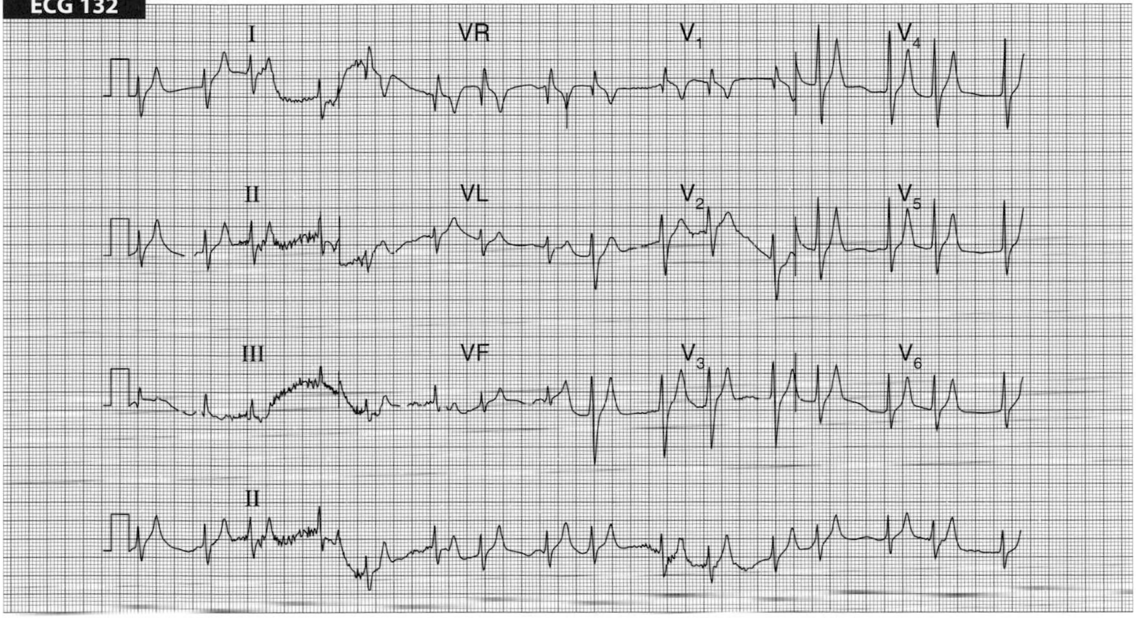

This ECG was recorded from a 30-year-old woman admitted to hospital with diabetic ketoacidosis. Any comments?

ANSWER 132

This is not a technically good record, and exhibits considerable artefacts. However, the ECG shows:

- The rhythm is probably sinus, with coupled junctional extrasystoles
- P waves difficult to identify, but there are probably flattened P waves before the first of each pair of QRS complexes, best seen in lead VR
- Probably normal PR interval
- Normal axis
- Narrow QRS complexes, so this is a supraventricular rhythm
- QRS complexes apparently in pairs, which are identical
- QRS complex duration at the upper limit of normal (120 ms)
- ST segment not easy to identify
- T waves sharply peaked in all leads

Clinical interpretation

These changes are characteristic of hyperkalaemia, which of course is likely to be present in diabetic ketoacidosis.

What to do

This ECG should alert you to check the serum potassium level immediately: in this patient it was found to be 7.1 mmol/l. It settled rapidly with treatment of the diabetes.

Summary ★★★
Hyperkalaemia.

ECG ME See p. 101, 8E

ECG IP See p. 331, 6E

ECG 133

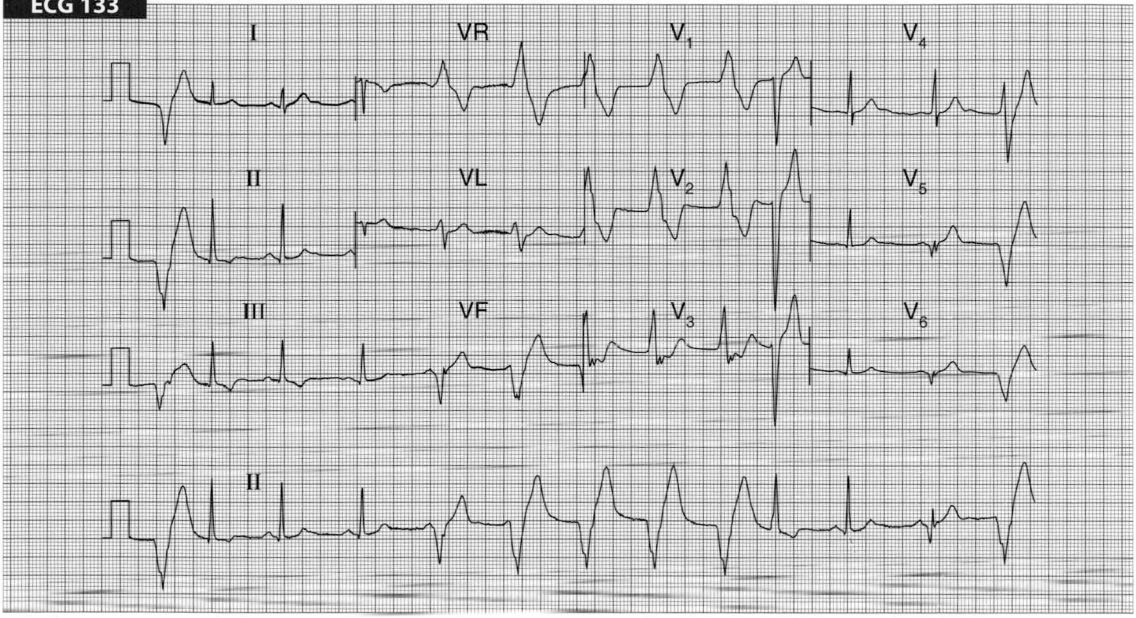

This ECG was recorded as part of the health screening of an asymptomatic 40-year-old man. How would you proceed?

ANSWER 133

The lead II rhythm strip at the bottom of the record shows that the rhythm changed during the recording, so it is necessary to try to identify the normal complexes (if any) in each lead. There are normal beats in the second and third complexes in leads I, II and III; in the first complex in leads VR, VL and VF; in the last complex in leads V_1–V_3; and in the first complex in leads V_4–V_6. The ECG shows:

- Sinus rhythm at about 77/min, with ventricular extrasystoles at the beginning and end of the record, and a six-beat run of a broad complex rhythm in the middle of the record
- The first complex of the run of broad complexes differs from the others, and is probably a fusion beat (a combination of a sinus beat and the ectopic rhythm)
- Normal axis when in sinus rhythm
- Normal QRS complexes in sinus rhythm
- Inverted T waves in lead III, but not VF

Clinical interpretation

The run of broad complexes represents accelerated idioventricular rhythm. This is quite common following a myocardial infarction, but in a healthy subject it is probably of no significance. The T wave inversion in lead III is not important because the T wave is upright in lead VF.

What to do

If the individual has no symptoms and the physical examination is normal, no further action is needed. Accelerated idioventricular rhythm should not be treated.

Summary ★★★

Sinus rhythm and accelerated idioventricular rhythm.

ECG ME See p. 60, 8E

ECG IP See p. 102, 6E

ECG 134

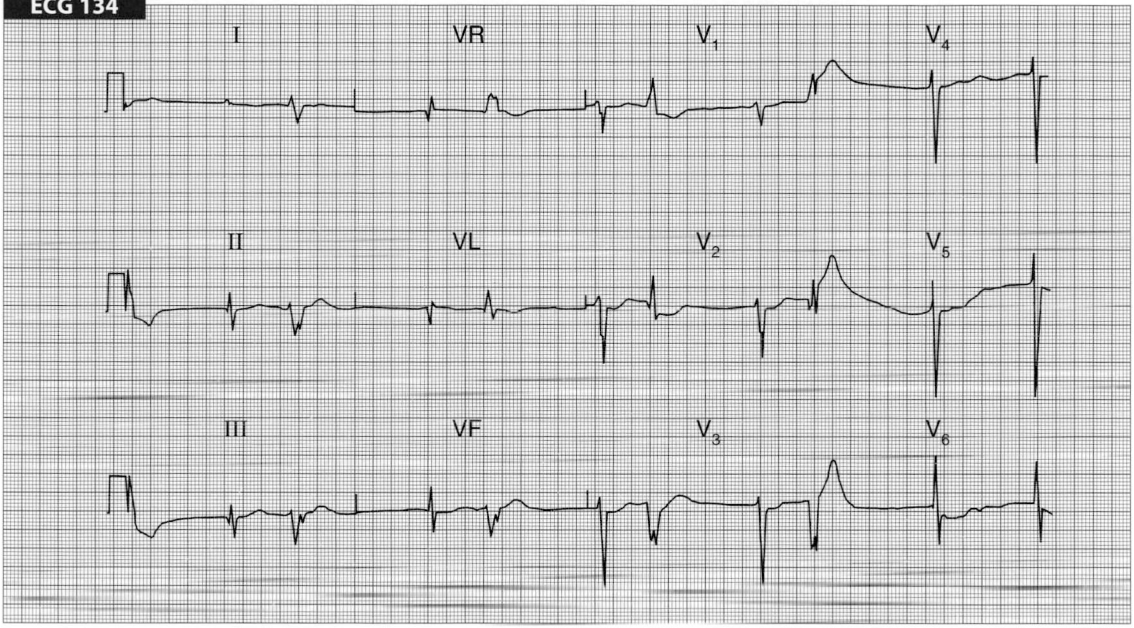

A 60-year-old woman, with long-standing heart failure of uncertain cause, complains of anorexia, weight loss, and general weakness and lethargy. Does this ECG help with her diagnosis and management?

ANSWER 134

The ECG shows:

- Atrial fibrillation
- Coupled ventricular extrasystoles
- Q waves in lead VL (in the supraventricular beats)
- ST segment depression in lead V_6
- Flattened T waves and prominent U waves (best seen in lead V_4)

Clinical interpretation

A patient with heart failure with atrial fibrillation will probably be receiving digoxin and diuretics. The history of anorexia and weight loss suggests digoxin toxicity, and the weakness could be due to hypokalaemia. The ECG supports this. Lead V_6 shows digoxin effect, and coupled ventricular extrasystoles are a feature of digoxin toxicity. The flat T waves and prominent U waves suggest hypokalaemia.

What to do

Remember that hypokalaemia potentiates the effect of digoxin. Therefore, stop the digoxin, check the electrolytes, and give oral potassium supplements. Do not give antiarrhythmic agents. Treat the heart failure with vasodilators.

This woman improved dramatically when her digoxin dose was reduced and she was given oral potassium. Then she was prescribed an angiotensin-converting enzyme inhibitor and a reduced dose of diuretics.

Summary ★★★

Atrial fibrillation with ventricular extrasystoles; probable digoxin toxicity and hypokalaemia.

ECG ME See p. 191, 8E

ECG IP See p. 335, 6E

ECG 135

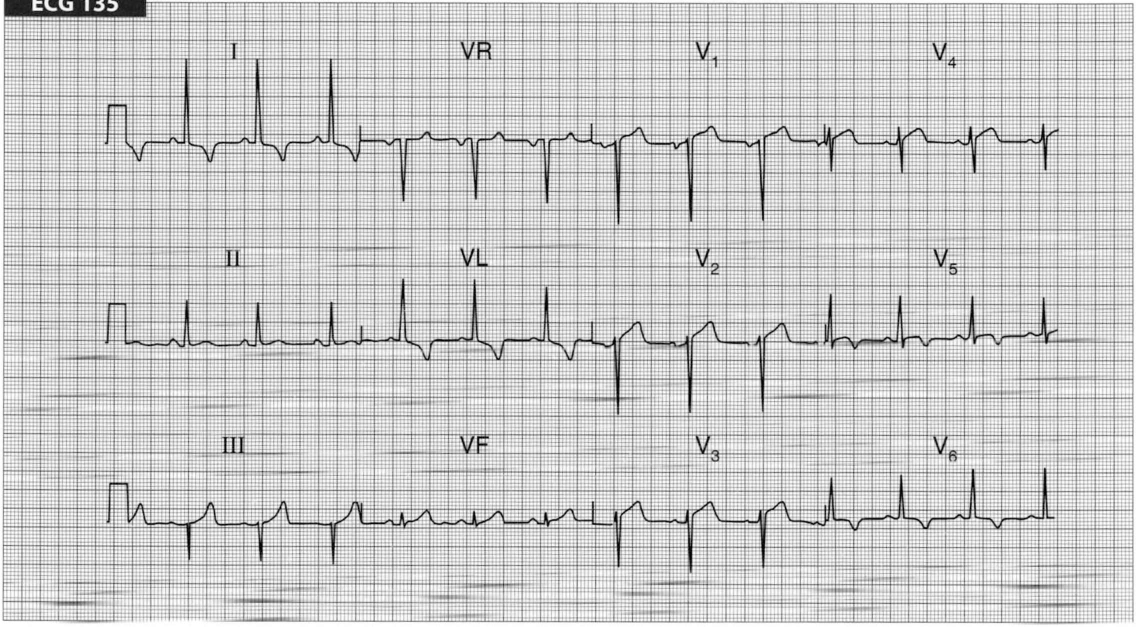

A 50-year-old man complains of typical angina. His blood pressure is 150/90, and he has an aortic ejection systolic murmur. This is his ECG. What is the probable cause of his angina, and what would you do?

ANSWER 135

The ECG shows:

- Sinus rhythm, rate 77/min
- Normal axis
- Normal QRS complexes
- Raised ST segments following S waves in leads V_4–V_5
- Inverted T waves in leads I, VL, V_5–V_6

Clinical interpretation

The raised ST segments in leads V_4–V_5 are due to 'high take-off' and are not important. The lateral T wave inversion could indicate left ventricular hypertrophy or ischaemia, and this patient could have aortic stenosis or coronary disease. In the absence of tall R waves, lateral ischaemia seems more likely than left ventricular hypertrophy, but it is often difficult to distinguish between these on the ECG.

What to do

Echocardiography will show whether the patient has significant aortic valve disease. Remember that anaemia can cause systolic murmurs and angina, though probably not this degree of T wave inversion. The patient had coronary disease.

Summary ★★★

Probable lateral ischaemia, but possible left ventricular hypertrophy.

ECG ME See p. 91, 8E

ECG IP See p. 256, 6E

ECG 136

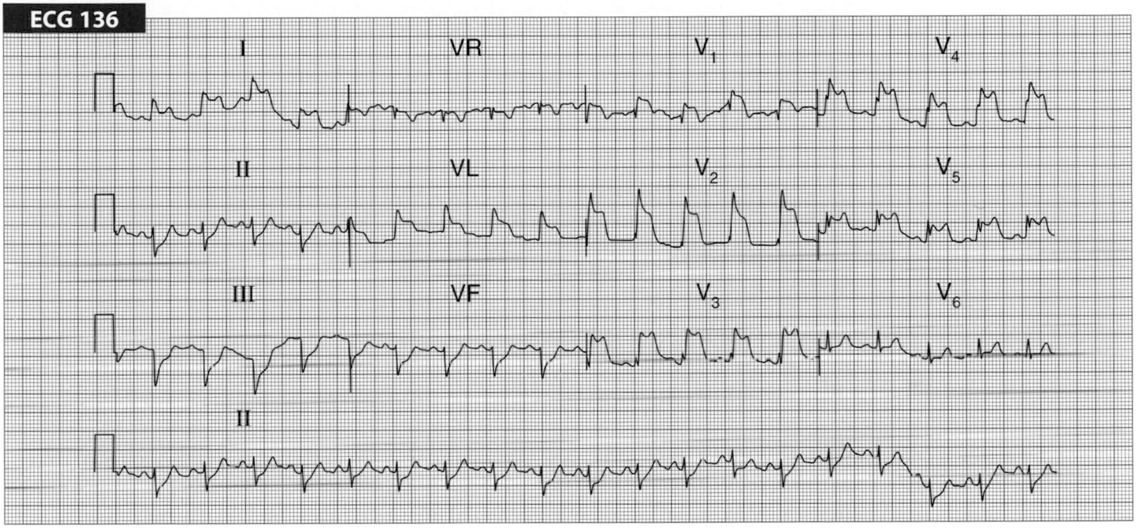

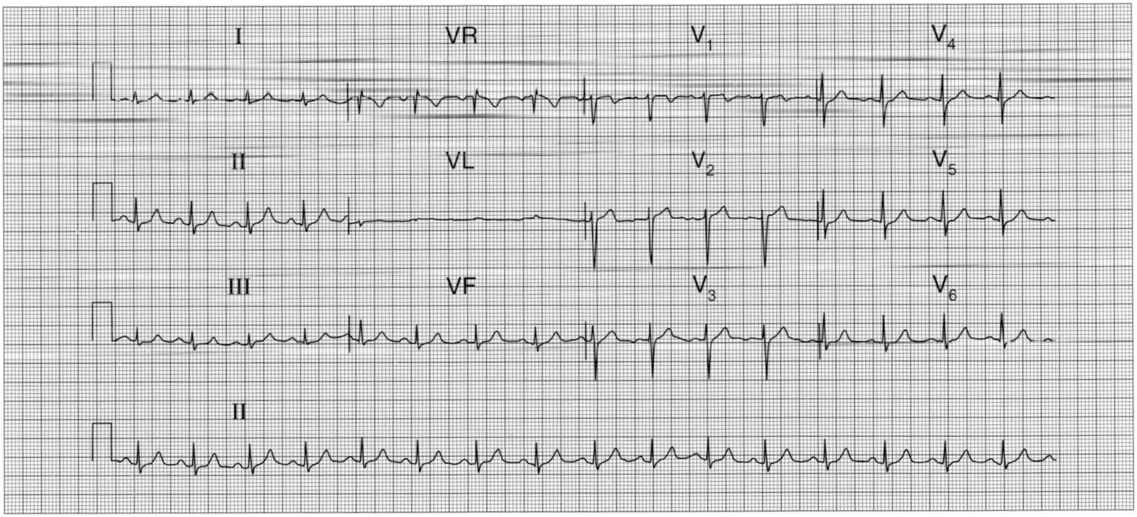

The upper ECG was recorded by paramedics from a 50-year-old woman who had had episodes of chest pain for several years, and who called an ambulance because of a severe attack. By the time she reached the A & E department, when the lower ECG was recorded, her pain had gone. What had happened?

ANSWER 136

The upper ECG shows:

- Sinus rhythm, average rate 111/min
- Left axis deviation
- QRS complexes probably normal, but partly obscured by the ST segments
- Raised ST segments in leads I, VL, V_1–V_5
- T waves probably normal

The lower ECG shows:

- Sinus rhythm, rate 97/min
- Normal axis
- Normal QRS complexes, ST segments and T waves

Clinical interpretation

The first ECG seems to indicate an acute anterolateral myocardial infarction. An alternative explanation, given the widespread changes, would be pericarditis. The second ECG is normal. Because the ECG reverted to normal when the pain cleared, it seems likely that the changes in the initial ECG represent Prinzmetal's variant angina.

What to do

Prinzmetal's variant angina was first described in 1959. It occurs at rest, and the characteristic raised ST segments seen in the ECG are not reproduced by exertion. It has been shown by angiography during pain to be due to spasm of one or more coronary arteries. Relatively few patients with this type of angina have totally normal arteries, and spasm may occur at the site of atheromatous plaques. Coronary angiography is indicated. Nifedipine and nitrates may be helpful, but the condition is difficult to treat.

Summary ★★★

Prinzmetal's variant angina.

ECG IP See p. 247, 6E

ECG 137

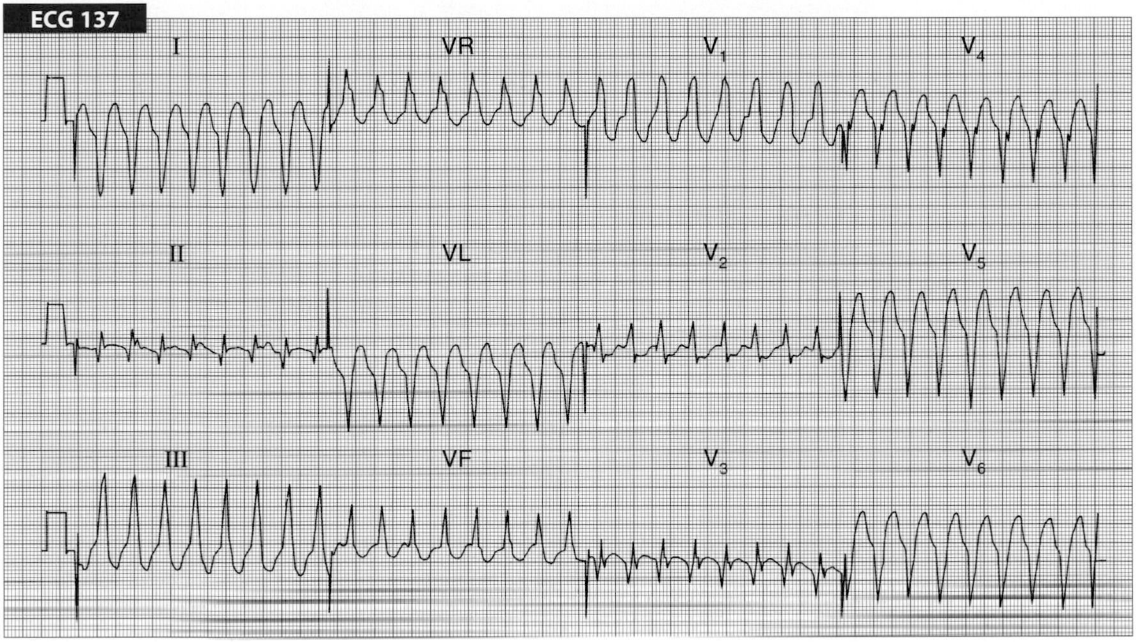

A 45-year-old man was admitted to hospital with a history of 2 h of ischaemic chest pain. His blood pressure was 150/80, and there were no signs of heart failure. What does his ECG show, and how would you treat him?

ANSWER 137

The ECG shows:

- Broad complex tachycardia, rate 180/min
- No P waves
- Right axis deviation
- QRS complex duration about 140 ms
- Right bundle branch block (RBBB) pattern, with the R peak taller than the R^1 peak in lead V_1 – best seen in the fifth complex
- Non-concordant QRS complexes, with a negative pattern in lead V_6 (i.e. complexes are upwards in lead V_1 but downwards in lead V_6)

Clinical interpretation

This is either ventricular tachycardia or supraventricular tachycardia with RBBB. In favour of the former are the relatively wide QRS complexes and the fact that the R peak is greater than the R^1 peak in lead V_1 (i.e. this is not the typical RBBB pattern). Against ventricular tachycardia are the right axis deviation and the different directions of the QRS complexes in the chest leads.

What to do

The problem is to decide whether the patient had a myocardial infarction complicated by ventricular tachycardia, or whether the arrhythmia is causing the anginal pain. Since he is haemodynamically stable, he needs pain relief, carotid sinus pressure, intravenous adenosine and intravenous lidocaine, in that order. If in doubt, or if his blood pressure were to fall or he were to develop heart failure, the safest course of action would be DC cardioversion.

This patient needed cardioversion, and the ECG then showed an anterior infarction. The rhythm was probably ventricular tachycardia.

Summary ★★★

Broad complex tachycardia of uncertain origin.

ECG ME See p. 166, 8E

ECG IP See p. 145, 6E

ECG 138

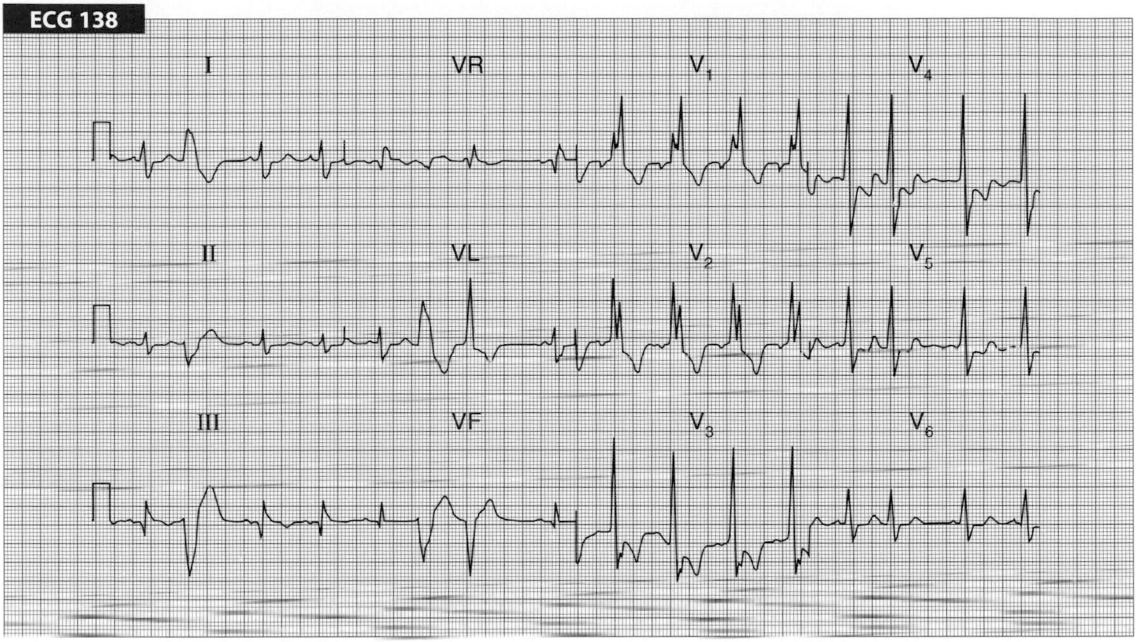

This ECG was recorded from a 65-year-old man who complained of breathlessness and who showed the physical signs of moderate heart failure. What does the ECG show? Does it have implications for treatment?

ANSWER 138

The ECG shows:

- Sinus rhythm, rate 97/min
- Multifocal ventricular extrasystoles and one supraventricular extrasystole
- Q waves in the sinus beats in leads III, VF
- Right bundle branch block (RBBB)

Clinical interpretation

The presence of Q waves in the inferior leads suggests an old infarction. Ischaemic disease is therefore probably the cause of the extrasystoles and the RBBB.

What to do

Control of the heart failure may well cause the extrasystoles to disappear; the extrasystoles should not be treated with antiarrhythmic drugs. The presence of multifocal extrasystoles should alert you to consider electrolyte abnormalities and digoxin toxicity.

Summary ★★

Multifocal ventricular extrasystoles, RBBB and probable old inferior myocardial infarction.

ECG ME See p. 43, 8E

ECG IP See p. 115, 6E

ECG 139

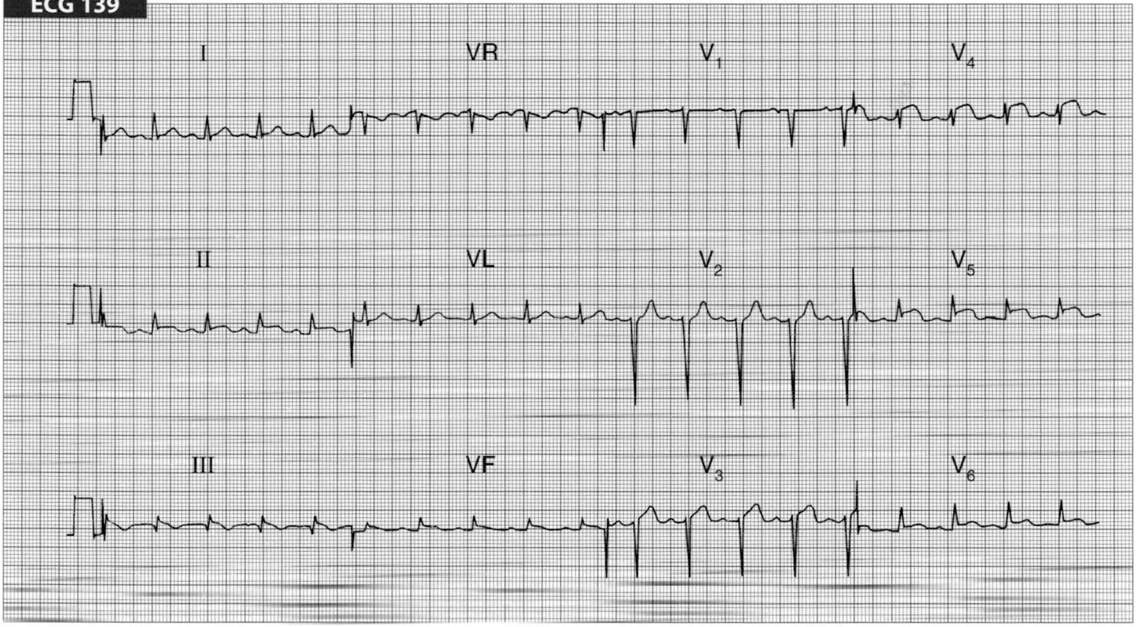

This ECG was recorded in the A & E department from a 25-year-old man with severe chest pain. No physical abnormalities had been detected, but having seen the ECG what would you look for and what would you do?

ANSWER 139

The ECG shows:

- Sinus rhythm, rate 105/min
- Normal axis
- Normal QRS complexes
- Raised ST segments in leads I–III, VF, V_4–V_6

Clinical interpretation

The raised ST segments in leads I and V_4 follow S waves, and are therefore 'high take-off' and of no significance. The ST segment elevation elsewhere could indicate an acute infarction, but since the change is so widespread, pericarditis seems more probable.

What to do

In a 25-year-old, pericarditis is a much more likely diagnosis than infarction, and thrombolysis must be avoided. The diagnosis is made by lying the patient flat, when a pericardial rub will become much easier to hear. Echocardiography will show a pericardial effusion if one is present.

Summary ★★★
Widespread ST segment elevation, suggesting pericarditis.

ECG ME See p. 96, 8E

ECG IP See p. 251, 6E

ECG 140

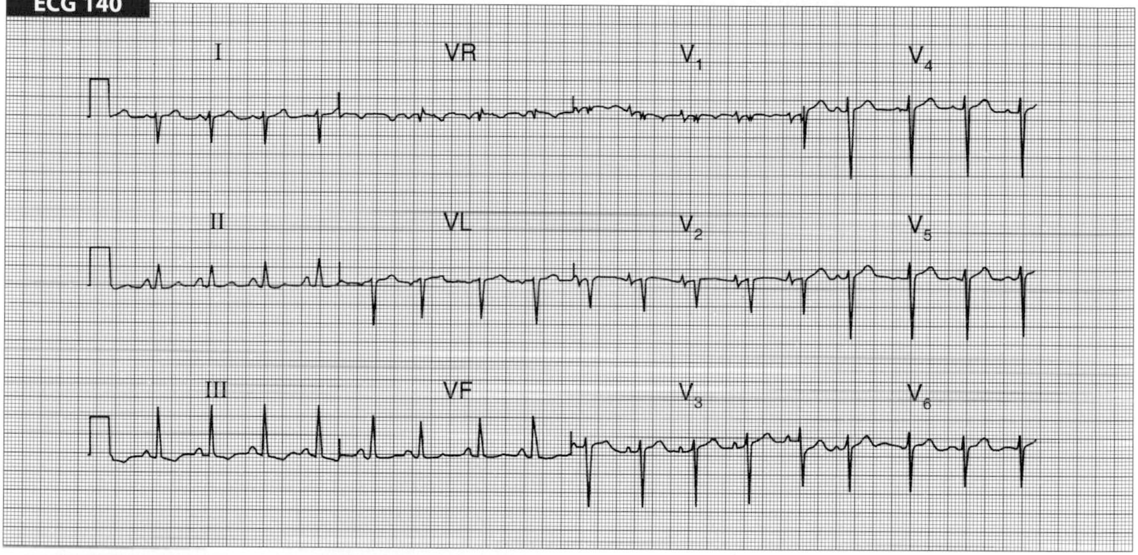

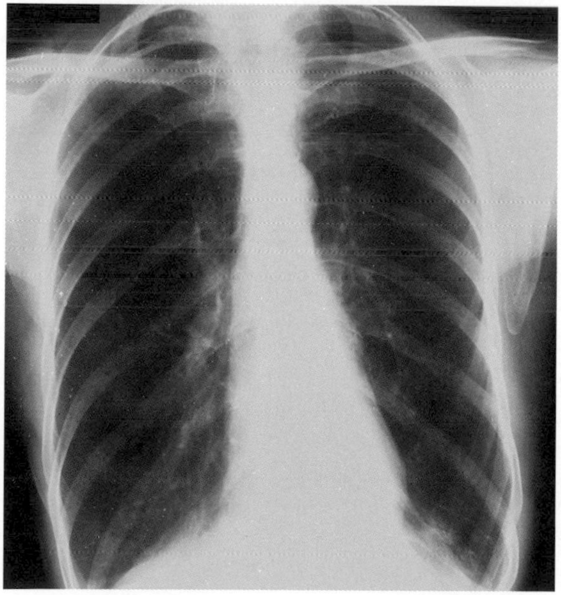

This ECG and chest X-ray were recorded from a 70-year-old man who complained of breathlessness. What abnormalities do they show and what is the most likely diagnosis?

X-ray reproduced with permission from Corne J & Pointon K (eds), *100 Chest X-Ray Problems*, Elsevier, 2007

ANSWER 140

The ECG shows:

- Sinus rhythm, rate 102/min
- Peaked P waves, best seen in leads V_1–V_2
- Right axis deviation (deep S waves in lead I)
- RSR^1 pattern with normal QRS complex duration in lead V_1 (partial right bundle branch block (RBBB))
- Deep S waves in lead V_6, with no left ventricular pattern

The chest X-ray shows a long and thin mediastinum, with no increase in heart size but possible prominence of the pulmonary arteries. The lung fields appear essentially black, which is a feature of emphysema. This is the picture of chronic obstructive pulmonary disease.

Clinical interpretation

Peaked P waves suggest right atrial hypertrophy. The partial RBBB pattern is not significant. Right axis deviation may be seen in tall, thin people with normal hearts, but with the deep S waves in lead V_6 it suggests right ventricular hypertrophy. The lack of development of a left ventricular pattern in the V leads (i.e. deep S waves persisting into lead V_6) results from the right ventricle occupying most of the precordium. This is sometimes called 'clockwise rotation' (looking at the heart from below) and is characteristic of chronic lung disease.

What to do

Lung function tests will be more helpful than echocardiography.

Summary ★★

Right atrial hypertrophy and chronic obstructive pulmonary disease.

ECG ME See p. 137, 8E

ECG IP See p. 21, 6E

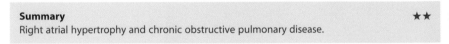

ECG 141

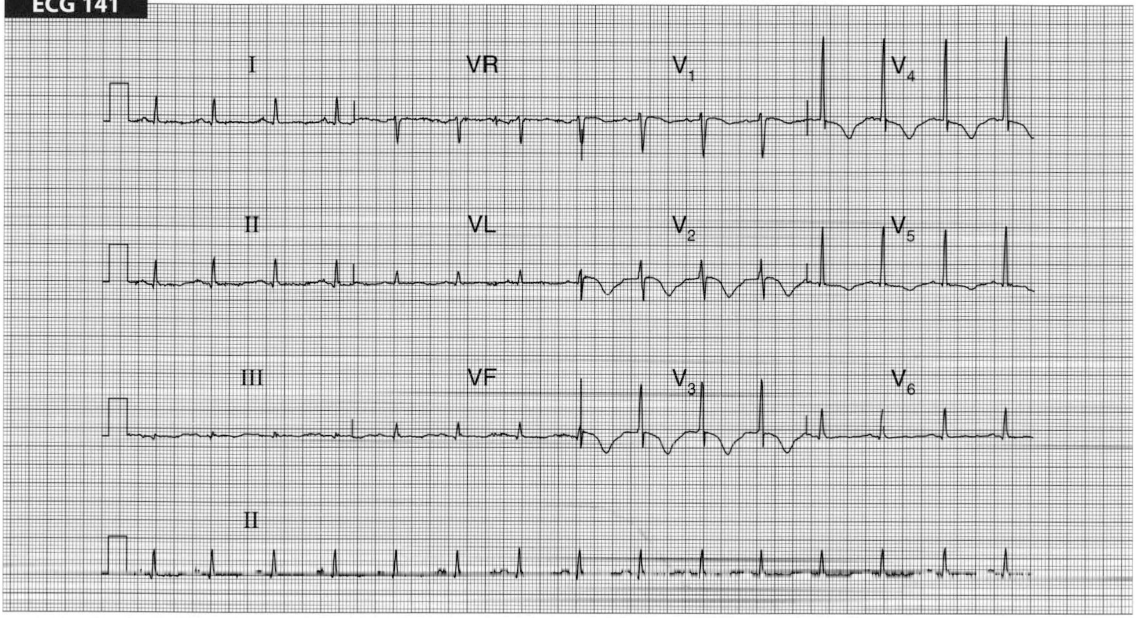

This ECG was recorded from a 15-year-old boy who collapsed while playing football. His brother had died suddenly. What does the ECG show and what clinical possibilities should be considered?

ANSWER 141

The ECG shows:

- Sinus rhythm, rate 91/min
- Normal PR interval
- Normal axis
- Normal QRS complexes
- Prolonged QT interval (QT = 492 ms; QT_c = 598 ms)
- Inverted T waves in leads V_2–V_5

Clinical interpretation

This is clearly a very abnormal ECG, with a markedly prolonged QT interval and abnormal T waves.

What to do

The family history suggests that this may well be an example of one of the congenital forms of prolonged QT interval: the Jervell–Lange–Nielson syndrome or the Romano–Ward syndrome. These are characterized by episodes of loss of consciousness in children, often at times of increased sympathetic nervous system activity, and beta-blockers are the immediate form of treatment. The insertion of a permanent defibrillator may be necessary. Prolonged QT interval syndrome is also associated with antiarrhythmic drugs (quinidine, procainamide, disopyramide, amiodarone and sotalol) and with other drugs such as the tricyclic antidepressants and erythromycin. Electrolyte abnormalities (low potassium, magnesium or calcium levels) also prolong the QT interval.

Summary ★★★

Marked prolongation of the QT interval – long QT syndrome.

ECG ME See p. 157, 8E

ECG IP See p. 76, 6E

ECG 142

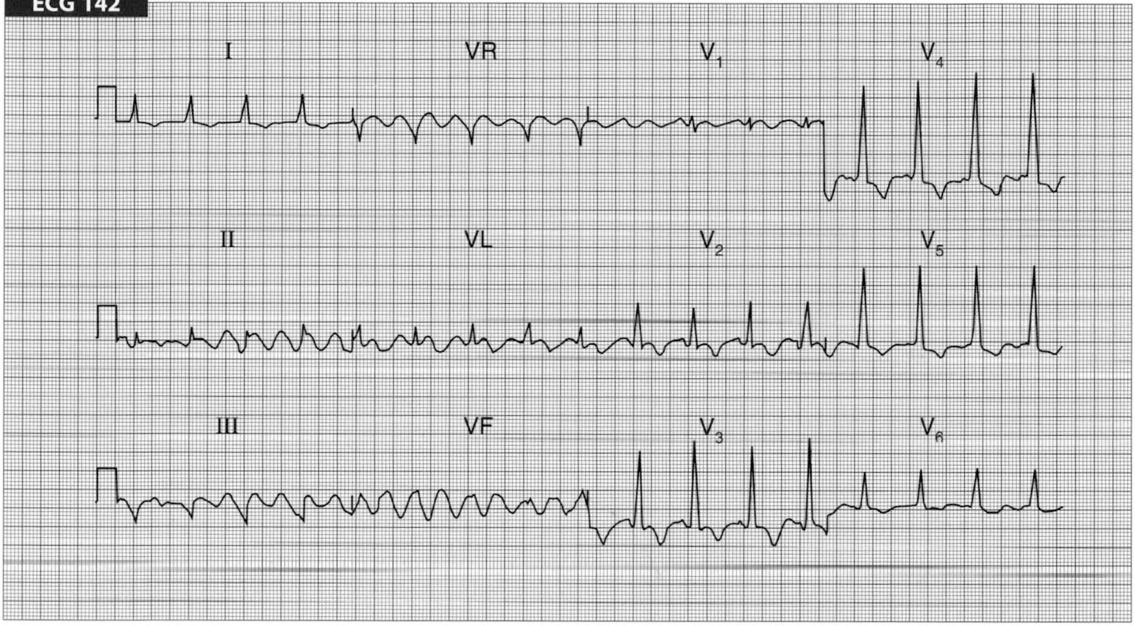

The house officer from the geriatric ward is puzzled by this ECG and requests your help. What questions would you ask him?

ANSWER 142

The ECG shows:

- Sinus rhythm, rate 100/min
- Slow rhythmic waves, the baseline in some ways resembling atrial flutter, but slower and coarser
- Short PR intervals
- Slurred upstroke of the QRS complexes, particularly in lead I
- T wave inversion in the anterior leads

Clinical interpretation

The slow rhythmic variation is due to muscle tremor, and is not cardiac in origin. The short PR intervals, slurred upstroke of the QRS complexes and inverted T waves are due to the Wolff–Parkinson–White (WPW) syndrome – the dominant R waves in the chest leads indicating type A.

What to do

Ask if the patient has Parkinson's disease: a Parkinsonian tremor would explain the baseline variation. Does the patient give a history of palpitations or syncope? This would be the only significant problem that the WPW syndrome might cause in an elderly patient.

Summary ★★★
Muscle artefact, possibly Parkinson's disease; the WPW syndrome type A.

ECG ME See p. 27, 8E

ECG IP See p. 316, 6E

ECG 143

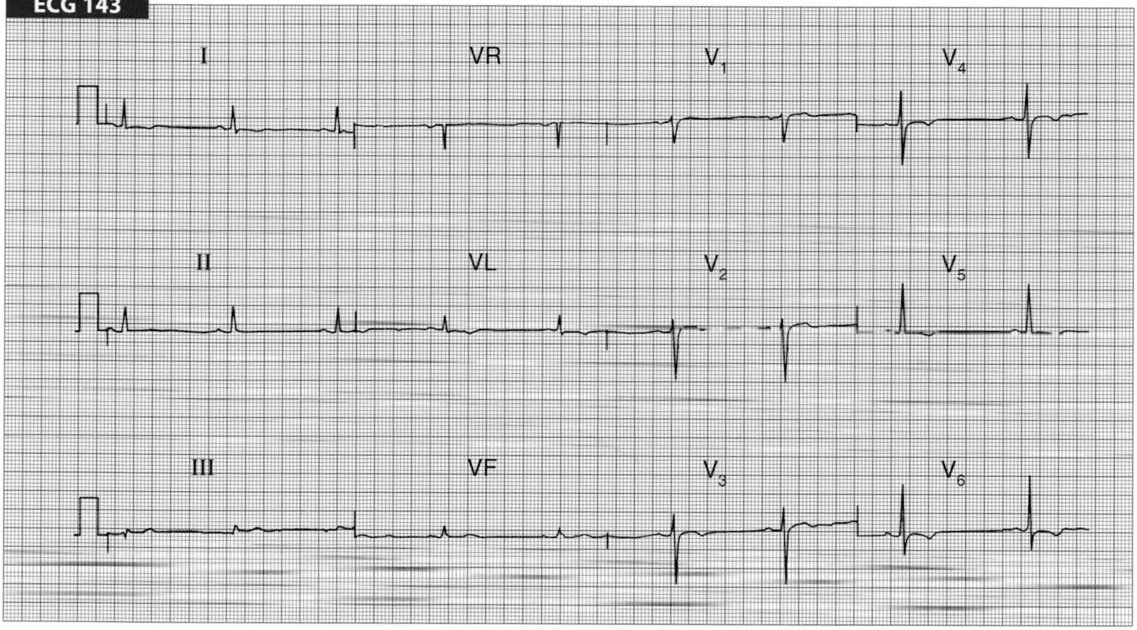

A 30-year-old woman, who had been treated for depression for several years, was admitted to hospital as an emergency following deliberate self-harm involving a small number of aspirin tablets. There were no abnormalities on examination but this was her ECG. Does it worry you?

ANSWER 143

The ECG shows:

- Sinus rhythm, rate 50/min
- Normal axis
- Normal QRS complexes
- T wave inversion in leads I, VL, V_4–V_6

Clinical interpretation

Anterolateral T wave inversion is most commonly due to ischaemia, but this seems unlikely in a young woman with no evidence of heart disease. A cardiomyopathy would be another possibility, but repolarization (T wave) abnormalities can be caused by lithium therapy.

What to do

As always when a diagnosis is not clear, find out what drugs the patient is taking. This patient was taking lithium, and exercise testing and echocardiography showed no evidence of heart disease.

Summary ★★★

Anterolateral T wave inversion due to lithium therapy.

ECG IP See p. 341, 6E

ECG 144

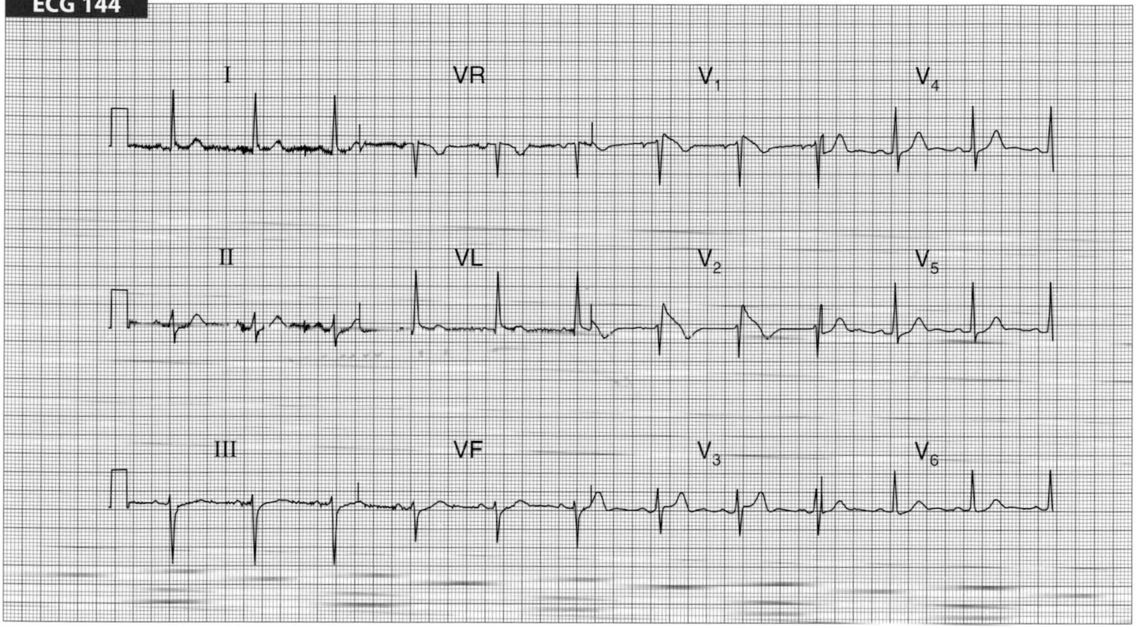

This ECG was recorded from a 40-year-old man who was admitted to hospital after collapsing in a supermarket. By the time he was seen he was well, and there were no abnormal physical signs. Would you pass this ECG as normal?

ANSWER 144

The ECG shows:

- Sinus rhythm, rate 70/min
- Normal PR interval and QRS complex duration
- Normal axis
- QRS complexes in leads V_1–V_2 show an RSR^1 pattern
- ST segments elevated, and downward-sloping, in leads V_1–V_2

Clinical interpretation

This is not a normal ECG. The appearances in leads V_1–V_2 are characteristic of the Brugada syndrome.

What to do

The Brugada syndrome involves a genetic abnormality that alters sodium transport in the myocardium, and predisposes to ventricular tachycardia and fibrillation. This patient's collapse may well have been due to an arrhythmia. The syndrome is often familial. The ECG changes are not constant, and on the day after admission this patient's ECG was perfectly normal. The ECG changes can be induced, and ventricular tachycardia caused, by antiarrhythmic drugs. The only treatment is an implanted defibrillator.

Summary ★★★
The Brugada syndrome.

ECG IP See p. 81, 6E

ECG 145

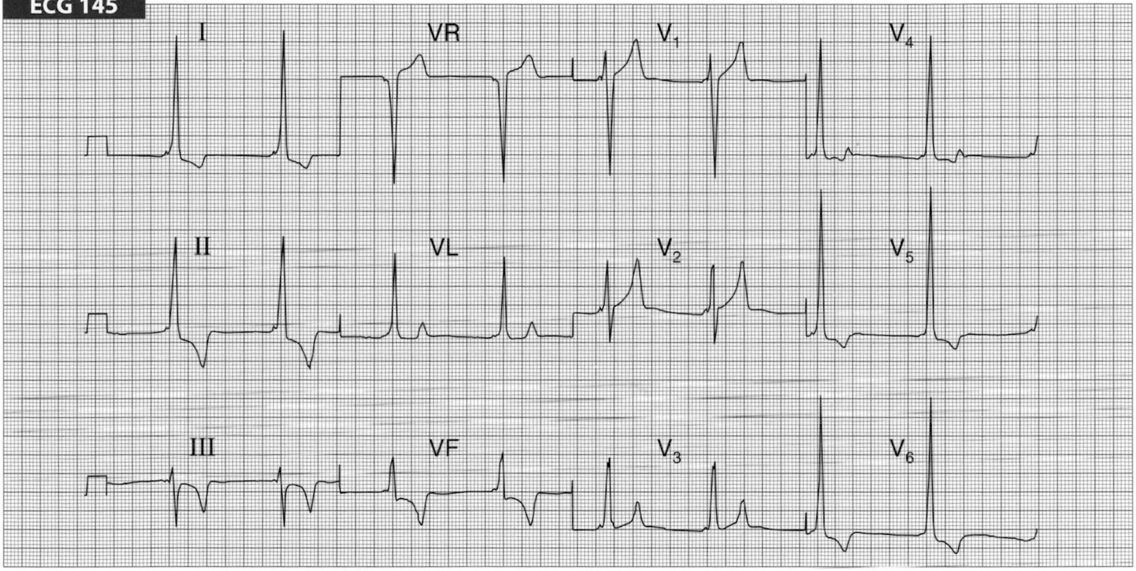

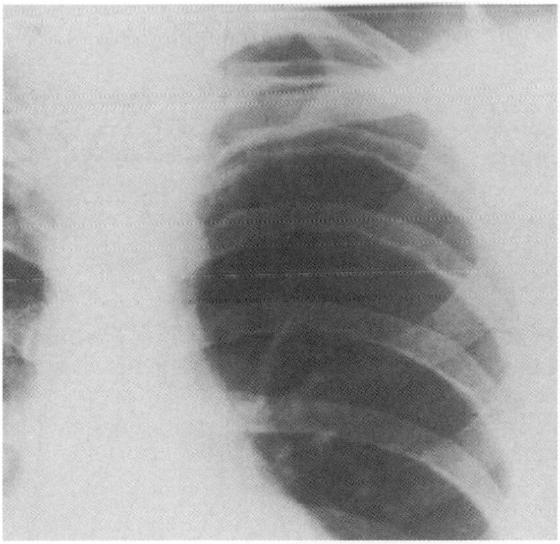

This ECG was recorded from a 35-year-old man who had no symptoms, but who had been found at a routine examination to have a blood pressure of 180/105. An enlarged part of the chest X-ray is also shown. What do the ECG and X-ray show and what action would you suggest?

ANSWER 145

The ECG (*note*: leads at half sensitivity) shows:

- Sinus rhythm, rate 50/min
- Very short PR interval
- Normal axis
- Slurred upstroke to QRS complexes – delta wave
- QRS complex duration prolonged (200 ms)
- Very tall QRS complexes in the lateral leads
- Inverted T waves in leads I–III, VF, V_5–V_6

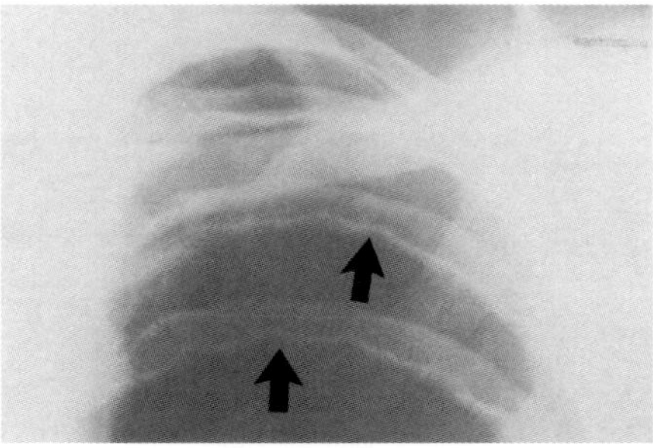

The chest X-ray shows rib notching (arrowed), due to collaterals that have developed because of a coarctation of the aorta.

Clinical interpretation

The ECG shows an example of the Wolff–Parkinson–White (WPW) syndrome type B. In a patient with high blood pressure the tall QRS complexes and inverted T waves in the lateral leads would raise the possibility of left ventricular hypertrophy. However, the changes here are too gross for that, and they are compatible with this pre-excitation syndrome. The rib notching shows that the high blood pressure is due to coarctation of the aorta, which is completely unrelated to the WPW syndrome.

What to do

If the patient has no symptoms to suggest a paroxysmal tachycardia, no further action is necessary – many patients with an ECG consistent with a pre-excitation syndrome never have an episode of tachycardia. The chance finding of an unrelated coarctation of the aorta is more important, and surgical correction of this must be considered.

See p. 154, 8E ECG ME

See p. 299, 6E ECG IP

Summary ★★★
The WPW syndrome type B, and an unrelated coarctation of the aorta.

ECG 146

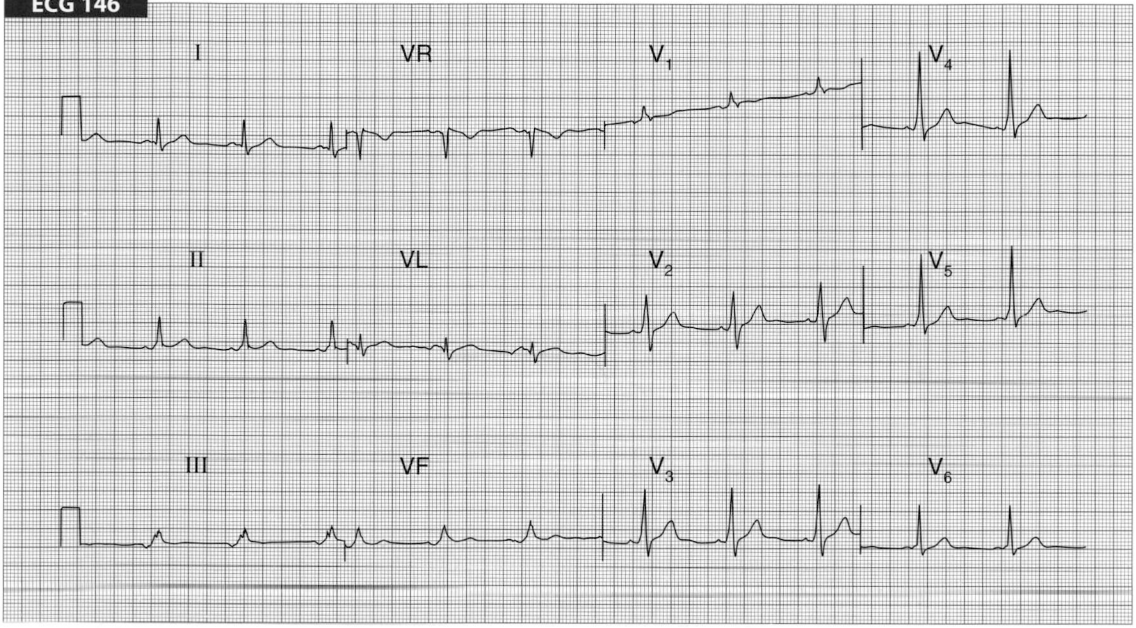

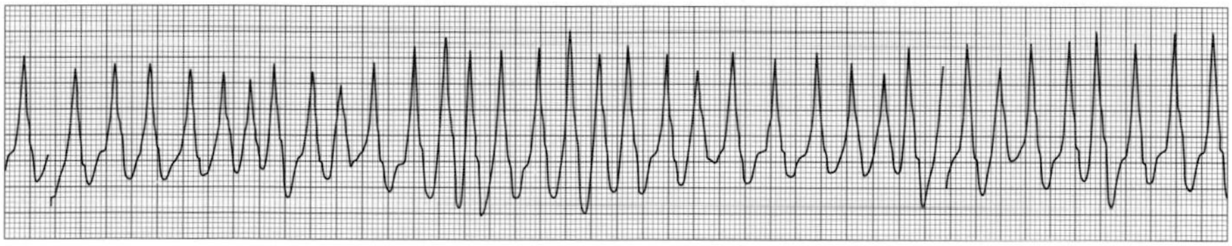

A 30-year-old woman complains of episodes of palpitations associated with dizziness and breathlessness. These begin and stop suddenly. She has had them for many years, but they are becoming more frequent and more severe. The upper ECG was recorded at rest; the lower ECG is part of an ambulatory record, during which she had a typical attack. What do these ECGs show and what would you do?

ANSWER 146

The upper ECG shows:

- Sinus rhythm, rate 64/min
- Short PR interval, best seen in leads V_4–V_5
- Normal axis
- Dominant R waves in lead V_1
- Slurred upstroke (delta wave) in the QRS complexes

The lower ECG (rhythm strip) shows:

- A broad complex tachycardia
- Rate about 230/min
- The rhythm is irregular
- There is a slurred upstroke in some of the beats, suggesting pre-excitation

Clinical interpretation

This is the Wolff–Parkinson–White (WPW) syndrome, involving a short PR interval and a widened QRS complex. This pattern, with a dominant R wave in lead V_1 and where there is a left-sided accessory pathway, is called 'type A'. It can easily be mistaken for right ventricular hypertrophy. The patient's palpitations are due to atrial fibrillation; an irregular broad complex tachycardia is characteristic of atrial fibrillation in the WPW syndrome.

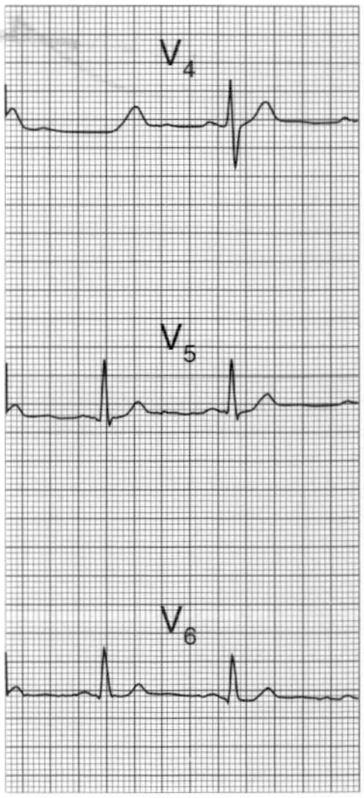

What to do

Atrial fibrillation in association with the WPW syndrome is extremely dangerous. The patient needs an immediate electrophysiological study with a view to ablation of the accessory pathway. An ECG was recorded after the ablation (see right – leads V_4–V_6 shown): the PR interval is now normal and there is no widening of the QRS complex.

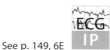

See p. 152, 8E

See p. 149, 6E

Summary ★★

The WPW syndrome type A, with paroxysmal atrial fibrillation.

ECG 147

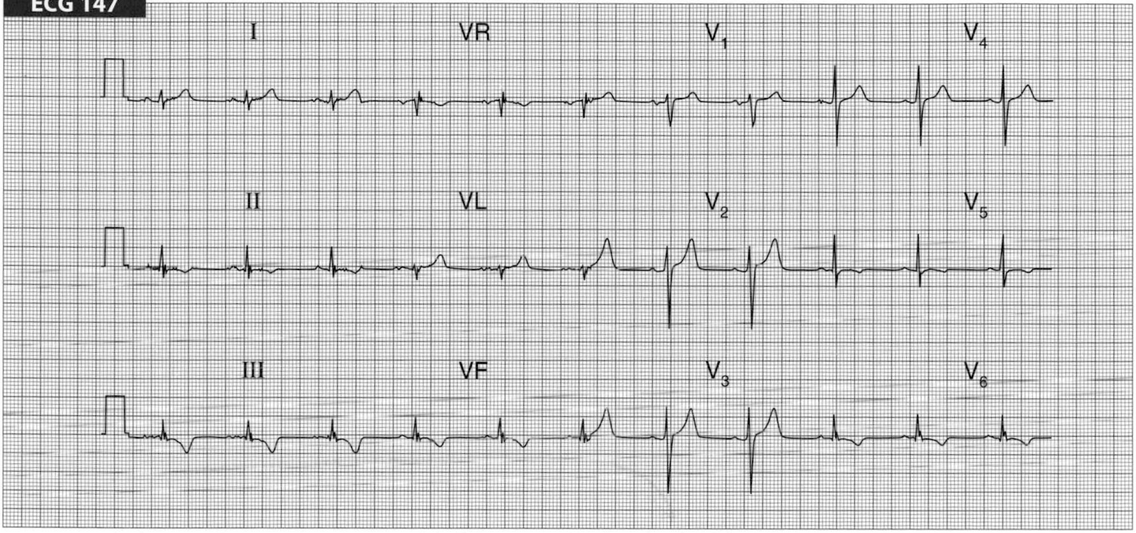

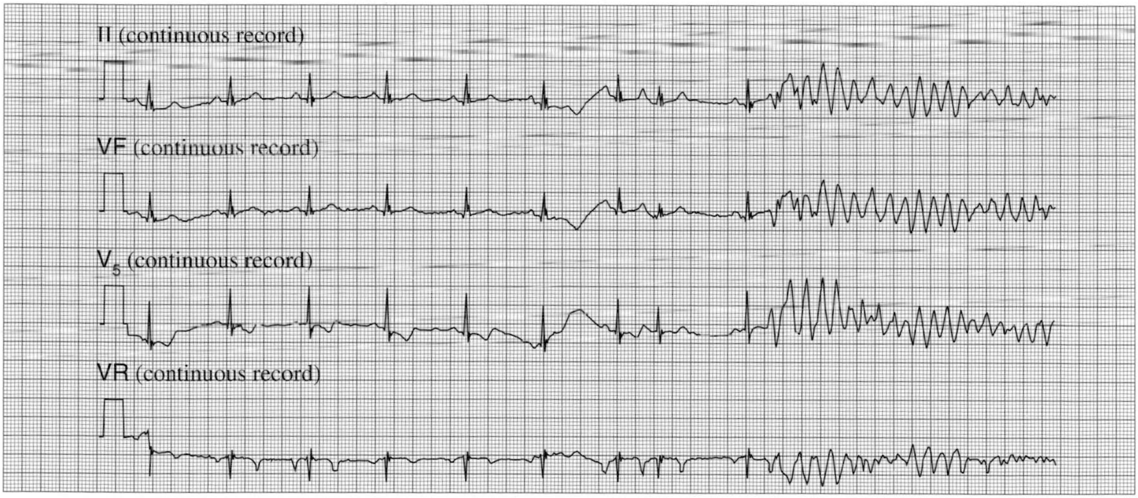

A 50-year-old man, who had had exertional chest pain for some months, was seen in the A & E department with persistent central chest pain which had commenced 1 h earlier. These are his ECGs. What does the upper ECG show and what would you do? The lower ECG shows what happened when an exercise test was performed.

ANSWER 147

The top ECG shows:

- Sinus rhythm, rate 65/min
- Normal axis
- 'Splintered' QRS complex in leads II–III, VF, V_6 – otherwise normal QRS complexes, duration 100 ms
- T waves inverted in leads II–III, VF, V_5–V_6

Clinical interpretation

The 'splintered' QRS complex in the inferior leads is probably of no significance. The T wave inversion in the inferior and lateral leads suggests a non-ST segment elevation myocardial infarction (NSTEMI).

What to do

This patient clearly has an acute coronary syndrome. Thrombolysis is not indicated. Pain relief is essential. He needs aspirin and clopidogrel, and a glyocoprotein IIb/IIIa inhibitor if angiography is contemplated. He also needs a beta-blocker and nitrates (intravenous or buccal). The ECG should be recorded every half-hour to see if ST segment elevation appears. The plasma troponin level should be measured 12 h after the onset of pain. The patient may well need early coronary angiography with a view to coronary intervention (percutaneous coronary intervention (PCI) or coronary artery bypass graft (CABG)). Exercise testing is commonly performed before the patient is discharged from hospital in an attempt to prioritize those who need an angiogram urgently.

Exercise test

The lower ECG, recorded in stage 2 of the Bruce protocol, after 4 min and 41 s, shows:

- Sudden onset of ventricular fibrillation

What to do

See p. 144, 8E

Immediate resuscitation, and early coronary angiography as soon as the patient is stable. Above all, remember that exercise testing is not totally free of risk.

See p. 282, 6E

Summary ★

Inferolateral NSTEMI; ventricular fibrillation during exercise testing.

ECG 148

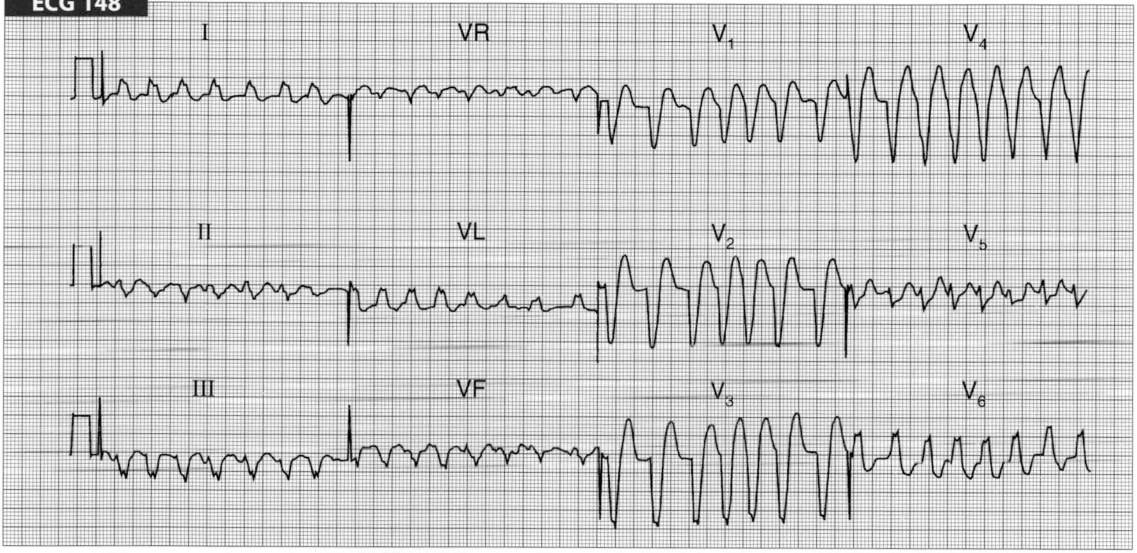

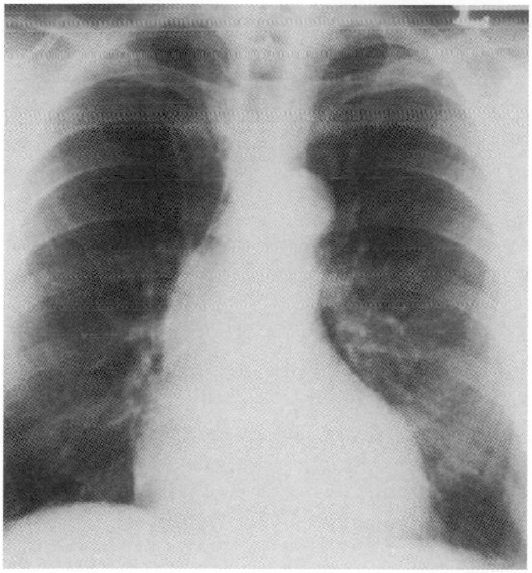

An 80 year old man was admitted to hospital because of a sudden onset of palpitations associated with breathlessness. He had congestive cardiac failure and a heart murmur suggestive of aortic regurgitation. What do this ECG and the chest X-ray show and how would you treat him?

ANSWER 148

The ECG shows:

- Broad complex tachycardia
- Irregular rhythm, rate 130–200/min
- No clear P waves but irregular baseline, best seen in lead VL
- QRS complex duration 160 ms, with 'M' pattern in lead V_6, indicating left bundle branch block (LBBB)

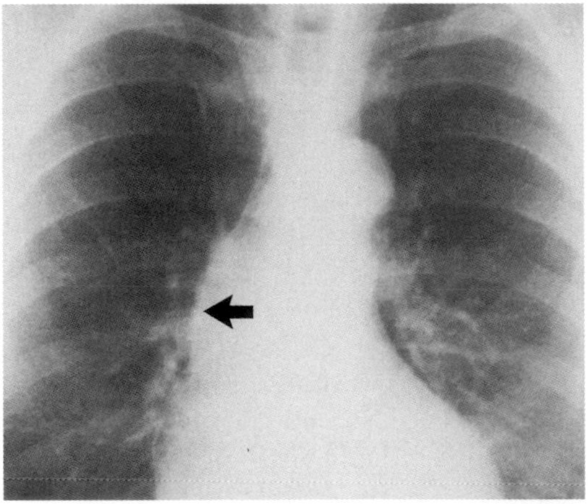

The chest X-ray shows left ventricular enlargement with dilatation of the ascending aorta. There is calcification in the aortic wall (arrowed). These changes suggest aortic regurgitation due to old syphilitic aortitis.

Clinical interpretation

The marked irregularity of rhythm, coupled with the irregular baseline glimpsed in one beat in lead VL, shows that this is atrial fibrillation with LBBB.

What to do

Aortic valve disease is commonly associated with LBBB. An echocardiogram is needed, to ensure that there is no significant aortic stenosis – in which case vasodilators must be used with extreme caution. The heart failure can be treated with diuretics, and digoxin will control the ventricular rate. Even at the age of 80 years, aortic valve replacement might be considered.

See p. 176, 8E ECG ME

See p. 127, 6E ECG IP

Summary ★★★

Atrial fibrillation with LBBB; aortic regurgitation due to syphilitic aortitis.

ECG 149

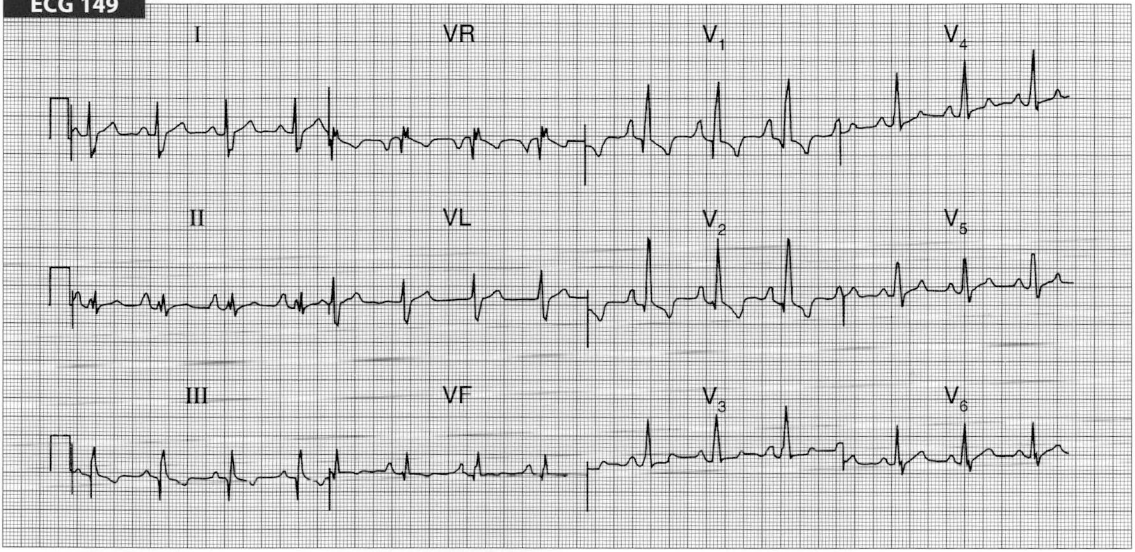

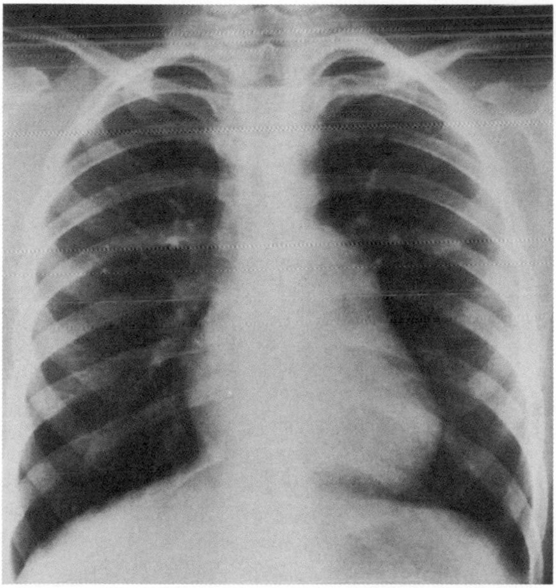

This ECG and chest X-ray were recorded from a 17-year-old girl who was breathless, had marked ankle swelling with signs of right heart failure, and who had been known to have a heart murmur since birth. She was acyanotic. What ECG abnormalities can you identify, and can you suggest a diagnosis?

ANSWER 149

The ECG shows:

- Sinus rhythm, rate 81/min
- Markedly peaked P waves (best seen in leads II, V_1)
- Normal axis
- Dominant R wave in lead V_1

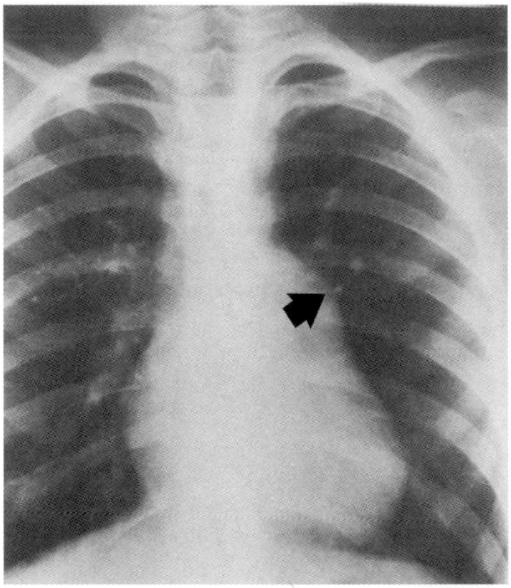

The chest X-ray shows a high and prominent cardiac apex, consistent with right ventricular hypertrophy, and a prominent pulmonary artery (arrowed) which is due to post-stenotic dilatation as a result of pulmonary stenosis.

Clinical interpretation

The ECG shows right atrial and right ventricular hypertrophy.

What to do

Right atrial hypertrophy is seen with pulmonary hypertension of any cause, tricuspid stenosis, and Ebstein's anomaly. Right ventricular hypertrophy is seen with pulmonary stenosis and pulmonary hypertension. These conditions can all be diagnosed by echocardiography. This patient had pulmonary stenosis.

See p. 86, 118, 8E

See p. 305, 6E

Summary ★★

Right atrial and right ventricular hypertrophy.

ECG 150

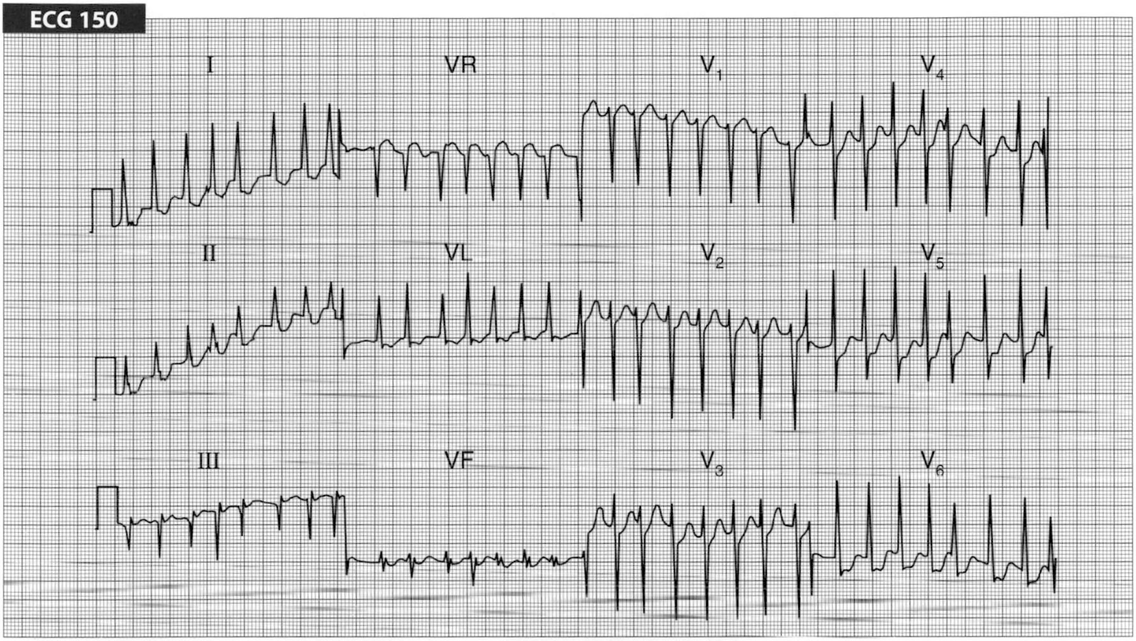

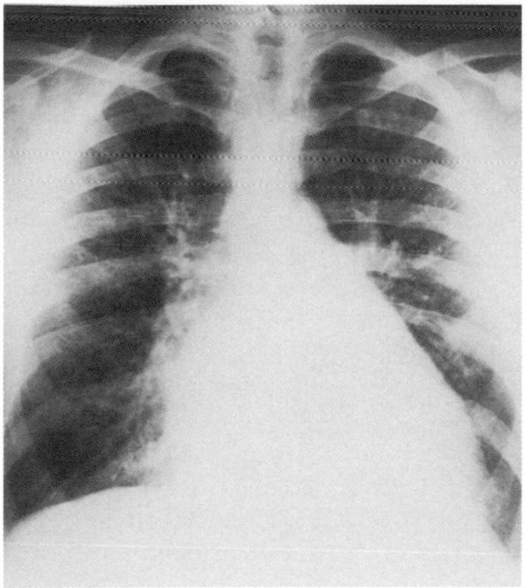

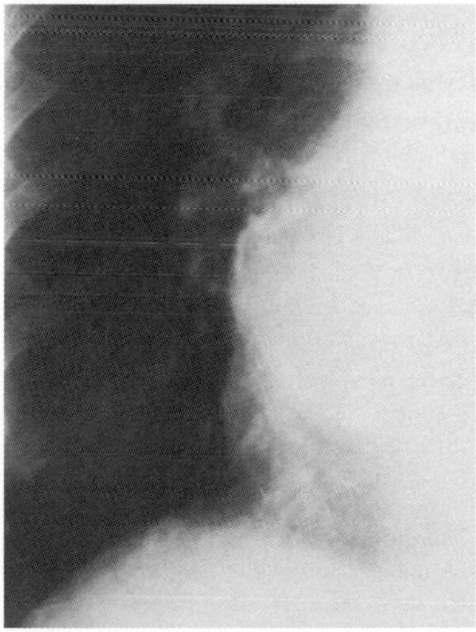

A 50-year-old woman came to the A & E department because of the sudden onset of palpitations and severe breathlessness. What abnormalities do the ECG and chest X-rays show, and what condition might be responsible? The X-ray on the right shows an enlargement of a penetrated view of the right heart border.

ANSWER 150

The ECG shows:

- Atrial fibrillation
- Normal axis
- Irregular QRS complexes with a ventricular rate of up to 200/min
- Otherwise normal QRS complexes, apart from an RSR[1] pattern in lead VF
- ST segments depressed in leads V_4–V_6, suggesting ischaemia
- Normal T waves

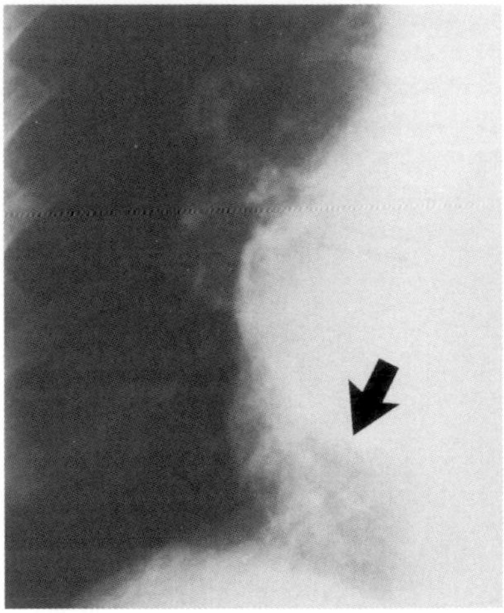

The chest X-ray shows an enlarged heart with a straight left heart border, which is due to left atrial (LA) enlargement. LA enlargement also causes a double shadow near the right heart border (arrowed).

Clinical interpretation

Atrial fibrillation with an uncontrolled ventricular rate. The ischaemic changes in leads V_4 and V_5 are probably related to the heart rate.

What to do

Ischaemia may have been the cause of the atrial fibrillation, or the rapid ventricular rate itself may be responsible for the ischaemic changes. Ischaemia is not a likely primary diagnosis in a 50-year-old woman, and the things to think about are rheumatic heart disease (particularly with mitral stenosis), thyrotoxicosis, alcoholism, and other forms of cardiomyopathy. Immediate treatment of the heart failure with diuretics may be necessary, but the ventricular rate is best controlled by digoxin, which can be given intravenously if necessary. DC cardioversion may be necessary if the patient is in severe heart failure. Remember that a patient with atrial fibrillation probably needs anticoagulants on a long-term basis. Echocardiography confirmed that this patient had mitral stenosis.

See p. 76, 8E

Summary ★★

Atrial fibrillation with a rapid ventricular rate and ischaemic changes, in a patient with mitral stenosis.

See p. 125, 6E

Index

Note: Numbers refer to PAGE NUMBERS, not question numbers; numbers in **bold** refer to ECG traces

A

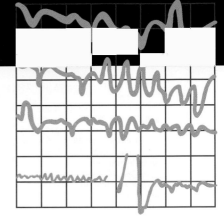

D

E

M

N

P

Q

R

S

T

U

V

W